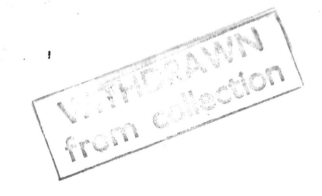
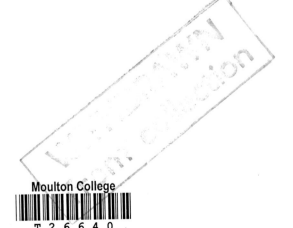

Veterinary Psychopharmacology

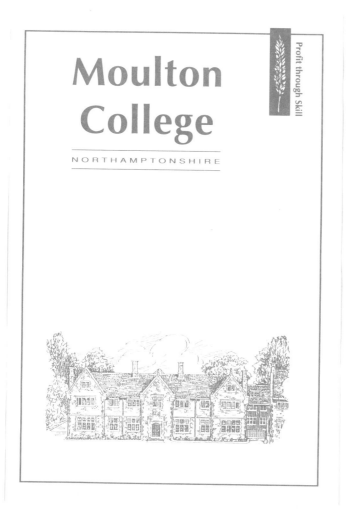

Moulton
College

NORTHAMPTONSHIRE

Profit through Skill

Veterinary Psychopharmacology

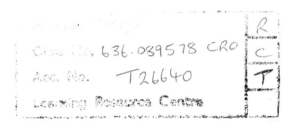
by
Sharon Crowell-Davis
and Thomas Murray

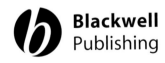
Blackwell
Publishing

Blackwell Publishing Professional
2121 State Avenue, Ames, Iowa 50014, USA

Orders: 1-800-862-6657
Office: 1-515-292-0140
Fax: 1-515-292-3348
Web site: www.blackwellprofessional.com

Blackwell Publishing Ltd
9600 Garsington Road, Oxford OX4 2DQ, UK
Tel.: +44 (0)1865 776868

Blackwell Publishing Asia
550 Swanston Street, Carlton, Victoria 3053, Australia
Tel.: +61 (0)3 8359 1011

Authorization to photocopy items for internal or personal use, or the internal or personal use of specific clients, is granted by Blackwell Publishing, provided that the base fee of $.10 per copy is paid directly to the Copyright Clearance Center, 222 Rosewood Drive, Danvers, MA 01923. For those organizations that have been granted a photocopy license by CCC, a separate system of payments has been arranged. The fee codes for users of the Transactional Reporting Service are ISBN-13: 978-0-8138-0829-1; ISBN-10: 0-8138-0829-4/2005 $.10.

First edition, 2006

Library of Congress Cataloging-in-Publication Data

Crowell-Davis, Sharon L.
    Veterinary psychopharmacology / by Sharon Crowell-Davis and Thomas Murray.— 1st ed.
        p. cm.
    Includes bibliographical references.
    ISBN-13: 978-0-8138-0829-1 (alk. paper)
    ISBN-10: 0-8138-0829-4 (alk. paper)
    1. Veterinary psychopharmacology. I. Murray, Thomas (Thomas F.) II. Title.

    SF756.84.C76 2005
    636.089′578—dc22

                                                                    2005012241

The last digit is the print number: 9 8 7 6 5 4 3 2 1

Dedication

For my father, Wallace Davis, whose lifelong dedication to science inspired me to follow in his footsteps, although on a very different path; my mother, Ruth Davis, who raised me to believe in myself; my husband, William Crowell-Davis, who has stood beside me through thick and thin; and for our two wonderful children, James Michael and Kristina Crowell-Davis, who grew up with a mother who always had animals around the house and was sometimes distracted by her work. Also for Prince, "the best dog in the history of the world," and my childhood friend, who no doubt initiated my love of animals.

Sharon Crowell-Davis 2005

To my wife, Cristina Wojcik, and daughter, Lia Lorraine Murray, for their patience with psychopharmacology during events such as a honeymoon and holiday vacation.

Thomas Murray 2005

Contents

Contributors

Sharon L. Crowell-Davis, DVM, PhD (Chapters 1, 3, 5, 6, 8, 10, 11, 13–15)
Diplomate, American College of Veterinary Behaviorists
Professor of Veterinary Behavior
The University of Georgia
College of Veterinary Medicine
Department of Anatomy and Radiology
Vet Med 1
Athens, GA 30602

Thomas Murray, BS, PhD (Chapters 2, 4, 7, 12)
Distinguished Research Professor and Head
The University of Georgia
College of Veterinary Medicine
Department of Physiology and Pharmacology
2223A Vet Med 1
Athens, GA 30602

Lynne M. Seibert, BS, DVM, MS, PhD (Chapter 9)
Diplomate, American College of Veterinary Behaviorists
Veterinary Behavior Specialist
VCA Veterinary Specialty Center
20115 - 44th Avenue West
Lynnwood, WA 98036

Acknowledgments

First, I would like to thank the many veterinarians who called me with questions about psychoactive medications, because it was their calls that triggered the realization that the general practitioner needed a resource that helped them to arrive at good decisions about drug selection and to better understand the drugs they were using. Without their eagerness to gain knowledge in this field, this book would not have been written.

Many people besides the authors contributed to the substantial work involved in bringing together the information presented in this first edition. Of particular assistance were Linda Tumlin, Wendy Simmons, and Lucy Rowland. In their capacity as librarians and reference librarians they were invaluable in locating and obtaining much of the information provided between these covers.

Information on drug costs was obtained through the able assistance of the University of Georgia Behavior Service Technician, Melissa Christian, and Sharon Campany, Certified Pharmacy Technician.

Students always challenge a professor to clarify and explain their decisions. In this context, the hundreds of veterinary students to whom I have taught the field of veterinary behavior over the last 27 years were significant contributors. Even more so were my first three residents, Dr. Lynne Seibert, an author in this book, Dr. Terry Curtis, and Dr. Mami Irimajiri. Drs. Seibert and Curtis also assisted in the teaching of our first continuing education course on psychopharmacology for veterinarians to graduate veterinarians. It was in the planning sessions for the organization of that course that much of the organization of this book developed. The course would not have taken place without the able assistance of Sandi Kilgo, who coordinated the details of the everyday running of the course.

I could not have developed the behavior program and the behavior service at the University of Georgia to its current strength if I had not had the continuing support of various administrators over the years. Dr. Royce Roberts, my department head of many years, has been particularly helpful. Dr. David Anderson, Dr. Keith Prasse, Dr. Bob Lewis, and Dr. Jack Munnell have also facilitated my continuing work in this field.

Sharon L. Crowell-Davis, 2005

Preface

This book grew out of a series of phone calls I received over the years from various veterinarians wanting information about their patients' behavior problems and the psychoactive medications that might help them. What were appropriate drugs for given problems? What were appropriate doses? What side effects should be watched for? The first answer to this steadily accumulating set of questions was a continuing education course in psychopharmacology specifically organized for veterinarians. The course was first presented at the University of Georgia in November of 2001 and is now presented biannually. Dr. Murray and I co-taught the course, with assistance from the clinical residents in behavior at the time, Dr. Lynne Seibert and Dr. Terry Curtis. The approach of coverage of the basic science of the molecular activity of the brain, followed by coverage of clinical applications (i.e., what drugs have been used in veterinary patients to affect that particular molecular activity and how well have they worked to treat behavior problems), was well received. The logical next step was a textbook so that practicing veterinarians would have a resource to turn to for the answers to their various questions.

Information on the effects of various psychoactive drugs in dogs, cats, and other veterinary patients comes from two major sources. First, animals were often used to test and study the actions of various drugs during their initial development. Thus, the reader who peruses the references will find papers published as early as the 1950s, when major breakthroughs in psychopharmacology were being made. The second set of information is much more recent. With the establishment of the American College of Veterinary Behaviorists in 1993 and the overall rapid development of the field of veterinary behavior over the last three decades, there has been increasing research on the efficacy of various medications on the treatment of various behavioral disorders of companion animals, zoo animals, and other nonhuman animals.

There are often huge gaps in our knowledge, and the reader may note them throughout the book. While we can glean bits and pieces of pharmacokinetic and other data from studies done on dogs and cats during early drug development, the quality and quantity of the information is highly variable. Studies of teratology and carcinogenicity are typically done in rats, mice, and rabbits, while comprehensive studies of all aspects of pharmacological activity in the body are done only in humans, the species that has historically been of interest. It is hoped that, as interest in this field continues to evolve, more comprehensive data will become available; new data will be supplied in future editions.

Sharon Crowell-Davis, DVM, PhD
Diplomate, American College of Veterinary Behaviorists
Professor of Veterinary Behavior
The University of Georgia

Veterinary
Psychopharmacology

Chapter One
Introduction

The term *psychopharmacology* derives from three Greek words. *Psyche* means soul or mind. *Pharmacon* means drug. Finally, the term *logos* means to study. Thus, psychopharmacology, in a basic sense, is the study of drugs that affect the soul or mind. We are interested in such drugs because psychoactive medications produce changes in behavior and/or motivation. They have been used with varying efficacy in human psychiatry for several decades, and efficacy has improved over time as we have come to better understand the complex interrelationships between brain chemistry, internal emotional states, and overt behavior. We are also developing an improved understanding of the neuroanatomy of various major behavior problems such as aggression (e.g., Krishnan 1999). Nevertheless, much remains to be discovered. While a great deal is understood about what happens on cell surfaces, the exact mechanism by which receptors and the molecules that interact with them affect mood and overt behavior remains an enigma (Burke 2004).

While we can never truly understand the animal soul or mind, we can measure changes in animal behavior that occur as a consequence of the administration of various drugs that enter the brain. We can also place those changes within the context of species-typical social organization and communication to interpret what is likely happening in terms of changes in the emotional and motivational state of the animal. The use of psychoactive medications has been rapidly integrated into the practice of veterinary clinical behavior because they can often be of tremendous assistance in the treatment of the serious behavior problems that are routinely encountered in this field.

Psychoactive medications can be extremely useful in the treatment of behavior problems in animals, but it is rare for medication alone to provide a cure. In most cases, treatment is most effective if medication is used in combination with environmental management and behavior modification, such as desensitization and counterconditioning. The most common protocols for behavior modification are defined and discussed briefly in this chapter and are mentioned throughout the book. It is suggested, however, that the practitioner read one or more books that focus on this area.

While data on the effect of psychoactive medications on behavior problems observed in the pet population are increasing yearly, much of the available data on actual efficacy for specific problems are derived from human psychiatric use and extrapolated to use in veterinary behavior. When using a medication with little historical use in pets, it must be remembered that sometimes medications have different efficacy and different side effect profiles in different species. A medication that works well in humans may work better or worse in a cat or dog, and those species may exhibit side effects never observed in humans. Wherever possible, data from studies on the use of a given medication in domestic species are provided. Beyond this, drugs that are commonly used by practitioners of veterinary behavior, but about which there is little published data, are discussed with reference to use in humans. Some medications have been used little or not at all in the pet population, but based on their use in humans, might reasonably be tried in pets that have been refractory to better-tested treatments when the owner is willing to take the chance that their species of pet will have a side effect that has not been observed in humans. In all cases, the species from which specific information on clinical use of a medication has been derived will be specified.

Prescribing in the United States: Animal Medicinal Drug Use Clarification Act (AMDUCA 1994)

As this book goes to press, the use of most psychoactive medications in veterinary medicine is extra-label. The only label uses of psychoactive medication for the treatment of behavior problems in animals are Clomicalm (clomipramine) for separation anxiety in dogs and Anipryl (L-deprenyl) for cognitive dysfunction in elderly dogs. Extra-label use means that the medication has not been approved by the Food and Drug Administration (FDA) for the specific problem and the specific species for which it is being prescribed. Thus, use of Clomicalm for separation anxiety in cats or storm phobia in dogs would be extra-label use. Use of all other psychoactive medications for any behavior problem on any species constitutes extra-label use.

This does not mean that use of medications other than clomipramine or L-deprenyl is contraindicated for behavioral problems in animals or that the extra-label use of clomipramine or L-deprenyl is contraindicated. In veterinary behavioral medicine, the off-label status of most drugs means that the substantial safety and efficacy trials required by the FDA for on-label use have not been conducted. In many cases, for economic reasons such trials will never be conducted, despite substantial scientific evidence that a given drug has a real usefulness, with minimal side effects, for a particular problem.

There are specific requirements for extra-label use of any medication, psychoactive or otherwise. First and foremost, there must be a valid veterinarian-client-patient relationship. The veterinarian must have personally examined the patient and, based on their own knowledge of the patient's physical and behavioral status, determined that extra-label use of medication is appropriate and may be beneficial. To come to this determination, the veterinarian must conduct a physical exam and take both a medical and behavioral history. While some behaviors cannot be observed in the examination room, objective information about the patient's behavioral history can be gathered by interviewing the owner and other persons who have personally witnessed the pet's behavior.

Because of widespread use and some degree of knowledge of psychoactive medications in society at large, it is not uncommon for persons who are not qualified or licensed to make decisions regarding medications to attempt to make these decisions. Dog trainers, behaviorists who are not veterinarians, and others, may attempt to convince a pet's owner and/or the pet's veterinarian to use a particular drug that the veterinarian does not feel is appropriate. Likewise, news shows that mention use of a particular drug in a pet may result in many calls to veterinarians in the area requesting that the drug be prescribed. In all cases, it must be remembered that the decision regarding which drug to use for a given problem in a given pet is the veterinarian's responsibility and therefore the veterinarian's decision. It is likewise the veterinarian's responsibility to remain current in his or her understanding of the use of medication for various behavioral problems in pets. When a prescription is written for a given medication, the veterinarian must have a specific rationale for the use of that medication in that patient, and its use must be accepted under current standards of sound medical and behavioral practice.

Because some psychoactive medications are used very commonly and to good effect for behavior problems, it can be easy to slip into habits of treating such medications as if their use was on-label. In all cases of extra-label use of medication, however, clients must be informed of the extra-label status of the drug. If necessary, explain to the client what extra-label means. Clients should be informed of known side effects and the risk of novel side effects occurring in their pet. An informed consent statement that describes the extra-label status of the drug, explains why the medication is being prescribed, lists known side effects, and states the risk of novel side effects should be provided to the client. One copy should be provided to the client to take home for reference and a signed copy kept in the patient's medical records.

When prescribing psychoactive medications, one should keep in mind that some have the potential for human abuse. For example, diazepam, which can be very helpful for a variety of phobias, is a schedule IV drug that has a rapid onset of effect and is addictive. Methylphenidate, used in dogs with true hyperkinesis is a Schedule II drug that is sold illegally on the street. It is essential that detailed records be kept of the exact prescription and that the patient be monitored closely for response.

Also, the practitioner must follow specific state laws regarding prescribing such medications. For example, in Georgia, as of 2003, U.S. Drug Enforcement Administration (DEA) Class II medications must be prescribed in writing only. Telephone prescriptions can be done on an emergency basis, but there must be a written follow-up within one week. DEA Class III–IV drugs can have five refills or up to six months' prescription written. Laws covering these details will vary from state to state and country to country. Some of the drugs discussed in this book cannot be used legally in certain countries. In all cases, it is the veterinarian's responsibility to be aware of both national and local laws that apply to the individual's practice.

Because of the nature of behavior problems in pets, it is often not advisable to provide prescriptions for long periods. As a matter of routine, the University of Georgia Behavior Service requires that all patients on psychoactive medication come in for an outpatient recheck at least every three months for medication to be continued. At this time, progress is assessed and the medication may be changed, the dose increased or decreased, or the medication be continued as during the previous three months.

Cost

Unlike human medicine, where cost issues are often of low priority when making a decision as to which medication to use, cost is often a significant issue in all areas of veterinary medicine, including behavior. Therefore, in order to aid practitioners in the process of advising their clients, we are providing information on relative cost. In all cases it must be remembered that prices vary with region, over time, and with source.

Large chain pharmacies can often offer significantly lower prices than small, individually operated and owned pharmacies. However, the latter are sometimes the only viable source of special compounding that may be needed for particular patients. The cost of a daily dose can also vary with how much medication is purchased at one time, especially if some degree of compounding is required. Thus, the information given should be considered only a rough guideline and should necessarily be considered less accurate with the passage of time.

The numbers given are for a 30-day supply of medication for a 20-kg dog and a 5-kg cat, respectively. A 30-day supply for smaller or larger animals may cost only a little more or less or a great deal more or less, depending on the medication. This information is supplied only to give the practitioner a general idea of the relative cost of various medications. In the case of medications given "as needed," it is assumed that it is needed daily for 30 days. In most cases, this will not be what actually happens, so that the 30-day supply may actually last for a much longer period, depending on the situation.

Costliness is indicated by one to six dollar signs (Table 1.1). In all cases, if the price range varies across a boundary, for example, a 30-day supply will cost $20–$30 depending on the pharmacy used, the lower price is used. Often, medication is less expensive if bought in bulk, for example a 90-day supply as opposed to a 30-day supply. The dollar values given are appropriate for purchase of a 30-day supply only. For cats and parrots, many medications must routinely be compounded or, for cats, if tablets are available they can be reasonably split into smaller doses than allowed by the scoring. If the medication is available in a tablet that can be quartered, and if this method of dosing is less expensive than compounding into a liquid, then the number of dollar signs given is based on prescribing the number of tablets needed for a month's supply of such splitting. If the medication must be compounded, the number of dollar signs given assumes compounding into a liquid form, rather than into many small-dose capsules. The latter technique is likely to be much more expensive than compounding into a solution, because labor fees for placing small amounts of medication into many small capsules can be large.

For some patients that can be pilled but that refuse to consume flavored liquids, and will even spit them out, compounding into small capsules will be necessary. While initial purchases should be small in order to allow time to determine if the pet does not exhibit serious side effects and does respond positively to the medication, clients may obtain considerable savings over the long term if a bulk purchase is made once long-

Table 1.1 Codes indicating relative cost of a 30-day supply of medication for a 20-kg dog or a 5-kg cat

Code	Cost for a 30-day supply
$	Less than $10
$$	$10–25
$$$	$25–50
$$$$	$50–75
$$$$$	$75–100
$$$$$$	More than $100

Note: See text for further explanation.

term use is expected. Because many psychoactive medications are expensive, it is recommended that the practitioner be aware of the relative costliness of these medications at pharmacies in their area and via legitimate mail order pharmacies and that clients contact multiple pharmacies to get price quotes for their specific prescription.

Drug Selection

Specific information on drug selection will be given in the chapters on various classes of drugs; however, there are certain general considerations that will be discussed here. First, it is important to remember that our understanding of drug selection for specific behavior problems is changing rapidly as new clinical trials are completed. Thus, some statements made in this book will become outdated as a result of new research findings. It is important for the practitioner to keep up with research publications.

Each patient is a unique individual. At this time, we can only choose what to use based first on the species, the diagnosis, and the health status of the individual patient in a combination of evidence regarding the efficacy of various medications for that patient's problem. However, if the first medication used is not effective or generates unacceptable side effects, it is not necessarily the case that no medication will work. Sometimes a different medication in the same class of drugs will work well, even if the first medication was totally ineffective. Sometimes a medication from a totally different class is required. Sometimes combinations are required. For example, if a patient has not improved, as expected, on a serotonin (5-hydroxytryptamine or 5-HT) reuptake inhibitor alone, it may be the case that the patient's production of 5-HT is low. In such a situation the addition of a 5-HT agonist may be efficacious. Using combinations in particular requires that the clinician understand exactly how each medication works in the brain so that overdosing and drug interactions do not occur. Details of using combinations of drugs are discussed in chapter 15, as well as throughout the discussion of specific medications.

When choosing a drug, selectivity of mechanism is an issue that has at times been considered advantageous in human psychiatry. However, the topic is controversial and will not be discussed in depth in this book. In general, a potential advantage to multiple mechanisms of action in a single drug, for example, norepinephrine reuptake inhibition and serotonin reuptake inhibition, is possible increased robustness of efficacy. This presupposes that both or all of the multiple mechanisms of action in some way benefit the particular patient's problem. A potential problem is a greater possibility of multiple side effects. Better decision-making protocols on this issue will be more feasible when very exact relationships are discovered between specific behaviors or behavior problems in a given species and a particular molecular action in the brain.

The following should always be considered when choosing a medication.

1. What is the species and signalment?
2. What is the diagnosis?
3. Is the drug being considered indicated for that species, signalment, and diagnosis?
4. How experienced are you with the drug?
5. Are there any large studies published on actual efficacy for this diagnosis? If so, what is the actual efficacy?

6. What is the side effect profile?
7. What is the health status of the patient? Does the patient have any conditions that are contraindicated with this drug?
8. How much is cost an issue of concern for the client? How expensive is the drug?
9. What other drugs have been tried, and how did the patient respond?
10. How can the patient be medicated? If special forms of dosing are required, can the drug be provided in those forms, for example, a palatable liquid to be hidden in food?

Medicating the Patient

Often there are issues of the patient being resistant to taking medication. This is particularly problematic if the medication has unpleasant taste, which is the case with undisguised tricyclic antidepressants. Also, many medications must be given daily for a long period of time. For the patient that is fearful and/or aggressive, which are common problems, the difficulties are compounded. Owners may not be able to handle the pet without frightening it, and they may also run the risk of being bitten if they attempt to force-pill the patient. Different approaches are helpful for dogs and cats, but in general developing some routine of food intake prior to beginning medication can be useful.

Many dogs gulp highly palatable foods without pausing to taste. This is especially the case if a routine has been established with a highly palatable food. If the owner and dog do not already have such a routine, it can be initiated by first offering a highly palatable, small, semifirm amount of food. This can be a piece of hot dog or a ball of cheese or canned dog food that is not too moist. It should be offered in whatever fashion works best for the patient. Tossing works well for some dogs, who will catch the treat and gulp it. Other dogs will respond best if they are hand-fed or if the treat is offered on a small plate. In all cases, a routine with a highly palatable treat coming at the same time of day should be established. Once the dog consumes the treat rapidly and without pausing to chew, a pill or capsule can be hidden in it.

While some cats respond well to the approach used in dogs, a different approach is required for many cats. If a pill is essential and the cat is not yet trained to take a pill, but is not a biter or afraid of humans, the owner can train it to take a pill at a particular location. Begin by calling the cat to a particular site, briefly holding the head, then giving the cat a treat. When the cat responds readily to being called to the site and tolerates the brief restraint of the head, the owner should briefly open the cat's mouth before giving it the treat. Continue this until the cat's mouth can be briefly opened with no resistance. Then the owner should open the cat's mouth, briefly stick a finger in, and give the cat a treat. Finally, the owner can pill the cat and give it a treat. Pilling should always be followed by the reward of a highly palatable treat.

For the cat that cannot be pilled at all, it may be necessary to hide the medication in palatable food. First, identify a food that the cat finds very desirable, such as tuna fish, a particular brand of canned food, or shredded chicken. Begin offering the cat a small amount of the food on a regular routine. Have the medication compounded as a liquid that is compatible in flavor with the treat, for example, tuna juice. Then begin mixing the medication in with the treat. If the cat rejects a full dose, it may be necessary to initially mix in a partial dose. The dose can then be gradually increased over several days until the cat is eating the complete dose.

Transdermal medication of cats that are difficult to medicate would be desirable if it was effective. However, research to date on azapirones, selective serotonin reuptake inhibitors (SSRIs), and tricyclic antidepressants has invariably identified this method of medication to be ineffective. Blood levels of drugs administered transdermally are substantially lower than blood levels of drugs administered orally (Ciribassi et al. 2003; Mealey et al. 2004). Raising the level of drug in the transdermal medication to levels that produce comparable blood levels results in dermatitis.

Because of difficulty in medicating veterinary patients, slow-release forms of various medications are desirable so that a single action of medicating the patient can result in long action of the drug. Slow-release forms of several medications have been developed for humans. However, in all cases remember that the medications have been designed for the human digestive tract, which is substantially different physiologically from that of the carnivorous cat and dog and the herbivorous rabbit and horse. Thus, rates of absorption are likely to vary substantially in these species from the rates that occur in humans.

Competition Animals

Treating nonhuman animals that are shown in conformation or performance classes or that are raced presents special ethical and legal issues.

Many organizations that oversee the racing, conformation competition, and performance competition of purebred animals specifically prohibit the use of psychoactive medications, at least during competition. It is because of the problem of illegally doping racehorses with psychoactive medications during racing that we have data on the pharmacokinetics of several drugs in the horse. Other organizations, especially small, breed-specific organizations that foster interest in a breed or activity in which there are not large amounts of money at stake, allow medication, at least under certain situations. Such situations might include the treatment of a behavior problem diagnosed by a veterinarian and with notification of the judge that the animal is on medication for the diagnosed problem. When treating purebred animals that are placed in any form of competition, it is important to communicate openly with the owner and, as appropriate, the organization sponsoring the competition, as to whether or not certain medications are allowed. The owner may have to make a choice between continuing to enter their animal in competitions or using medication in the treatment of its behavior problem. Sometimes it is legal and desirable to remove the patient from competition for a period of a few months while the behavior problem is treated, after which it might be legally returned to competition once all traces of medication have been metabolized and cleared from its system.

The existence of serious behavior problems in animals owned for competition of any sort also begs the question of breeding that animal. If the problem can be clearly identified as being due to an event or a series of events that might reasonably be expected to cause behavior problems in any animal, for example, being beaten, having lightning strike a tree only a few feet away, etc., then the question of genetic influence is not an issue. However, if such experiences cannot be clearly identified, the question remains of how much genetics has made the patient predisposed to serious behavior problems.

Taking the Behavioral History

As discussed above, a diagnosis must be arrived at before a decision is made on which drug or drugs to use. Coming to a diagnosis requires that a behavioral history be taken. This applies to cases that are entirely behavioral in nature as well as cases that involve an interaction between behavior problems and medical problems or behavior problems and physical injury. An example of the latter might be a traumatic injury that the patient licks at and mutilates even when the original injury has healed entirely.

Behavioral histories can be collected in two major fashions. First, a standardized form can be provided for the client to fill out. This technique can be particularly useful in the case of a client who brings up a serious behavior problem during a routine exam for which 10 or 15 minutes of the veterinarian's time have been scheduled. This will not be adequate time to address a serious problem. However, the moment can be used to verify that the client's pet has a serious problem that needs some serious time with the veterinarian in order to address it. The client can be given the history form and instructed to make an appointment to return for a behavioral evaluation for the pet and then to fill out the form completely and bring it back upon their return visit. Ideally, the client should mail the form back in advance so that the veterinarian has the time to review the form before the client and patient return. The other way that information can be collected is by a direct interview. The direct interview has the disadvantage that some clients will digress at length, requiring skillful interviewing techniques to tactfully bring them back to the problem at hand. The advantage is that information can often be obtained that is not likely to come out on the written form.

A blended technique involves using both means of collecting history. Have the client fill out the written form in advance and either mail it to you or turn it in upon arrival for the appointment. Read the written answers before entering the room with the client. From those responses, develop a list of questions that build on the information you have obtained from the initial document.

The history needs to include the following seven areas: signalment, problem behavior, current environment, early history, training, miscellaneous behaviors, and medical history.

The signalment gives information about probabilities of certain diagnoses with given chief complaints. For example, if the complaint is owner-directed aggression in a dog, dominance aggression syndrome is more likely in a young, intact male adult than in an old, intact female. Herding-based aggression is more likely in a herding breed than in a non-herding breed. If the complaint is elimination in the house, cognitive dysfunction is more likely in a 12-year-old than in a 7-year-old, while it does not occur in a 2-year-old. If the complaint is owner-directed aggression in a cat, play aggression is more likely in a 2-year-old than in a 12-year-old.

A great deal needs to be learned about the problem behavior or chief complaint. First, it is necessary to get a good description of what behavior it is that the owner perceives as a problem. Owners often initially give their subjective interpretation of the behavior, rather than describing what the pet is actually doing. It is necessary to get a specific description of exactly what is happening. For example, the owner may say that their dog "gets angry" whenever they get near the food bowl while it is eating. In the author's experience, the following diversity of scenarios may lead to the use of this phrase.

1. My dog lowers his head and tucks his tail between his legs whenever I get near while he's eating. Then he'll just cringe and stare at the floor so long as I'm near. If I stay for long, he may start growling.
2. My dog stops eating whenever anyone gets near him. If I stand by his food bowl, he'll walk away.
3. Once I put the food bowl down, I leave the kitchen. If I don't leave fast enough, my dog will chase after me, barking and growling. I've been bitten twice when I didn't leave fast enough. Everyone knows to stay out of the kitchen while he's eating.

These three dogs clearly have three very different problems. However, owners may use the same subjective language in interpreting those problems. Since the veterinarian needs to make a diagnosis based on facts, not opinions and interpretations, it is essential to get descriptions of what the patient is doing that is a problem. A phrase that can be helpful in leading the client into this is "Can you describe what (your pet) does that makes you say he/she is angry (or sad, jealous, spiteful, depressed, etc.)?" Most people will understand what is needed once this question has been posed two or three times and will begin giving objective descriptions. A few will say things like "Oh, you know. He just acts jealous." At this point, it may be helpful to ask the client to pretend that they were a neutral observer, totally uninvolved in the situation, or to pretend that they witnessed the pet's behavior on TV. Again, from this point of view, ask them to describe what the problem pet and other involved people and animals actually did. It may require the description of multiple specific incidents for any underlying patterns to become clear. In the case of aggression, get complete, detailed descriptions of every incident of aggression that the client can recall. It may be necessary to get information from multiple people, because the client may not have personally witnessed some of the important incidents. For this reason, it is often desirable to have the entire family, or at least multiple family members, present for the interview.

Beyond a good description of what is actually occurring, several specific pieces of information are needed. When did the problem begin? As a general rule, problems of long duration are more difficult to resolve than problems of recent onset. Thus, duration of the problem may affect prognosis. Also, problems of long duration are likely to have undergone progressive changes. For example, a feline elimination behavior problem that began as avoidance of the dirty litter and/or separation anxiety when the owners were absent on vacation may have evolved into a location preference for the carpet under the dining room table and, most recently, into a generalized carpet preference. Changes over time in manifestation of the problem and in probable causes of the problem need to be examined carefully throughout the history-taking procedure.

The examining veterinarian also needs to know the frequency of the problem behavior and the circumstances in which the problem occurs. The frequency is needed in order to have baseline information from which to evaluate response to treatment. Spraying three times a week can be good or bad, depending on whether the patient was spraying 2 times a month or 10 times a week at the beginning of treatment. Information about the circumstances in which the problem behavior occurs can lead to improved understanding of the motivation for the behavior and, possibly, to identification of circumstances that the owner needs to avoid with environmental management. For example, if an aggressive cat is particularly prone to attacking a woman when she is wearing a broomstick skirt, it may be necessary for her to discontinue wearing broomstick skirts when at home for a while.

Changes in the frequency or form of the problem that have happened over time also need to be identified. Changes generally happen for a reason; understanding why the change has occurred will lead to a better understanding of the problem and, hence, identification of a specific treatment.

It is important to know what has been done so far to attempt to correct the problem. Clients may have read books in the library or gotten information off the Internet. Again, find out exactly what they actually did, and do not rely on client familiarity with behavioral jargon. The author has frequently had clients tell her that they had already tried "desensitization," only to learn that, in fact, they had not done so. Either the technique had been incorrectly described to them, or they had not understood the technique, or they had not adapted the technique to their pet's specific needs. In contrast, if they have been trying something that seems to be working and that is appropriate, instruct them to continue. Sometimes a technique has been working, but has stopped working because the pet has reached a stage at which it needs a modification of the technique in order for progress to resume. Find out the specific dosages and dosing schedules that have been prescribed by other veterinarians. Find out exactly what the client did, as well, because they may have modified the original instructions for various reasons. It is not uncommon to find that a suitable medication has been previously prescribed, but at only the lowest dose, and the client discontinued the medication when it didn't work at that dose. Alternatively, the client may have given the medication more or less frequently or at a lower or higher dose than prescribed without telling the veterinarian who originally prescribed the drug. The author has found it to be important, as a matter of routine, to ask referring veterinarians exactly what dosage schedule they prescribed and to also ask the client the exact schedule by which they medicated their pet.

Client education about what to expect from psychoactive medications and how to dose is critical. For example, SSRIs may not take effect for four to six weeks with daily dosing. However, many of my clients have been giving them only on an as-needed basis and decided from that schedule that the medicine doesn't work. Also verify exactly what side effects the patient has experienced with a particular medication. This information may tell you that the medication is contraindicated with this particular patient or that the client needs further education about the medication. For example, some pets experience transient, mild sedation of a few days' duration when first put on a SSRI. Usually, they recover from this in one to two weeks and return to normal levels of activity. Clients who have not been warned of this potential side effect may have taken their pet off medication or decreased the dose too early in the treatment and done so without telling their veterinarian.

A different area for discussion is the question of whether there are other behavior problems besides the chief complaint that caused them to bring their pet to you in the first place. While some clients will state that the pet is "perfect" except for that one problem, others will have a short or long list of other behaviors they do not like. In some cases, the other problems will be even more serious than the presenting complaint. The client may have brought the pet in for the original complaint because they heard through some means, for example, the television, that this problem was treatable. The client may have assumed that the other problems were untreatable and would not have brought them up except for your specifically asking. Sometimes the client will not have mentioned other problems because he or she considers them minor. If it turns out that the pet has multiple problems, it is good to make a problem list and have the client prioritize them as to which he or she most wants to have treated first. Sometimes it is not possible to treat two particular problems at once because there is some degree of conflict in the treatment techniques for the two problems. More often, the problems cannot all be addressed at once simply because even the most dedicated client has a finite amount of time they can spend helping their pet.

The patient's current environment has many facets, any or all of which can affect behavior and the behavior problem. Major categories are (1) the humans in the environment, (2) other animals in the environment, and (3) the physical environment, which includes all aspects of housing and management.

Regarding the human environment, it is important to know who lives with the pet or is a frequent visitor. This will include all family members who live in the home, but may also include housekeepers, babysitters, gardeners, and other domestic personnel. Identify when individuals are typically at the house and how they interact with the patient or are involved with the patient's care. Also ask if there have been any significant departures, especially around the time the problem began. Examples would include older children leaving for college and spouses who have departed due to separation or divorce.

Also find out what other animals, typically but not necessarily household pets, interact with the pet. The species, gender, age, and behavioral relationship with the patient should be identified for all household pets. An example of non-pet animals that may be of importance would include neighborhood cats or dogs that frequently visit the yard or even house. This is of potential significance with urine marking and any stress-induced behavior problem. A different example would be a large number of squirrels living outside that cause frequent arousal in a patient that has arousal-induced aggression.

The degree and type of detailed information about the environment that will be needed will necessarily vary somewhat with species and chief complaint. The following basic information should always be obtained: (1) a description of the housing the patient lives in, for example, the size of the house and what areas of the house the patient has access to and, in the case of dogs, whether or not the backyard is fenced; (2) information about diet and feeding schedules; (3) the entire daily routine for handling and caring for the patient. In the case of cats, identify how many litter boxes there are in the house, whether or not they are hooded, what type of litter is in them, where they are located in the house, and how often they are cleaned. Much of this information will be important background information that you will need in designing your total treatment program.

Learning the early history is not often useful in coming to a diagnosis or designing a treatment program. However, sometimes useful information is identified that may help the owners better understand their pet. If there is a background of abandonment, owners are likely to be more sympathetic to their pet's current difficulty with being left alone. Information to obtain includes the source of the pet, the age when obtained, and any information that is available about previous owners, including the pet's possible experiences with them, such as abuse, and their reports about the pet's early behavior.

Learning about training and other structured learning experiences the patient has had is important with all species, but especially with species that typically undergo extensive formal training, such as the dog and the horse. The veterinarian needs to be familiar not only with ethical and appropriate training techniques, but also with commonly used abusive training techniques. While there are many ethical and competent animal trainers, there are also, unfortunately, some unethical and abusive animal trainers. Owners sometimes take their pet, in good faith, to a trainer whom they do not realize is using abusive and inappropriate techniques. Impressed by advertising and the charisma of the trainer, they may leave the pet with the trainer or do things to the pet under the trainer's directions that make them uncomfortable. In taking the history, first get a good description of exactly what has been done to the patient. If there are problems, explain objectively why they are problems. In cases of clear abuse, the trainer should be reported to the state veterinarian's office. Often, owners feel guilty about what has happened to the pet. This is especially likely to be the case if they stood by while the pet was mistreated and the mistreatment has now resulted in a major behavior problem, typically fear of people or fear-induced aggression. Some owners will become defensive, both of their own actions and of their trainer. In this case, calmly conducted client education about appropriate animal training techniques is essential.

Often, training is included in a treatment program, and understanding a pet's response to various training situations will be important. For example, the author once worked with an aggressive dog that was often tense during interactions with the family. However, the command "Gimme five," which meant to raise the paw to be touched by the palm of a human family member, consistently resulted in relaxation and an amicable interaction. The command "Gimme five," accompanied by a treat, was an important part of the initial phase of treatment.

Miscellaneous other behaviors that need to be touched on briefly or in depth, depending on the chief complaint, include sexual behaviors, maternal behaviors, and grooming. In particular, grooming, in all of its aspects of bathing, brushing the coat and teeth, clipping the nails, and cleaning the ears can be a source of historical problems that the family has simply accepted. However, identifying what parts of grooming result in behaviors of escape, fear, or aggression can be essential to understanding the patient. It is important to ask about the patient's behaviors of self-grooming, as well. Early cases of compulsive disorder, discussed below, may manifest as simple increased amounts of grooming with lesions just beginning to develop, which the clients will not have thought to mention.

If you have been the patient's veterinarian its entire life, you will know its medical history. Often, though, you will treat patients who have been previously cared for by one or more other veterinarians. If at all possible, obtain copies of the medical records from all previous veterinarians. Medical issues of particular relevance include (1) illness, injuries, or elective surgery that occurred around the time the problem began; (2) chronic medical problems; and (3) previous or current medication for the behavior or other problems.

The Behavioral Exam

While you are taking the history, even if it is a brief history to supplement a written history given to you by the owner, you will be able to conduct your initial direct behavioral exam of the animal. For horses and other large animals, it is ideal that this initial interview be conducted in a location where you can comfortably observe the patient as you talk with the client. You may be able to observe the actual problem, for example, cribbing or head shaking, but also discern such important information as whether or not the horse is constantly alert and never relaxes, avoids people, rushes people with its ears pinned back, approaches people and solicits attention, etc. Likewise, with dogs, which will usually be observed in the exam room, note what signaling the patient sends to the human family members, yourself, and your staff. If there are any concerns about aggression to you or your staff, the patient should be kept on a leash. Otherwise, allow the patient to wander freely around the exam room so that you can note its general demeanor, for example, hiding under a chair, curiously investigating the exam room and visiting you and your staff, or climbing into the owner's lap and soliciting attention. If there are serious concerns about possible biting incidents, the patient should be wearing an appropriately fitted basket muzzle. It is essential that a basket muzzle be used so that the patient can pant, drink, etc. Most patients can be trained to calmly accept the basket muzzle, or even voluntarily place their muzzles into it, by pairing wearing of the basket muzzle with receipt of delicious food treats.

In the case of other pets such as cats, parrots, and rabbits, again much can be learned by direct observation of the patient. Unless it is not safe to do so, allow the patient to move freely around the exam room while you interview the client.

Sometimes it is desirable to do a specific, direct exam of the behavioral responses of the patient to specific stimuli. Before doing this, carefully consider what you have learned from the owner and from direct observation of the pet's spontaneous behavior. Then, in considering special tests, assess whether it will be both safe and useful. For example, if you suspect that a dog specifically is aggressive to strangers reaching their hands toward it, but does not have a problem with strangers walking around it so long as they do not reach for it, you might ask the owner to restrain their dog, then attempt both behaviors while keeping at a distance that will not result in injury. If your suspicion is confirmed, you can then establish the initial starting place for a desensitization protocol by determining how much the hand has to move toward the dog before it exhibits aggression.

Finally, it is important to discuss with the owners what their specific goals are for their pet. Discuss whether or not the goals are realistic and potentially attainable and give an initial estimate of how long it is likely to take to achieve their goals. While we may think, based on prior discussion, that we understand the owner's goals, we may not.

Desensitization and Counterconditioning

Desensitization and counterconditioning are two techniques that are commonly used in behavioral therapy, either separately or together. While behavior modification is not the focus of this book, the terms are mentioned here for the benefit of individuals who are not familiar with them. In desensitization, the animal is exposed to a stimulus that elicits a given response, but at such a low level that the response is not elicited. Over time and successive repetitions, the intensity of the stimulus is gradually increased, ideally without eliciting the response. In counterconditioning, a response is elicited that is both behaviorally and physiologically incompatible with another response.

Duration of Treatment

Once a patient's problem has been diagnosed and a treatment plan devised, a common question is how long the treatment will take. Many owners are concerned that their pet will have to be on medication for the rest of its life. The exact duration will vary not only with the treatment, the species, and the problem, but with the individual patient. Also, the family's ability to follow through with management and behavior modification changes will affect duration of treatment. As a general rule, the goal is to eventually wean the patient off of medication. Nevertheless, behavior problems are not cured in a week or 10 days. Their resolution requires several weeks, at the least. Commonly, several months are required. Severe or refractory cases may take years or never resolve. When treatment is initiated, the author instructs the owner that our goal is, first, to identify and conduct treatments that entirely resolve the problem. After that, we will maintain treatment for two to three months after the problem appears to be resolved. This length of time is necessary to adequately confirm that the problem is, indeed, resolved. Once the patient has remained behaviorally well for two to three months, a gradual weaning process is initiated whereby drug doses are decreased and, eventually, discontinued entirely.

Common Categories of Major Behavior Problems

Problems of Anxiety, Fears, and Phobias

Fear is a normal behavior. It is the emotional component of the flight or fight response that facilitates animals in engaging in behaviors that are likely to facilitate their survival when faced with such phenomena as predators and natural disasters. It is when fear becomes excessive in frequency and intensity relative to the stimuli that are inducing the fear that it becomes a problem. Thus, whereas seeking shelter or hiding during a severe thunderstorm would be a normal and adaptive behavior for a wolf or feral dog, a house dog's whining, howling, shaking, urinating, pacing, and panting when there are dark clouds in the sky and a shifting barometric pressure is not normal. In this case, we would call such an intense response to such a mild stimulus a phobia.

In humans, anxiety is defined as "apprehension of danger and dread accompanied by restlessness, tension, tachycardia, and dyspnea unattached to a clearly identifiable stimulus" (*Stedman's Concise Medical Dictionary* 1997). In veterinary behavior, we cannot know if our patients are experiencing "apprehension" or "danger." The term is used to refer to behavior consistent with mild to moderate fear. Anxiety may occur in response to a specific stimulus or situation, or it may occur almost independently of external stimuli. When a patient is anxious most of the time, regardless of the situation it is in, it may have generalized anxiety disorder (GAD).

In identifying fear objectively, we look for combinations of signals. In cats and dogs this would include, but not be limited to, crouching, turning back the ears, lowering the tail, hiding, avoiding the object or individual causing the fear, trembling, pacing, lip licking, panting, salivating excessively, vocalizing (whining, crying), urinating, and defecating. Some behaviors indicative of fear, such as retraction of the commissure of the lips in dogs, are species specific. There may be other causes for specific behaviors, for example, panting occurs in both cats and dogs when they are hot. Thus, it is necessary to identify a combination of behaviors that are consistent with fear to come to this assessment of the patient's emotional status. Horses balk, shy, snort, defecate, avoid, and run away from the object inducing fear. Parrots scream, growl, hiss, raise the crest (in crested species), weave, and attempt to escape whatever is threatening them. Rabbits hide, crouch, whimper, grind their teeth, and thump.

In fear-induced aggression, the most common cause of aggressive behavior in many species, various signals of fear, such as those listed above, will be exhibited in conjunction with aggressive threats such as showing the teeth and growling (cats, dogs), hissing (cats, parrots), or pinning back the ears and threatening to kick (horses).

Phobias are fears of specific objects, animals, people, or situations. They are persistent over time, not just occurring once or twice. They are also consistent in terms of what causes the fear, although a given patient may have multiple phobias. They are also learned, irrational, and not adaptive. Phobias may result in intense behavioral responses that are best described as hysteria or panic. These would include screaming loudly or digging at a barrier so violently that the barrier is destroyed and the patient is severely injured in the process. Some phobic animals exhibit extremely decreased behavioral arousal and may become, in extreme cases, catatonic. The catatonic patient will be frozen in place and will show little response to stimulation.

A variety of factors, including genetics, early experience, and specific learning, contribute to the development of excessive and inappropriate fear.

Animals that have no genetic predisposition to easily become fearful, as well as animals that had appropriate early experiences, can become fearful due to the phenomenon of classical conditioning. Classical conditioning is also called *Pavlovian conditioning* because it was first described by Ivan Pavlov as a result of his experiments on the physiology of eating. He found that if a bell was rung as a subject was being presented with meat, salivation could eventually be elicited just by ringing the bell. The phenomenon of classical conditioning was subsequently found to be very widespread. It is particularly relevant to veterinary behavior because it is the cause of many chronic and severe phobias. In classical conditioning there is a stimulus, called the unconditioned stimulus (US), that naturally causes a response, the unconditioned response (UR). In this case, the USs would be anything that naturally elicits a fear response, or UR, such as being hit, screamed at, dropped, or otherwise being harmed or experiencing fright. Unfortunately, many animal training techniques involve the use of pain as a source of motivation. This practice quite commonly leads to fear.

Stimuli that are present at the time the animal is exposed to the US can become conditional stimuli (CSs). Visual, auditory, tactile, olfactory, gustatory, and other stimuli that

Table 1.2 Types of stimuli that commonly become CSs for fear responses

Visual	Colors, shapes, faces, garments (e.g. jeans, glasses, hats), objects being carried, structures
Auditory	Voices, thunder, firecrackers, vacuum cleaners
Olfactory	Specific perfumes
Tactile	Being touched in a certain place or manner
Other	Changes in barometric pressure, increasing levels of negative ions in the atmosphere

the animal can sense can become CSs (Table 1.2). The animal may discriminate very particular CSs that induce the fear response or generalize to broad categories that induce the fear response. An example of stimulus discrimination would be the dog that cringes and urinates only when it hears a particular man's voice. An example of stimulus generalization would be a dog that cringes and urinates when it hears any person speak.

Treatment of anxieties and phobias is generally greatly benefited by use of appropriate anxiolytic medications. In cases of mild phobias progress with behavior modification alone may be sufficient. However, in cases of moderate to severe phobias, use of anxiolytics will greatly facilitate the speed of response to treatment, increasing the compliance of the owner and decreasing the time that the patient spends in a state of fear. In the most severe cases, progress is not possible without the use of anxiolytics.

Problems of Aggression

Aggression is not a unitary phenomenon with a single motivation. On the contrary, it is a complex behavior, with many causes. When the terms *aggression* or *aggressive behavior* are used, both actual attempts to cause injury and threats to cause injury are included. While the teeth, claws, or hooves typically cause injury, animals may use other parts of their bodies to threaten, including the ears, head, eyes, and tail.

The term *affective aggression* is used to refer to aggression involving intense autonomic responses that include sympathoadrenal interactions. Animals give specific signs of threat, and if the individual threatened does not exhibit appropriate responses, they attack. In all cases, there is intense arousal, at least in the attack phase. The various types of affective aggression can be divided into offensive and defensive subtypes, which is of particular concern when deciding if a particular patient can be safely managed during treatment. Offensive aggression is typically a more dangerous phenomenon than defensive aggression. In common usage, affective aggression includes fear, dominance, territorial, possessive, and maternal aggression.

Predatory aggression is not considered a kind of affective aggression. Instead, it is a maintenance behavior of carnivores that is necessary for survival. While the carnivore may become highly aroused while attempting to kill a strong prey animal that is fighting off its attack, predatory aggression per se does not necessarily involve substantial arousal. Some behaviorists do not consider predatory aggression to be aggression at all, but simply food gathering. However, to the individual being bitten and clawed, it is certainly aggression and is particularly relevant in the context of predatory attacks by large dogs or packs of dogs on humans and small pets.

Serotonin is involved in the modulation of aggression; therefore, medications that increase central serotonergic activity should produce a decrease in affective aggression by decreasing the tendency to engage in sudden outbursts of aggression and increasing the threshold of tolerance to stimuli that might typically induce aggression. Because of this, medications that increase serotonin activity in the central nervous system are commonly and effectively used to treat many types of affective aggression (e.g., Coccaro et al. 1990; White et al. 1991; Markowitz 1992; Sanchez and Hyttel 1994). Conversely, medications that inhibit brain serotonin increase aggression, including predatory aggression (e.g., Katz 1980).

There is much supporting evidence for the role of serotonin in aggression. An inverse correlation between levels of hydroxyindole acetic acid (5-HIAA) in the cerebrospinal fluid (CSF) and the history of aggressive behavior has been found repeatedly in human, primate, and laboratory studies (e.g., Brown and Linnoila 1990; van Praag 1991; Coccaro et al. 1992; Mehlman et al. 1994; Kyes et al. 1995; Lee and Coccaro 2001). Dogs diagnosed with dominance aggression have significantly lower levels of 5-HIAA in their CSF than do control dogs (Reisner et al. 1996). Even small variation in levels, turnover, or metabolism of 5-HT, as well as activation, density, or binding affinity of receptor subtypes, affect aggression (Nelson and Chiavegatto 2001).

Male vervet monkeys given either tryptophan or fluoxetine, both of which enhance serotonin activity, exhibit increased affiliative behavior and dominance rank, with a concurrent decrease in aggressiveness. Male vervet monkeys given fenfluramine or cyproheptadine, both of which decrease serotonergic activity, exhibit decreased affiliative behavior and dominance rank and increased aggressiveness (Raleigh et al. 1991).

Furthermore, rats with a knockout mutation of the gene for 5-HT1B receptors fight incessantly and, when confronted with an intruder, attack the intruder faster and more intensely than non-knockout mice (Saudou et al. 1994; Ramboz et al. 1996).

Impaired synthesis or metabolism of serotonin has been repeatedly found to be associated with increased aggression (e.g., Brunner et al. 1993; Nelson et al. 1995; Nielsen et al. 1994; Sandou et al. 1994).

Fluoxetine and fluvoxamine, both medications that increase levels of serotonin in the central nervous system by inhibiting reuptake of the molecule, suppress defensive and biting reactions and territorial aggression in rodents (Oliver and Mos 1990; Fuller 1996).

Because predatory aggression is so dangerous, resulting in the deaths of many humans and large numbers of livestock every year, medications are not routinely used as treatment. Adequate restraint of predators, including cats in environments where birds and small mammals must be protected from them, and all dogs, is the mainstay of addressing problems of predatory aggression. Nevertheless, from a theoretical point of view serotonergic medications and γ-aminobutyric acid (GABA) agonists should be helpful with this problem.

In laboratory studies, serotonin and GABA have been found to have an inhibitory effect on predatory behavior (e.g., Eichelman 1987; Miczek and Donat 1989). Mouse-killing behavior in rats has been effectively attenuated by the use of serotonin agonists and SSRIs (Molina et al. 1987).

Compulsive Disorder

Obsessive-compulsive disorder is a common problem in the human population. It is a disorder in which the obsessions or compulsions take up significant amounts of time, cause distress to the individual affected by them, and interfere with normal life. The *DSM-IV* defines obsessions as "persistent ideas, thoughts, impulses, or images that are

Table 1.3 Common behaviors for several domestic species that may be due to compulsive disorder

Species	Commonly presented behaviors in compulsive disorder
Cat	Licking self or objects, chewing self or objects
Cattle	Kicking, bar licking, tongue rolling, inappropriate suckling
Dog	Licking self or objects, chewing self or objects, freezing, tail chasing, flank sucking, "checking" hindquarters, shadow chasing
Horse	Cribbing, wood chewing, stall circling, kicking, pawing, weaving, head shaking, flank biting
Parrot	Feather picking, feather chewing, self-mutilating, pacing, intention movements for flight
Pig	Chain rooting, chain chewing

Note: In all cases, the behavior may be due to compulsive disorder or to other causes, including learning, psychomotor seizures, or various dermatological conditions. Comprehensive behavioral and medical evaluation must be done to determine if the problem is due to compulsive disorder or another cause.

experienced as intrusive and inappropriate and that caused marked anxiety or distress." Compulsions are "repetitive behaviors (e.g., hand washing, ordering, checking) or mental acts (e.g., praying, counting, repeating words silently). . ." (American Psychiatric Association, 1994). In veterinary patients, we cannot ever know whether obsessions or mental compulsions occur, although we suspect they do. We can, however, observe behavioral compulsions, which take many forms. Therefore, the term compulsive disorder, rather than obsessive-compulsive disorder, is used in veterinary behavior.

Compulsive disorder takes many forms. It is characterized by the animal engaging in a repetitive, stereotyped behavior for significant amounts of time, at least one hour each day. As with humans, compulsive disorder also comes to interfere with normal maintenance and social behaviors. Compulsive disorder must be distinguished from learned behavior that has become more and more common because it results in owner attention and environment-induced stereotypic behavior. In the latter case, animals that have been confined to an understimulating or overstimulating environment may begin engaging in stereotypic behavior, but will discontinue the behavior once they are removed to an appropriate environment. Long-term maintenance in an inappropriate environment may result in a transition from a simple environment-induced stereotypic behavior to a true compulsive disorder. An example would be the horse that begins walking in a circle in its stall. If kept in the inappropriate environment of its stall for a sufficiently long period, it will eventually reach the point where, even if turned out on a large pasture, it will go to a specific point in the pasture and walk in a circle the same size as the circle walked in the stall. In all cases, underlying medical causes for the behavior must also be ruled out. For example, animals that constantly bite, chew, or lick themselves may be experiencing pain or itching, rather than manifesting a compulsive behavior.

Behaviors of compulsive disorder are derived from normal behaviors, because normal behaviors constitute the behavioral repertoire from which the animal can develop pathological behaviors. The various forms of compulsive disorder can generally be classified as locomotor, oral, grooming, aggressive, vocalization, and hallucinatory. An example of the latter would be the constant chasing of invisible mice or flies by dogs. Because behaviors of compulsive disorder are derived from normal behavior, there is species variation in what are considered to be common presentations for compulsive disorder (Table 1.3).

Posttraumatic Stress Disorder

Posttraumatic stress disorder (PTSD) is not currently referred to in the veterinary behavior literature, and it will be impossible to ever verify if animals do, in fact, experience flashbacks the way humans do. Nevertheless, the author has had a number of patients in her practice with a known or strongly suspected history of severe abuse that exhibit behaviors that suggest that this does happen. These patients may appear to be normal much of the time, but exhibit periods when their behavior suddenly and dramatically changes, often for reasons that the owner cannot discern. Someone putting on a jacket can suddenly result in a dog that was playing a moment earlier starting to scream, cry, and try to crawl under a piece of furniture. Sometimes pets exhibit acute onset of intense aggression with clear signaling of fear. Owners often describe their pet as appearing to "be in another world" or "not recognizing us." Seizure disorders must be ruled out in these cases, but these patients sometimes respond to the same medications effective in the treatment of human PTSD in which long-term changes in the chemistry of the central nervous system are believed to result from extremely traumatic events (e.g., Davidson et al. 1991; McDougle et al. 1991; Shay 1992; Nagy et al. 1993; Pearlstein 2000). Since abuse of dogs, cats, horses, and other animals is, unfortunately, an all too common phenomenon, modern methods of treatment of PTSD should be considered when treating animals that have been the victims of the darker side of human nature.

Using This Book

The general practitioner may find it most useful to look up information as cases arrive for which they need information about drug selection. Table 1.4 directs the practitioner to particular chapters based on the chief complaint or suspected diagnosis. Clinical chapters are indicated separately from basic science chapters for those who need to get directly to information that will help them make a decision, although it is recommended that the basic science chapter(s) that discusses action in the brain of the molecule affected by the drug prescribed be reviewed as well.

Table 1.4   Quick reference for what chapters to go to for given chief complaints or suspected diagnoses

Chief complaint or diagnosis	Basic information (Chapter)	Clinical information (Chapter)
Aggression	4	5, 6, 11, 14, 15
Anxieties, fears, and phobias; without aggression	2, 4, 7	3, 5, 6, 8, 11
Cognitive dysfunction in geriatric patients	7	8
Compulsive disorder	4, 12	5, 9, 11,13
Hyperkinesis or attention deficit disorder	7	10
Problems not responsive to initial treatment		15

Limitations

Information on FDA-approved and unique uses of medications in humans is given because, sometimes, this can be a valuable reference tool when considering what to attempt with a nonhuman patient. However, some cautions are in order. First, it is important to understand that the fact that Drug A and not Drug B is listed as approved for disorder X does not necessarily mean that Drug B is not useful for disorder X, or even that Drug A is better. It means that the company that owns the patent on Drug A has invested the money in the trials mandated by the FDA to prove that Drug A is better than placebo. It might be the case that Drug B is better for disorder X, but the company owning the patent for Drug B does not consider it economical to seek to obtain approval for disorder X. Or Drug B might be available generically, and there is no company willing to invest the large amounts of money necessary for FDA approval.

Additionally, while human psychiatric disorders and the research on their treatment can sometimes be considered to be models for animal behavior disorders, there is not always a good analogy. Looking to the literature on human obsessive-compulsive disorder, patients who are persistent handwashers may be useful in investigating possible best treatments for dogs that persistently lick their paws. In the long run, it may or may not turn out that treatment of human obsessive-compulsive disorder is a good model for treatment of canine compulsive disorder. It is probably a further stretch to look to treatments approved for social phobia in humans and assume that this is necessarily a good model for excessively shy cats. The underlying biology and learning processes may well be different. Nevertheless, until more trials are conducted comparing the efficacy of various drug treatments on specific populations, we must rely on the vast literature of human psychiatry as a starting point.

Not all drugs commercially available in a given class are covered in this book, and not all classes of psychiatric drugs are covered. Selection of specific drugs to be discussed is based on a combination of the authors' experience with the medication, published reports on the medication, communication with colleagues about their use of the medication, and current availability of the medication. Some of the newest drugs that have been developed for human psychiatric disorders may have great potential for veterinary patients but are not covered in this edition because of a lack of experience in veterinary populations. Future editions will doubtless include an expanded drug list.

Likewise, while there is some discussion of effects on mice and rats, the extensive and detailed information available in the literature on the various metabolic effects and behavioral changes that occur in laboratory testing are not covered comprehensively, because such coverage would double the size of this book without greatly increasing its usefulness to the veterinarian whose practice is directed to the care of privately owned animals rather than laboratory populations.

Clinical Examples

To further illustrate use of psychoactive medications in veterinary patients, short case reports are presented at the end of most of the clinical chapters. While actual cases are presented, the names of the patients have been changed.

References

American Psychiatric Association. 1994. *DSM-IV*. p. 418, American Psychiatric Association: Washington, DC.

Brown GL and Linnoila MI 1990. CSF serotonin metabolite (5-HIAA) studies in depression, impulsivity, and violence. *Journal of Clinical Psychiatry* 51(4)(suppl): 31–43.

Brunner HG, Nelen M, Breakefield XO, Ropers HH and Van Oost BA 1993. Abnormal behavior associated with a point mutation in the structural gene for monoamine oxidase A. *Science* 262 (5133): 578–580.

Burke WJ 2004. Selective versus multi-transmitter antidepressants: are two mechanisms better than one? *Journal of Clinical Psychiatry* 65(suppl4) 37–45.

Ciribassi J, Luescher A, Pasloske KS, Robertson-Plouch C, Zimmerman A and Kaloostian-Whittymore L 2003. Comparative bioavailability of fluoxetine after transdermal and oral administration to healthy cats. *American Journal of Veterinary Research* 64(8): 994–998.

Coccaro EF, Astill JL, Herbert JL and Schut AG 1990. Fluoxetine treatment of impulsive aggression in DSM-III-R personality disorder patients. *Journal of Clinical Psychopharmacology* 10(5): 373–375.

Coccaro EF, Kavoussi RJ and Lesser JC 1992. Self-and other-directed human aggression: the role of the central serotonergic system. *International Clinical Psychopharmacology* 6 (suppl 6):70–83.

Davidson J, Roth S and Newman E 1991. Fluoxetine in post-traumatic stress disorder. *Journal of Trauma Stress* 4:419–423.

Eichelman, B. 1987. Neurochemical and psychopharmacologic aspects of aggressive behavior. In *Psychopharmacology: the third generation of progress*, pp. 697–704, edited by HY Meltzer. Raven Press: New York.

Fuller RW 1996. Fluoxetine effects on serotonin function and aggressive behavior. In *Understanding aggressive behavior in children*, pp. 90–97, edited by CF Ferris and TT Grisso. *Annals of the New York Academy of Sciences* 794: New York.

Katz RJ 1980. Role of serotonergic mechanisms in animal models of predation. *Progress in Neuro-Psychopharmacology*. 4: 219–231.

Krishnan KR 1999. Brain imaging correlates. *Journal of Clinical Psychiatry* 60 (suppl 15): 50–54.

Kyes RC, Botchin MB, Kaplan JR, Manuck SB and Mann JJ 1995. Aggression and brain serotonergic responsivity: Response to slides in male macaques. *Physiology and Behavior* 57: 205–208.

Lee R and Coccaro E 2001. The neuropsychopharmacology of criminality and aggression. *Canadian Journal of Psychiatry* 46: 35–43.

Markowitz PI 1992. Effect of fluoxetine on self-injurious behavior in the developmentally disabled: A preliminary study. *Journal of Clinical Psychopharmacology* 12(1): 27–31.

McDougle CJ, Southwick SM, Charney DS and St James RL 1991. An open trial of fluoxetine in the treatment of posttraumatic stress disorder [letter]. *Journal of Clinical Psychopharmacology* 11(5): 325–327.

Mealey KL, Peck KE, Bennett BS, Sellon RK, Swinney GR, Melzer K, Gokhale SA and Krone TM. 2004. Systemic absorption of amitriptyline and buspirone after oral and transdermal administration to healthy cats. *Journal of Veterinary Internal Medicine* 18(1): 43–46.

Mehlman PT, Higley JD, Faucher I, Lilly AA, Taub DM, Vickers J, Suomi SJ, Linnoila M 1994. Low CSF 5-HIAA concentrations and severe aggression and impaired impulse control in nonhuman primates. *The American Journal of Psychiatry* 151(10): 1485–1491.

Miczek KA and Donat P 1989. Brain 5-HT systems and inhibition of aggressive behavior. In *Behavioral pharmacology of 5-HT*, pp. 117–144, edited by P Bevan, A Cools and T Archer, Lawrence Erlbaum Associates: Hillsdale, NJ.

Molina V, Ciesielski L, Gobaille S, Isel F and Mandel P 1987. Inhibition of mouse killing behavior by serotonin-mimetic drugs: effects of partial alterations of serotonin neurotransmission. *Pharmacology, Biochemistry, and Behavior* 27(1): 123–131.

Nagy LM, Morgan CA, Southwick SM and Charney DS 1993. Open prospective trial of fluoxetine for posttraumatic stress disorder. *Journal of Clinical Psychopharmacology* 13(2): 107–113.

Nelson RJ and Chiavegatto S 2001. Molecular basis of aggression. *Trends in Neurosciences* 24(12): 713–719.

Nelson DA, Demas GE, Huang PL, Fishman MC, Dawson VL, Dawson TM and Snyder S 1995. Behavioral abnormalities in male mice lacking neuronal nitric oxide synthase. *Nature* 378(6555): 383–386.

Nielsen DA, Goldman D, Virkkunen M, Tokola R, Rawlings R and Linnoila M 1994. Suicidality and 5-hydroxyindoleactic acid concentration associated with a tryptophan hydroxylase polymorphism. *Archives of General Psychiatry* 51: 34–38.

Olivier B and Mos J 1990. Serenics, serotonin and aggression. In *Current and future trends in anticonvulsant, anxiety, and stroke therapy,* pp. 203–230, edited by BS Meldrum and M Williams, Wiley-Liss, Inc.

Pearlstein T 2000. Antidepressant treatment of posttraumatic stress disorder. *Journal of Clinical Psychiatry* 61(7): 40–43.

Raleigh MJ, McGuire MT, Brammer GL, Pollack DB and Yuwiler A 1991. Serotonergic mechanisms promote dominance acquisition in adult male vervet monkeys. *Brain Research* 559: 181–190.

Ramboz S, Saudou F, Amara DA, Belzung C, Dierich A, LeMeur M, Segu L, Misslin R, Buhot MC and Hen R 1996. Behavioral characterization of mice packing the 5-HT1B receptor. *NIDA Research Monograph* 161: 39–57.

Reisner IR, Mann JJ, Stanley M, Huang Y and Houpt KA 1996. Comparison of cerebrospinal fluid monoamine metabolite levels in dominant-aggressive and non-aggressive dogs. *Brain Research* 714: 57–64.

Sanchez C and Hyttel J 1994. Isolation-induced aggression in mice: effects of 5-hydroxytryptamine uptake inhibitors and involvement of postsynaptic 5-HT$_{1A}$ receptors. *European Journal of Pharmacology* 264: 241–247.

Saudou F, Amara DA, Dierich A, LeMeur M, Ramboz S, Segu L, Buhot MC and Hen R 1994. Enhanced aggressive behavior in mice lacking 5HT1B receptor. *Science* 265(5180): 1875–1878.

Shay J 1992. Fluoxetine reduces explosiveness and elevates mood of Vietnam combat vets with PTSD. *Journal of Traumatic Stress* 5: 97–101.

Stedman's concise medical dictionary for the health professions 1997. Williams and Wilkins, Baltimore, MD, p. 59.

Van Praag HM 1991. Serotonergic dysfunction and aggression control. *Psychological Medicine* 21: 15–19.

White SM, Kucharik RF and Moyer JA 1991. Effects of serotonergic agents on isolation-induced aggression. *Pharmacology Biochemistry & Behavior* 39: 729–736.

Chapter Two
Amino Acid Neurotransmitters: Glutamate, GABA, and the Pharmacology of Benzodiazepines

Introduction

In addition to their role in intermediary metabolism, certain amino acids function as small molecule neurotransmitters in the central and peripheral nervous systems. These specific amino acids are classified as excitatory or inhibitory, based on the characteristic responses evoked in neural preparations. Application of excitatory amino acids such as glutamic acid and aspartic acid typically depolarize mammalian neurons, while inhibitory amino acids such as γ-aminobutyric acid (GABA) and glycine characteristically hyperpolarize neurons. Glutamate, aspartate, and GABA all represent amino acids that occur in high concentrations in the brain. The brain levels of these amino acid transmitters are high (micromoles per gram) relative to biogenic amine transmitters (nanomoles per gram) such as dopamine, serotonin, norepinephrine, and acetylcholine. In mammals, GABA is found in high concentrations in the brain and spinal cord, but is present in only trace amounts in peripheral nerve tissue, liver, spleen, or heart (Cooper et al. 1996). These observations reveal the enrichment of this amino acid in the brain and suggest an important functional role in the central nervous system (CNS).

Glutamatergic Synapses

Glutamate and aspartate produce powerful excitation in neural preparations, and glutamate is generally accepted as the major excitatory transmitter in the brain. The establishment of glutamate as a neurotransmitter in the brain has been difficult due to its role in general intermediary metabolism. Glutamate is also involved in the synthesis of proteins and peptides and also serves as the immediate precursor for GABA in GABAergic neurons. The enzyme glutamic acid decarboxylase converts glutamate to GABA in these GABAergic neurons. In contrast to GABA, the glutamate content of the brain outside of glutamatergic neurons is high as a consequence of its role in intermediary metabolism and protein synthesis. An array of neurochemical methods has accordingly demonstrated that all cells contain some glutamate, and in the brain all neurons contain measurable amounts of glutamate.

In neurons glutamate is primarily synthesized from glucose through the pyruvate→ acetyl-CoA→2-oxoglutarate pathway and from glutamine that is synthesized in glial

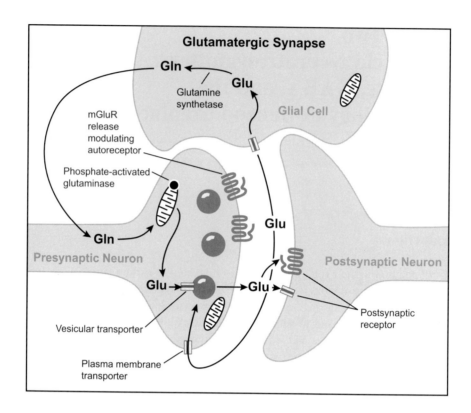

Figure 2.1 Schematic representation of a glutamatergic synapse. Glutamine (Gln) is converted to glutamate (Glu) by mitochondrial glutaminase in glutamatergic neurons. Glutamate is released into synaptic cleft where it may activate both pre- and postsynaptic receptors. Glutamate in the synaptic cleft is recaptured by neuronal and glial plasma membrane transporters that terminate the synaptic actions of the excitatory transmitter. Glial glutamate is converted to glutamine by the enzyme glutamine synthetase. This glutamine is then shuttled back to glutamatergic neurons to replenish glutamate. Glutamate receptors include both G protein-coupled (mGluRs) and ligand-gated ion channel (AMPA, NMDA, and kainite) receptors.

cells, transported into nerve terminals, and converted by neuronal glutaminase into glutamate. In terminals of glutamatergic neurons, glutamate is stored in synaptic vesicles from which Ca^{2+}-dependent release in response to depolarization occurs. This synaptically released glutamate is taken up, in part, by glial cells and converted to glutamine by the enzyme glutamine synthetase. This glutamine is then transported back to neurons where glutamate is regenerated through the action of glutaminase (see Figure 2.1).

Extracellular glutamate concentrations are maintained within physiological levels by a family of transmembrane proteins known as excitatory amino acid transporters (EAATs). At least five EAATs have been identified with individual subtypes differing with respect to their pharmacology and distribution within the central nervous system (CNS). Two of these EAATs are localized primarily on glial cells in the CNS, with the other three EAAT subtypes being localized to neurons. The two glial glutamate transporters have been shown to be the primary regulators of extracellular glutamate in the

CNS (Amara and Fontana 2002). There is some evidence that neuronal EAATs are localized predominantly outside the synapse where they control extrasynaptic, rather than synaptic, glutamate concentration. This extrasynaptic glutamate may function to activate pre- and postsynaptic metabotropic glutamate receptors (mGluRs). Presynaptic mGluRs are involved in the feedback regulation of synaptic glutamate release.

In the normal brain the prominent glutamatergic pathways are the cortico-cortical pathways, the pathways between the thalamus and the cortex, and the extrapyramidal pathway (the projections between the cortex and striatum). Other glutamate projections exist between the cortex, substantia nigra, subthalamic nucleus, and pallidum. Glutamate-containing neuronal terminals are ubiquitous in the CNS, and their importance in brain function and neurotransmission is therefore considerable. Estimates of the fraction of neurons in the brain that use glutamate as a neurotransmitter range from 60 to 75%.

Glutamate receptors are categorized into two main classes, namely, ionotropic glutamate receptors (iGluRs) and mGluRs. The iGluRs were originally classified using a pharmacologic approach that led to identification of three subtypes bearing the names of selective agonists: the AMPA, kainate (KA) and N-methyl-D-aspartate (NMDA) receptors. These glutamate receptor subtypes are often described as being either NMDA or non-NMDA (AMPA and kainate) receptors based on their sensitivity to the synthetic aspartate analog NMDA. All of these iGluRs represent ligand-gated cation channels permeable to Na^+ and K^+ with differing permeabilities to Ca^{2+}. Activation of these receptors by glutamate or selective agonists at normal membrane potentials allows Na^+ to enter the cell with attendant membrane depolarization; this is the underlying mechanism for the rapid excitatory response of most neurons to glutamate. In addition to Na^+ permeability, NMDA receptors also display high permeability to Ca^{2+} and a voltage-dependence of inward currents carried by Na^+ and Ca^{2+} ions. The voltage dependence of the inward ionic current through the NMDA receptor arises from Mg^{2+} blockade of this channel at normal resting membrane potentials. This channel-blocking action of extracellular Mg^{2+} is relieved when the cell is depolarized. Thus, the NMDA receptor requires depolarization of the cell through the excitatory actions of non-NMDA receptors before this ligand-gated ion channel can produce an inward current. This property of NMDA receptors has led to this channel being termed a coincident detector due to the requirement for simultaneous activation of NMDA receptors and excitatory input to a cell as a precondition for the passage of ionic current through NMDA receptor ion channels.

A molecular classification of glutamate receptors has confirmed the subdivision based on pharmacological profiles of receptor subtypes. Molecular cloning techniques have identified gene families corresponding to each functional subtype of glutamate receptor. NMDA receptors are formed by assemblies of three gene families, including NR1, NR2A-D, and NR3A/3B (Mayer and Armstrong 2004). Functional NMDA receptors exist as heteromers containing two NR1 and two NR2 subunits (Erreger et al. 2004). NMDA receptors can also contain NR3A or NR3B subunits that modulate channel function. AMPA receptors comprise assemblies from the GluR1-GluR4 gene family, whereas kainate receptors are assemblies of GluR5-7 and KA1 and KA2 subunits.

In addition to the iGluRs, there are mGluRs that are members of the large family of G protein–coupled receptors. These mGluRs are therefore not ligand-gated ion channels, but rather change cell physiology through an interaction with G proteins that in turn regulate the activity of enzymes and/or ion channels involved in cell-signaling cascades. These mGluRs are widely distributed in the brain where they mediate a variety of effects including the modulation of glutamate release from glutamatergic neurons. These presynaptic mGluRs therefore function as autoreceptors.

Pharmacology of Ketamine and Tiletamine

Ketamine is an anesthetic agent that was first introduced in clinical trials in the 1960s. It is a dissociative anesthetic, which is a term originally introduced by Corssen and Domino in 1966 to describe the unique state of anesthesia produced by ketamine in which the subject is profoundly analgesic while appearing disconnected from the surrounding environment. Domino and coworkers attributed this unique anesthetic state to a drug-induced dissociation of the electroencephalogram (EEG) activity between the thalamocortical and limbic systems. It was demonstrated that the cataleptic anesthetic state induced by intravenous ketamine (4 mg/kg) in cats was associated with an alternating pattern of hypersynchronous δ wave bursts and low-voltage, fast wave activity in the neocortex and thalamus. Subcortically, the δ wave bursts were observed prominently in the thalamus and caudate nucleus, and the EEG patterns of thalamic nuclei were closely related phasically to the δ waves of the neocortex. In contrast to the marked δ wave bursts in the neocortex, thalamus, and caudate nucleus, prominent δ waves were not observed in the cat hippocampus, hypothalamus, or midbrain reticular formation. The hippocampus showed θ "arousal" waves despite the appearance of high-voltage, hypersynchronous δ wave bursts in the thalamus and neocortex. Thus, ketamine was demonstrated to produce a functional dissociation of the EEG activity between the hippocampus and thalamocortical systems.

Ketamine and the newer dissociative anesthetic tiletamine act as noncompetitive antagonists of NMDA receptors in the CNS (Figure 2.2). The discovery by Lodge et al (1983) of the capacity for ketamine and related arylcyclohexylamines to antagonize specifically the neuronal excitation mediated by NMDA provided a pivotal advance in our understanding of the mechanism of action of dissociative anesthetics. Based on the earlier observation that ketamine selectively reduced polysynaptic reflexes in which excitatory amino acids were the transmitter, Lodge and coworkers investigated the action of ketamine on the excitation of cat dorsal horn interneurons by amino acids used in the classification of excitatory amino acid receptors, namely N-methyl-D-aspartate (NMDA), quisqualate, and KA. The microionotophoretic or intravenous administration of ketamine selectively reduced the increased firing rate of dorsal horn neurons evoked by focal application of NMDA. The excitatory responses elicited by quisqualate and KA remained little affected. The selective NMDA-blocking effect was not restricted to ketamine inasmuch as the dissociative anesthetics, phencyclidine (PCP) and tiletamine, had similar actions that paralleled their relative anesthetic potencies. The primary molecular target for ketamine-induced analgesia and anesthesia therefore appears to be brain NMDA receptors. The inhibitory concentration for ketamine antagonism of NMDA responses in rat cortical preparations range from 6 to 12 μM. These values are comparable to the plasma concentration (20–40 μM) obtained in rats following intravenous anesthetic doses. It therefore appears likely that a large

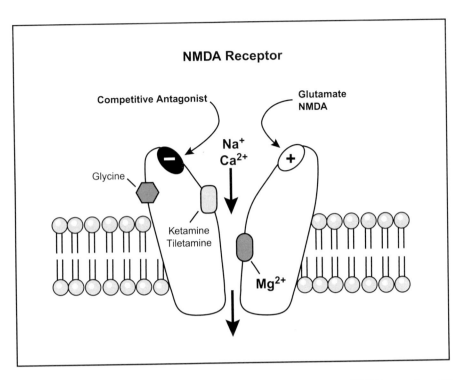

Figure 2.2 Schematic of the NMDA subtype of glutamate receptors. NMDA receptors possess binding sites for the transmitter glutamate and the coagonist, glycine. Competitive antagonists bind to the glutamate site, whereas noncompetitive antagonists such as ketamine and tiletamine bind to a site in the ion channel domain. Mg^{++} exerts a voltage-dependent block of the ion channel.

fractional occupancy of NMDA receptors may be required for ketamine induction of anesthesia (Murray 1994).

Subanesthetic doses of ketamine produce a spectrum of psychoactive actions in humans, including mood elevation, distortions in body image, hallucinations, delusions, and paranoid ideation. These effects resemble those of PCP and are responsible for the illicit use of ketamine. The availability of ketamine in veterinary medicine has resulted in numerous case reports of ketamine abuse by veterinarians. Similar to the anesthetic and analgesic actions of ketamine, the psychoactive properties appear to be related to the noncompetitive antagonism of NMDA receptors.

GABAergic Synapses

Of all the putative neurotransmitters in the brain, γ-aminobutyric acid (GABA) is perhaps the one whose candidacy rests on the longest history of investigation. Glutamic acid decarboxylase (GAD), the enzyme that catalyzes the formation of GABA, appears to be largely restricted to GABAergic neurons and therefore affords a suitable marker for this population of neurons. In brain regions such as the hippocampus, histochemical studies have repeatedly demonstrated that GAD is distributed in the neuropil with highest concentrations between cell bodies reflecting the presence of GABAergic neuron terminals. The abundance of GABAergic interneurons and projection neurons in the brain has been estimated to represent 17–20% of the neurons in the brain (Somogyi et al. 1998). Upon stimulation, these GABAergic neurons release GABA from presynaptic terminals into the synaptic cleft. The concentration of GABA in the synaptic cleft is controlled by the high-affinity uptake into presynaptic terminals and glial cells.

GABA represents the major inhibitory transmitter in the brain, and this inhibition is mediated by GABA binding to postsynaptic receptors. GABAergic systems serve important regulatory functions in the brain, such as vigilance, anxiety, muscle tension, epiletogenic activity, and memory. In brain areas such as the cerebral cortex and hippocampus, GABAergic neurons are predominantly interneurons that function as primary regulators of the activity of the projecting glutamatergic pyramidal neurons. The activity of these GABAergic interneurons is largely driven by glutamatergic afferents arising from either projecting afferents or recurrent glutamatergic collaterals. (See Figure 2.3.)

It is now generally recognized that GABAergic-mediated inhibition results from GABA activation of $GABA_A$ receptors. These ligand-gated ion channels open a Cl^- channel when activated by GABA, thereby facilitating the diffusion of this ion according to its concentration gradient. Thus, $GABA_A$ receptor activation may depolarize or hyperpolarize membranes depending on the difference in Cl^- concentration of the postsynaptic neuron and extracellular milieu. Although excitatory responses to GABA have been described in embryonic cells that maintain high intracellular Cl^- concentrations, the typical response of an activated $GABA_A$ receptor is hyperpolarization that is mediated by Cl^- influx. $GABA_A$ receptors are pentameric ligand-gated ion channels assembled from members of seven different subunit classes, some of which have multiple isoforms: α (1–6), β (1–3), γ (1–3), δ, ϵ, θ, and ρ. A pentameric assembly could theoretically be composed of over 50 distinct combinations of these subunits; however, $GABA_A$ receptor subunits appear to form preferred assemblies, resulting in possibly dozens of distinct receptor complexes in the brain (see Figure 2.4). Most $GABA_A$ receptor subtypes are presumed to be composed of α, β, γ subunits. Molecular studies have demonstrated that distinct $GABA_A$ receptor assemblies often have different physiologic and pharmacologic profiles, suggesting that subunit composition is an important determinant of pharmacological diversity in $GABA_A$ receptor populations.

$GABA_A$ receptors represent the molecular target for all of the characteristic pharmacological actions of benzodiazepines including sedation, muscle relaxation, seizure suppression, and anxiety reduction (anxiolysis). Benzodiazepines enhance the $GABA_A$ receptor opening frequency producing a potentiation of the GABA-induced inhibitory response (Rudolph et al. 1999). The benzodiazepine binding site is believed to be located at the interface between the α and γ_2-subunits of a pentameric $GABA_A$ receptor complex. There are six types of α subunit, α_1–α_6, and $GABA_A$ receptors containing the α_1, α_2, α_3, or α_5 subunits in combination with any β subunit and the γ_2 subunit are sensitive to benzodiazepines such as diazepam, alprazolam, and clonazepam (Möhler et al. 2002). $GABA_A$ receptors containing these four α subunits are most abundant in the brain, and the most prevalent receptor complex is composed of $\alpha_1\beta_2\gamma_2$ subunits. $GABA_A$ receptors that do not respond to benzodiazepines such as diazepam and clon-

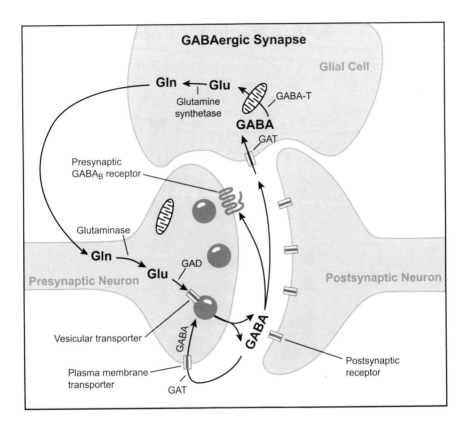

Figure 2.3   Schematic representation of a GABAergic synapse. Glutamate is the immediate precursor of GABA in these neurons where it is metabolized by the enzyme glutamic acid decarboxylase (GAD). The GABA is stored in and released from vesicles into the synaptic cleft. Synaptic GABA activates both pre- and postsynaptic receptors. The latter are primarily ligand-gated ion channels (GABA$_A$ receptors), whereas presynaptic GABA$_B$ receptors are G protein-coupled receptors involved in the regulation of neurotransmitter release. GABA in the synaptic cleft is recaptured by an active transporter (GAT) in the plasma membrane of both neurons and glia. GABA is metabolized by the mitochondrial enzyme GABA-transaminase (GABA-T) to succinic semialdehyde, which in turn is converted to succinic acid by the enzyme succinic semialdehyde dehydrogenase. Succinic acid exerts a negative feedback inhibition on glutamic acid decarboxylase. Succinic semialdehyde dehydrogenase is inhibited by the anticonvulsant sodium valproate.

azepam are less abundant in the brain and characterized by the presence of the α_4 and α_6 subunits (Möhler et al. 2002). The use of transgenic mice with mutated GABA$_A$ receptors has recently demonstrated that it may be possible to develop benzodiazepine-like drugs that are anxioselective, meaning that they may reduce anxiety in the absence of sedation and muscle relaxation (incoordination). The anxiolytic action of diazepam is selectively mediated by potentiation of GABAergic inhibition in a population of neurons expressing the α_2-GABA$_A$ receptor, which constitutes only 15% of all diazepam-sensitive GABA$_A$ receptors (Möhler et al. 2001). The α_2-GABA$_A$ receptor-expressing neurons in the cerebral cortex and hippocampus are therefore specific targets for the fu-

GABA$_A$ Receptor Pentamer

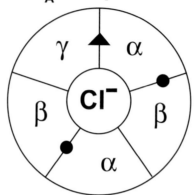

●   **GABA binding site**

▲   **Benzodiazepine (clonazepam) binding site**

Figure 2.4   Schematic structure of the GABA$_A$ receptor pentamer composed of two α subunits, two β subunits, and one γ subunit. The neurotransmitter GABA binds to a site at the interface between the α and β subunits (●) causing the Cl$^-$ channel to open. Benzodiazepines such as clonazepam and diazepam bind to a site at the interface of the α and γ subunits.

ture development of selective anxiolytic drugs. The sedative actions of benzodiazepines, in contrast, appear to be mediated by α subunit-containing GABA$_A$ receptors.

References

Amara SG and Fontana ACK 2002. Excitatory amino acid transporters: keeping up with glutamate. *Neurochemistry International* 41: 313–318.

Cooper JR, Bloom FE and Roth RH 1996. *The biochemical basis of neuropharmacology.* Oxford University Press, New York.

Corssen G and Domino EF 1966. Dissociative anesthesia: further pharmacologic studies and first clinical experience with the phencyclidine derivative CI581. *Anesthesia and Analgesia* 45: 29.

Erreger E, Chen PE, Wyllie DJA and Traynelis SF 2004. Glutamate receptor gating. *Critical Reviews in Neurobiology,* in press.

Lodge D, Anis NA, Berry SC and Burton NR 1983. Arylcyclohexylamines selectively reduce excitation of mammalian neurons by aspartate like amino acids. In *Phencyclidine and related arylcyclohexylamines: present and future applications*, p. 595, edited by J-M Kamenka, EF Domino, P Geneste. NPP Brooks, Ann Arbor.

Mayer ML and Armstrong N, 2004. Structure and Function of glutamate receptor ion channels. *Annual Reviews Physiology* 66: 161–81.

Möhler H, Crestani F and Rudolph U 2001. GABA$_A$-receptor subtypes: A new pharmacology. *Current Opinion in Pharmacology* 1: 22–25.

Möhler H, Fritschy JM and Rudolph U 2002. A new benzodiazepine pharmacology. *The Journal of Pharmacology and Experimental Therapeutics* 300: 2–8

Murray TF 1994. Basic pharmacology of ketamine. In *The pharmacologic basis of anesthesiology*, edited by TA Bowdle, A Horita and ED Karasch, Churchill Livingston, NY, pp. 337–355.

Rudolph U, Crestani F, Benke D, Brunig I, Benson JA, Fritschy JM, Martin JR, Bluethmann H and Möhler H 1999. Benzodiazepine actions mediated by specific γ-aminobutyric acid$_A$ receptor subtypes. *Nature (London)* 401: 796–800.

Somogyi P, Tamas G, Lujan R, and Buhl EH 1998. Salient features of synaptic organisation in the cerebral cortex. *Brain Research Brain Research Review*. 26 (2–3): 113–35.

Chapter Three
Benzodiazepines

Action

The benzodiazepines work by facilitating GABA in the central nervous system (CNS). They do this specifically by binding to $GABA_A$ receptors. The behavioral effects are due to action on the hypothalamus and the limbic system.

Overview of Indications

Benzodiazepines are anxiolytic medications with a rapid onset of action that lasts for a few to several hours, depending on the specific drug and the species. There are specific binding sites in the brain for benzodiazepines, with the highest density being in the central cortex, the cerebellum, and the limbic system (e.g., Braestrup and Squires 1977; Möhler and Okada 1977; Danneberg and Weber 1983). There are benzodiazepine receptors elsewhere in the body, for example, on bovine adrenal chromaffin cells (Brennan and Littleton 1991). Thousands of benzodiazepine molecules have been synthesized, although only a small segment of these are available commercially (Sternbach 1973). While thousands of papers have been published on laboratory studies of the effects of benzodiazepines on nonhuman animals and clinical studies of their effect on humans, few clinical studies or even case reports of their effect on nonhuman animals have been published. Fortunately, there are a few, and some of the laboratory studies conducted on animals provide useful information on such topics as toxicity, half-life and dose-response relationships.

Of the commercially available benzodiazepines, only alprazolam, chlordiazepoxide, clonazepam, clorazepate dipotassium, diazepam, flurazepam, lorazepam, oxazepam, and triazolam will be discussed in this chapter. Benzodiazepines are potentially useful for any problems involving anxiety, fear, or phobia in which a rapid onset of action is desired. Their immediate and discrete efficacy makes them particularly useful for fears that are induced by specific stimuli that can be predicted in advance. Examples of appropriate use include submissive urination, urine marking, cases of storm phobia or separation anxiety with panic, and fear of people (without aggression) in dogs; feather-picking and fear of people in birds; foal rejection due to fear in mares; urine marking, storm phobia, separation anxiety, and extreme timidity in cats. In humans, benzodiazepines reduce somatic symptoms of generalized anxiety disorder, but do not reduce cognitive symptoms, that is, chronic worry (Gorman 2003). Thus, they are probably not an ideal drug of choice for veterinary patients that exhibit chronic anxiety independent of external stimuli. Benzodiazepines, especially diazepam, should be used with caution in cats because of the rare possibility of medication-induced hepatic necrosis.

The use of benzodiazepines in cases involving aggression is controversial. When chlordiazepoxide and diazepam were first released in the early 1960s for use in psychiatry they were considered to have great potential in the treatment of aggression in humans because in various studies of laboratory animals it was noted that they had an effect of calming and taming "wild" or "vicious" animals (DiMascio 1973). However, the potential initially believed to be present did not turn out to be either consistent or reliable. Effect on aggression varies between species and between individuals and depends on the type of aggression being measured and how it is provoked, the specific benzodiazepine, the specific dose, and whether or not the benzodiazepine is given as a single, acute dose or whether it is given repeatedly over a period of days (see, for example, Randall 1960, 1961; Boyle and Tobin 1961; Heuschele 1961; Heise and Boff 1961; Horowitz et al. 1963; Scheckel and Boff 1966; Valzelli et al. 1967; Boissier et al. 1968; Fox and Snyder 1969; Hoffmeister and Wuttke 1969; Sofia 1969; Bauen and Possanza 1970; Christmas and Maxwell 1970; Cole and Wolf 1970; Fox et al. 1970; Guaitani et al. 1971; Langfeldt and Ursin 1971; Miczek 1974; Salzman et al. 1974; Kochansky et al. 1975; Miczek and O'Donnell 1980; Rodgers and Waters 1985; Mos et al. 1987; Mos and Olivier 1989; Olivier et al. 1991; Gao and Cutler 1993; Miczek et al. 1995; Tornatzky and Miczek 1995 for some examples of research on humans and animals that repeatedly identify these discrepancies). While benzodiazepines sometimes decrease aggressiveness, their use sometimes results in increased aggression.

Relief from anxiety can result in the loss of inhibition of behavior (e.g., Margules and Stein 1968). This results in modern textbooks of veterinary behavior being ambivalent on the subject of the use of benzodiazepines in the treatment of nonhuman aggression. For example, Landsberg et al. (2003) state that "Benzodiazepines can be considered for the treatment of any condition that may have a fear or anxiety component, including fear aggression . . ." but later in the same paragraph they point out that benzodiazepine's "disinhibition could lead to an increase in aggression." Clinically, just as alcohol or benzodiazepines can result in loss of inhibitions and consequent atypical behavior, including aggression, in humans, so can the use of benzodiazepines result in loss of normal inhibitions and consequent atypical behavior in animals. Also, benzodiazepines, particularly diazepam, appear to increase impulsivity (Thiébot 1985). Generally, lacking good clinical guidelines as to the specific aggression situations in which benzodiazepines might be helpful or risky, they should be avoided or used with extreme caution in cases involving aggressive animals.

The benzodiazepines may result in increases in affiliative behavior. For example, rhesus monkeys (*Macaca mulatta*) treated with chloridazepoxide, diazepam, or lorazepam exhibit increased social grooming, social approach, and social contact (Kumar et al. 1999).

All benzodiazepines are metabolized in the liver and excreted through the kidneys. Therefore, premedication blood work to assess the function of these organs is recommended.

Contraindications, Side Effects, and Adverse Events

Side effects include sedation, ataxia, muscle relaxation, increased appetite, paradoxical excitation, increased friendliness, anxiety, hallucinations, muscle spasticity, insomnia, and idiopathic hepatic necrosis in cats. The last has specifically been reported as a response to diazepam.

Overdose

Treatment of overdose is primarily supportive. Activated charcoal can be used to adsorb benzodiazepines within the gastrointestinal tract. In cats, vomiting can be induced with 0.05 mg/kg of apomorphine subcutaneously (SC) or 1 mg/kg xylazine SC. Flumazenil (Mazicon), a benzodiazepine receptor antagonist, can be given to partially or fully reverse the effects. Three hours after ingestion, gastric lavage or induction of vomiting is not recommended, because benzodiazepines are rapidly absorbed from the gastrointestinal tract. By this time, gastric lavage or induction of vomiting is not useful and sedation or convulsions will make these procedures counterproductive. Hypothermic patients should be kept in a warm environment. Intravenous fluids can help increase the rate of excretion of the benzodiazepine.

In a study of benzodiazepine poisoning in companion animals, specifically dogs and cats, the 10 most common signs observed in dogs were, in order of prevalence, ataxia, prostration, agitation, vomiting, hyperesthesia, muscle tremors, coma, hypersalivation, aggressiveness, and paresis. In cats, the 10 most common signs were prostration, ataxia, muscle tremors, agitation, coma, mydriasis, polypnea, decubitus, bradypnea, and vomiting (Bertini et al. 1995).

Clinical Guidelines

Benzodiazepines are DEA Schedule IV drugs. While they are available by prescription, there is potential for human abuse due to both psychological and physical dependency.

Benzodiazepines are excreted through the milk and pass through the placenta. They therefore should be used with caution and generally avoided, in pregnant or lactating females.

While benzodiazepines are good anxiolytics, they can have an amnesic effect and sometimes interfere with learning. Thus, they may be more useful in situations in which the control of intense fear is more important than ongoing learning. Nevertheless, the fact that they can have an amnesic effect does not mean that they always do, and research on the ability to learn while under the influence of benzodiazepines exhibits as much variation as research on the effect of benzodiazepines on aggression (e.g., Iwasaki et al. 1976; Vachon 1984; Hodges and Green 1987). The author has had numerous cases in which learning that was subsequently retained long-term clearly occurred while the patient was given a benzodiazepine.

There is wide variation in the optimum dose for a given patient. It is best to have the client give the pet a test dose in the low range of the dosage schedule at a time when they will be home to watch the pet for several hours. In this way they can observe whether their pet has such side effects as paradoxical excitement or sedation at that dose. Paradoxical excitement generally occurs at a specific window of dosage. Therefore, if paradoxical excitement occurs, the dose should be increased, while if sedation occurs, the dose should be decreased. If the patient exhibits no side effects, the medication can then be tried at that dose in the situation that induces fear. If the low dose used at the beginning is insufficient to alleviate the fear, steadily increase the dose until fear is alleviated or side effects are encountered.

Withdrawal of patients that have been frequently dosed with benzodiazepines over a period of several weeks should be gradual. This allows the identification of a specific dose that may still be required to control the problem behavior. Also, sudden termination in a patient that has been continuously on a benzodiazepine for several weeks can result in rebound, that is, a resumption of symptoms that may be more intense than they were before treatment. While specific schedules for decreasing medication will vary with the patient, a general rule is to decrease no faster than 25–33% per week. Many patients will require that the decrease occur more slowly.

In addition to the above considerations, all benzodiazepines have the potential to produce physical addiction. Different benzodiazepines produce different kinds of physical dependence. In studies of flumazenil-induced abstinence in dogs that had been treated chronically with diazepam, nordiazepam, flunitrazepam, alprazolam, oxazepam, halazepam, and lorazepam, it was found that oxazepam and lorazepam resulted in a less-intense physical dependence than did the other benzodiazepines (Martin et al. 1990). Therefore, if it is anticipated that a dog will need to be regularly medicated with a benzodiazepine for an extended period of time, oxazepam or lorazepam may be a better choice than the other benzodiazepines. Dogs made dependent on diazepam by prolonged administration of 60 mg/kg/day and acutely withdrawn by administration of flumazenil exhibit tremor, rigidity, decreased food intake, and tonic, clonic convulsions (McNicholas et al. 1983).

Tolerance is a phenomenon that also occurs with these medications; that is, when a patient is on a benzodiazepine for an extended period of time, steadily greater doses may be required to achieve the same behavioral effect (Danneberg and Weber 1983).

Benzodiazepines can safely be used with a variety of other psychoactive medications. Details of these combinations are discussed further in chapter 15.

The doses and comparative costs of the various benzodiazepines are shown in Tables 3.1, 3.2, and 3.3.

Specific Medications

I. Alprazolam

Chemical Compound: 8-Chloro-1-methyl-6-phenyl-4H-*s*-triazolo [4,3-α] [1,4] benzodiazepine

DEA classification: Schedule IV drug

Preparations: Generally available as 0.25-, 0.5-, 1.0-, and 2.0-mg tablets. Also available as a 1 mg/mL oral solution. The extended release form comes in 0.5-, 1-, 2-, and 3-mg tablets.

Table 3.1 Doses of various benzodiazepines for dogs and cats

Medication	Dogs	Cats
Alprazolam (Xanax)	0.02–0.1 mg/kg q4h	0.0125–0.25 mg/kg q8h
Chlordiazepoxide (Librium)	2.0–6.5 mg/kg q8h	0.2–1.0 mg/kg q12h
Clonazepam (Klonopin)	0.1–0.5 mg/kg q8–12h	0.015–0.2 mg/kg q8h
Clorazepate dipotassium (Tranxene)	0.5–2.0 mg/kg q4h	0.5–2.0 mg/kg q12h
Diazepam (Valium)	0.5–2.0 mg/kg q4h	0.1–1.0 mg/kg q4h
Flurazepam (Dalmane)	0.1–0.5 mg/kg q12h	0.1–0.4 mg/kg q12h
Lorazepam (Ativan)	0.02–0.5 mg/kg q8–12h	0.03–0.08 mg/kg q12h
Oxazepam (Serax)	0.04–0.5 mg/kg q6h	0.2–1.0 mg/kg q12–24h

Note: All doses given are orally and are given as needed until the desired effect is reached. The hourly schedules are the maximum frequency at which the medication should be given. As a general rule, start at the lowest dose and titrate upward if needed. See text for further explanation.

Source: Scherkl et al. 1985; Dodman and Shuster 1994; Simpson and Simpson 1996; Overall 1994b, 1997, 2004; Simpson 2002; Crowell-Davis et al. 2003; Landsberg et al. 2003.

Table 3.2 Dose of diazepam for parrots, horses, and rabbits

Parrot	Horse	Rabbit
Two drops of 5 mg/ml solution per ounce of drinking water	10–30 mg q8h	0.1–0.6 mg/kg

Source: Ryan 1985; Crowell-Davis 1986.

Table 3.3 Comparative cost of various benzodiazepines for a one-month supply for a 20-kg dog and a 5-kg cat

Medication	Cost for dog	Cost for cat
Alprazolam	$$	$$
Chlordiazepoxide	$$	
Clonazepam	$$	
Clorazepate dipotassium	$$$$	$$$$
Diazepam	$$	$$
Oxazepam	$$$	

Note: See chapter 1 for a complete explanation.

Clinical Pharmacology

Alprazolam is readily absorbed following oral administration. In humans, peak concentrations occur in the plasma at 1–2 hours, and the plasma levels are proportionate to the dose given. Mean plasma elimination half-life in healthy humans is about 11.2 hours. However, in humans, changes in absorption, distribution, metabolism, and excretion occur in various disease states, for example, impaired hepatic or renal function. This is no doubt also the case in nonhuman animals. Doses should be decreased in old or obese veterinary patients and in those with impaired liver or renal function (Pharmacia and Upjohn 2001).

The two most common metabolites are α-hydroxy-alprazolam and a benzophenone. The benzophenone is inactive, but α-hydroxy-alprazolam has about half the activity of alprazolam. Metabolism is initiated by hydroxylation that is catalyzed by cytochrome P450 3A. Therefore, any drugs that inhibit the activity of this metabolic pathway are likely to result in decreased clearance of alprazolam (Pharmacia and Upjohn 2001).

In humans, extended-release tablets are absorbed more slowly than non-extended-release tablets, resulting in steady-state concentration that is maintained for 5–11 hours after dosing. Time of day, consumption of a meal, and type of meal affect the absorption rate (Pharmacia and Upjohn 2001). Since the digestive physiology and typical diet of veterinary patients differs significantly from the digestive physiology and diet of humans, it is likely that there is substantial variation from the human data.

In African green monkeys, the mean elimination half-life is 5.7 hours (Friedman et al. 1991).

Uses in Humans

In humans, alprazolam is approved for use in general anxiety disorder, anxiety with depression, and panic disorder with or without agoraphobia. Effective treatment of panic disorder requires several months, and withdrawal must be very gradual, taking at least eight weeks, in order to avoid rebound (Pecknold et al. 1988).

Contraindications

Alprazolam is contraindicated in patients with known hypersensitivity to benzodiazepines, glaucoma, or severe liver or kidney disease. It is also contraindicated in pregnant or lactating females. It should not be given with medications that significantly impair the oxidative metabolism of cytochrome P450 3A, such as the antifungal agents ketoconazole or itraconazole (Pharmacia and Upjohn 2001).

Side Effects

Side effects typical of the benzodiazepines, including sedation, ataxia, muscle relaxation, increased appetite, paradoxical excitation, and increased friendliness may occur.

Rats treated with 3–30 mg/kg/day of alprazolam over a two-year period showed a dose-related tendency to develop cataracts in females and corneal vascularization in males. Lesions appeared after at least 11 months of treatment. Rats given doses of alprazolam up to 30 mg/kg/day and mice given doses up to 10 mg/kg/day for a period of two years showed no evidence of increased cancer. Alprazolam has not been shown to be mutagenic in rats. In rats given alprazolam at doses up to 5 mg/kg/day, fertility was unimpaired. The LD_{50} (the dose that kills half of the animals tested) in the rat is 331–2171 mg/kg (Pharmacia and Upjohn 2001).

Overdose

Clinical signs reported in dogs that had consumed overdoses of up to 5.55 mg/kg alprazolam included ataxia, disorientation, depression, hyperactivity, vomiting, weakness, tremors, vocalization, tachycardia, tachypnea, hypothermia, diarrhea, and increased salivation. In 38% of the cases, clinical signs developed within 30 minutes of ingestion. Ataxia typically resolved within 9 hours, but some dogs were ataxic for up to 24 hours. Depression lasted 10–31 hours. There was no correlation between the dose consumed and paradoxical excitement (Wismer 2002).

Treat an overdose with gastric lavage and supportive treatment, including fluids. Flumazenil may be given for complete or partial reversal; however, administration of flumazenil to a patient that has received alprazolam daily for several weeks may result in convulsions.

Doses in Nonhuman Animals

Initiate treatment at the lowest dose. If no undesirable side effects occur, titrate dose up to the desired effect.

Discontinuation

If a patient has been receiving alprazolam daily for several weeks, discontinuation should be gradual, and conducted over a period of at least one month.

Other Information

While liver failure has not been reported in cats or other veterinary patients given alprazolam for behavior problems, it has occurred in humans. While it is a rare event even in humans, liver failure should always be considered as a possible sequela to medication with alprazolam.

Dogs given alprazolam at an escalating dose over 18–26 days until a dose of 12 mg/kg four times a day (q.i.d.) is attained, then maintained on that dose for about three weeks, become physically addicted, as demonstrated by flumazenil-precipitated abstinence (Sloan et al. 1990). These doses are much higher than would be given for the clinical treatment of anxiety disorders. Acute withdrawal of an addicted dog may result in seizures. Other sequelae to withdrawal reported in humans include insomnia, abnormal involuntary movement, headaches, muscle twitching, and anxiety. Dogs addicted to alprazolam that underwent acute withdrawal due to administration of flumazenil exhibited wild running, barking and lunging at nonexistent objects, and uncontrolled splaying, rigidity, and jerking of the limbs (Martin et al. 1990). As with humans, veterinary patients that have been on alprazolam daily for several weeks should have their dose gradually decreased.

As with other benzodiazepines, alprazolam is particularly noted for its rapid action. For example, in the treatment of humans with panic disorder, patients treated with alprazolam respond within the first week of treatment, while patients treated with imipramine, a tricyclic antidepressant, respond, but not until the fourth week of treatment (Charney et al. 1986). This rapid response has been observed clinically in veterinary patients, making alprazolam a good choice for dogs that exhibit panic behaviors to the degree that rapid improvement is essential.

Effects Documented in Nonhuman Animals
Cats

While the use of alprazolam to treat behavior problems in cats is mentioned in several textbooks, the author is unaware of any papers presenting results of clinical use in this species.

Dogs

Crowell-Davis et al. (2003) used alprazolam as part of a treatment protocol for dogs with storm phobia. Alprazolam is most likely to be effective if it is given 30–60 minutes before the occurrence of the earliest stimuli that elicit fear responses, for example, the sound of rain or strong winds. To do this, owners of storm-phobic pets must monitor weather conditions closely. As a general rule for patients with severe signs of this phobia, medication should be given if there is any likelihood that weather conditions that induce fear responses will occur. If, however, the fear-inducing stimuli have already begun and the patient is showing fear when the owner realizes there will be a problem, alprazolam should still be administered. For alprazolam-responsive patients, fear is likely to be somewhat abated, although a higher dose may be required for full relief from signs of fear.

Dogs chronically dosed with increasing quantities of alprazolam until they began losing weight did so at doses of 48 mg/kg by day 18–28 of the increasing regimen (Martin et al. 1990).

II. Chlordiazepoxide HCl

Chemical Compound: 7-Chloro-2-(methyl-amino)-5-phenyl-3H-1,4-benzodiazepine 4-oxide hydrochloride
DEA Classification: Schedule IV drug
Preparations: Generally available in 5-, 10-, and 25-mg capsules

Clinical Pharmacology

Chlordiazepoxide HCl acts on the limbic system of the brain, modifying emotional responses. It has antianxiety, appetite-stimulating, and sedative effects. It is also a weak analgesic. It does not have an autonomic blocking effect, so moderate doses do not affect blood pressure or heart rate (Randall et al. 1960). It crosses the blood–brain barrier, is highly bound to plasma proteins, and is metabolized by the liver. Metabolites generated in the liver include desmethyldiazepam (nordiazepam), demoxepam, desmethylchlordiazepoxide, and oxazepam (Schwartz and Postma 1966; Kaplan et al. 1970; ICN Pharmaceuticals 1996). These metabolites are active and typically have long half-lives. In humans, peak blood levels are not reached until several hours after taking the medication. Chlordiazepoxide has a half-life in humans of 24–48 hours, and plasma levels decline slowly over several days. Chlordiazepoxide is excreted in the urine, with only 1–2% in unchanged form (ICN Pharmaceuticals 1996).

In dogs, plasma levels peak around 7–8 hours after a single dose of 4 mg/kg or 20 mg/kg of chlordiazepoxide. Plasma levels are about half the peak value after 24 hours and chlordiazepoxide is still being excreted in the urine 96 hours after administration.

This dose causes mild sedation with high plasma levels for 24 hours in this species. When dogs are redosed daily, there is no cumulative effect on blood levels or sedation. Dogs given doses of 50 mg/kg by mouth (PO) for six months have shown no adverse effects (Randall 1961). Doses of 10–40 mg/kg may produce ataxia, while doses of 80 mg/kg produce sleep when dogs are not stimulated (Randall et al. 1960). Doses of 2.5 to 20 mg/kg have an appetite-stimulating effect (Randall et al. 1960).

When dogs are given a single dose of 0.5–0.8 mg/kg PO, peak plasma levels occur earlier, just 2–5 hours after dosing, and the half-life is likewise shorter, 12–20 hours (Koechlin and D'Arconte 1963). Seven days after administration of a single dose of 4 mg/kg, 44% of the dose is recovered through the urine, while five days after the same dose an additional 44% is recovered in the feces. Urinary excretion rate peaks at 10 hours after oral administration (Koechlin et al. 1965).

In the dog, demoxepam, one of the metabolites of chlordiazepoxide, has a half-life of 10–20 hours, with substantial individual variation. Some of the demoxepam is subsequently converted to oxazepam (Schwartz et al. 1971). Slightly over 1% (1.1%) of chlordiazepoxide given as a single 26-mg/kg dose PO or as a daily dose of 5 mg/kg PO for nine weeks is ultimately excreted in the urine as oxazepam, while an additional 1.3% is excreted in the feces on either regimen (Kimmel and Walkenstein 1967).

Electroencephalographic studies in the cat have shown that the peak drug effect for chlordiazepoxide when given at 1.25 mg/kg intraperitoneally (IP) occurs within 90 minutes (Fairchild et al. 1980).

The LD_{50} in mice is 123 ± 12 mg/kg IV and 366 ± 7 mg/kg intramuscularly (IM). In rats the LD_{50} is 120 ± 7 mg/kg IV and more than 160 mg/kg IM (ICN Pharmaceuticals 1996). The oral dose LD_{50} is 590 mg/kg in rabbits, 1315 mg/kg in rats, and 620 mg/kg in mice (Randall et al. 1965). In cats, a dose of 200 mg/kg PO was fatal in five days (Randall and Kappell 1973).

Uses in Humans

Chlordiazepoxide is used in the treatment of various anxiety disorders, for short-term relief of symptoms of anxiety, for example, preoperatively, and for relief from symptoms of alcoholism.

Contraindications

Chlordiazepoxide is contraindicated in patients with known sensitivity to this or other benzodiazepines. Avoid or use with extreme caution in patients with a history of aggression, because chlordiazepoxide, like all benzodiazepines, may cause loss of learned inhibitions.

Reduced doses should be used in geriatric patients and patients with mild to moderate liver or kidney disease.

Chlordiazepoxide crosses the placental barrier and enters the milk. There is an increased risk of congenital malformations when chlordiazepoxide is given during the first trimester of pregnancy. Therefore, its use should be avoided in pregnant as well as lactating females.

Side Effects

Various side effects, including sedation, ataxia, paradoxical excitation, and rage may occur. In humans, there have been isolated reports of effects on blood coagulation in patients receiving chlordiazepoxide at the same time that they are given anticoagulants. Blood dyscrasias, jaundice, and hepatic dysfunction occasionally occur in humans (ICN Pharmaceuticals 1996). Any veterinary patient that is maintained on chlordiazepoxide for an extended period of time should have complete blood counts and blood chemistries conducted regularly. Tolerance may develop, particularly to the sedative effects (Goldberg et al. 1967).

Two out of six dogs given chlordiazepoxide at 127 mg/kg died with evidence of circulatory collapse, as did six out of six given 200 mg/kg/day. Dogs given 80 mg/kg exhibited nonspecific toxic changes (Wyeth Laboratories 1999b).

Rat pups of mothers given 10, 20, and 80 mg/kg during conception and pregnancy had normal growth and showed no congenital anomalies. Lactation of the mothers was unaffected. When rats were given 100 mg/kg, there was a significant decrease in fertilization rate. There was also a decrease in the viability and body weight of the pups. These problems were attributed to the sedation induced at this dose, which resulted in less mating activity and decreased maternal care. Some of the offspring also exhibited skeletal defects at this dose (ICN Pharmaceuticals 1996).

Overdose

In case of overdose, conduct gastric lavage immediately, then provide general supportive therapy. Administer intravenous fluids and maintain an adequate airway. If excitation occurs, do not use barbiturates. Flumazenil is indicated for the complete or partial reversal of the sedative effects of chlordiazepoxide.

Doses in Nonhuman Animals

Initiate treatment at the lowest dose. If no undesirable side effects occur, titrate dose up to the desired effect.

Discontinuation

As with other benzodiazepines, if the patient has been receiving chlordiazepoxide daily for several weeks, discontinuation should be gradual and conducted over at least a one-month period of time.

Other Information

Chlordiazepoxide has been shown to cause delayed reversal learning and failure to accomplish successive discrimination learning in the rat, although it does not disrupt simultaneous discrimination (Iwahara and Sugimura 1970; Iwasaki et al. 1976).

Effects Documented in Nonhuman Animals

Taming effects have been noted in multiple species, including monkeys, rats, tigers, lions, dingos, and squirrels at doses that did not induce sedation (e.g., Harris 1960; Heise and Boff 1961; Scheckel and Boff 1966).

Cats

Laboratory cats given chlordiazepoxide intraperitoneally at doses ranging from 1.25 to 5 mg/kg exhibited dose-related stimulation and decreased sleep. They were also observed to be playful or mildly aggressive on this medication, although what form of aggression was exhibited is not specifically described (Fairchild et al. 1980). At 10 mg/kg PO, cats exhibit muscle relaxation when suspended by the scruff of the neck (Randall 1961).

Dogs

Angel et al. (1982) treated a strain of nervous pointer dogs with chlordiazepoxide or placebo at 3.5 mg/kg in the morning for seven consecutive days. The dogs' avoidance of humans was significantly attenuated with the chlordiazepoxide treatment, but not the placebo. The dogs behavior returned to baseline four days after discontinuation of medication (Angel et al. 1982).

Five of eight laboratory beagle dogs with abnormal withdrawn and depressed behavior exhibited improvement when given 5 mg/kg daily of chlordiazepoxide, while the behavior of all three of three such beagles given 2.5 mg/kg daily of chlordiazepoxide was resolved (Iorio et al. 1983).

Chlordiazepoxide has an appetite stimulation effect in dogs, with a single low dose increasing food intake of fasted dogs. Chronic treatment with chlordiazepoxide for 90 days results in weight gain (Randall et al. 1960).

Monkeys

Chlordiazepoxide has been used to tame monkeys at a dose of 1 mg/kg (Zbinden and Randall 1967).

Within social colonies of rhesus monkeys, chlordiazepoxide (2.5–5.0 mg/kg PO daily) produces dose-dependent increases in social grooming, approach, contact, self-grooming, feeding, and resting with the eyes open. There is also decreased vigilance and aggression (Kumar et al. 1999).

Zoo Animals

A number of zoo animals changed from being aggressive or intensely frightened to being calm, nonaggressive, and even friendly when given chlordiazepoxide. These include a male European lynx (*Lynx lynx*; 6 mg/kg PO), a female dingo (*Canis familiaris dingo*; 3–7 mg/kg PO), a female Guinea baboon (*Papio papio*; 13 mg/kg PO), a male California sea lion (*Zalophus californianus*; 7 mg/kg PO), a male Burmese macaque (*Macaca nemestrina andamensis*; 5 mg/kg IM), a female red kangaroo (*Macropus rufus*; 11 mg/kg PO), a female mule deer (*Odocoileus hemionus*; 2.2 mg/kg IV), a male white-bearded gnu (*Connochaetes taurinus*; 4 mg/kg IM), a female gerenuk (*Litocranius walleri*; 5 mg/kg IM), and three golden marmosets (*Leontocebus rosalia*; 15 mg/kg PO)(Heuschele 1961).

Animals that did not respond as desired to chlordiazepoxide included a male klipspringer (*Oreotragus oreotragus saltatrixoides*), a female South American tapir (*Tapirus terrestris*), and a Hensel's cat (*Felis pardinoides*) (Heuschele 1961).

III. Clonazepam

Chemical Compound: 5-(2-Chlorophenyl)-1,3-dihydro-7-nitro-2H-1,4-benzodiazepin-2-one
DEA Classification: Schedule IV controlled substance
Preparations: Generally available as 0.5-, 1.0-, and 2.0-mg tablets

Clinical Pharmacology

Clonazepam is completely and rapidly absorbed following oral dosing. In humans, maximum plasma concentrations are reached in 1–4 hours, with an elimination half-life of 30–40 hours. Dogs given 0.2 mg/kg IV exhibit an elimination half-life of 1.4 ± 0.3 hours. Most clonazepam is metabolized to various inactive metabolites. In humans, less than 2% is excreted in the urine in an unchanged form. Because extensive metabolism occurs in the liver, hepatic disease may result in impaired elimination. Thus, clonazepam is not the best choice for patients with liver disease. Pharmacokinetics are dose dependent throughout the dose range (Al-Tahan et al. 1984, Roche Laboratories 2001).

Cats given 1000 mg/kg clonazepam PO survived. In contrast, cats given bromazepam died at a dose of 1000 mg/kg, while several benzodiazepines proved fatal in cats at much lower doses (Randall and Kappell 1973).

In dogs given 0.5 mg/kg of clonazepam every 12 hours (q12h) for a period of three weeks, the elimination half-life of clonazepam increases with each passing week. In week one, the average half-life is about 2 hours, while by week three it is almost 8 hours. Acute withdrawal from clonazepam after three or more weeks of treatment has been shown to result in anorexia, hyperthermia, and weight loss (Scherkl et al. 1985). Plasma concentrations in the range considered to be therapeutic in humans can be maintained in dogs by dosing 0.5 mg/kg two times a day (b.i.d.) or three times a day (t.i.d.) (Al-Tahan et al. 1984).

Uses in Humans

Clonazepam is used to treat a variety of seizure disorders and panic disorder.

Contraindications

Clonazepam is contraindicated in patients with a history of sensitivity to benzodiazepines, severe liver or kidney disease, or glaucoma. Clonazepam should not be given to pregnant or lactating females.

Low doses should be used in patients with mild to moderate kidney or liver disease, because their ability to metabolize and excrete clonazepam will be compromised.

Side Effects

As with all benzodiazepines, clonazepam may result in sedation, ataxia, muscle relaxation, increased appetite, paradoxical excitation, increased friendliness, anxiety, and hallucinations.

Carcinogenicity of clonazepam has not been studied. Genotoxic studies are insufficient to conclude if clonazepam has any genotoxic potential. In rats given 10–100 mg/kg/day over two generations, there was a decrease in the number of pregnancies and the number of offspring that survived until weaning. With administration of clonazepam to pregnant rabbits during the period of organogenesis at doses ranging from 0.2 to 10.0 mg/kg/day, various malformations, including cleft palate, open eyelids, fused sternebrae, and defects of the limbs, occurred at a low, non-dose-related rate. Pregnant rabbits given 5 mg/kg/day or higher doses exhibited reductions in maternal weight gain, while reductions in embryo-fetal growth occurred at doses of 10 mg/kg/day. However, no adverse effects were observed on the mothers, embryos, or fetuses when mice and rats were given doses up to 15 mg/kg/day and 40 mg/kg/day, respectively (Roche Laboratories 2001).

Elimination of clonazepam from both plasma and cerebral cortex becomes slower with age (Barnhill et al. 1990).

Drug Interactions

Ranitidine and propantheline, which decrease stomach acidity, and fluoxetine, an SSRI, have little to no effect on the metabolism of clonazepam. Cytochrome P-450 inducers, including phenytoin, carbamazepine, and phenobarbital, facilitate clonazepam metabolism, resulting in a 30% decrease in clonazepam levels in humans. Strong P-450 3A inhibitors, such as oral antifungal agents, should be combined cautiously with clonazepam, because concurrent use may result in clonazepam overdose due to insufficient metabolism (Roche Laboratories 2001).

Overdose

Symptoms of overdose that are characteristic of CNS depressants may occur, including sedation, confusion, diminished reflexes, and coma. Gastric lavage should be initiated as soon as possible, followed by appropriate supportive treatment and monitoring of respiration, pulse, and blood pressure. Flumazenil, a benzodiazepine-receptor antagonist, can be used to partially or completely reverse the effects, but should be avoided in patients that have been treated with clonazepam daily for an extended period of time because seizures may be induced.

Doses in Nonhuman Animals

Initiate treatment at the lowest dose. If no undesirable side effects occur, titrate dose up to the desired effect.

Discontinuation

As with all benzodiazepines, clonazepam should be reduced gradually in patients that have been receiving it on a daily basis for several weeks.

Other Information

Clonazepam is not useful in the treatment of myoclonus caused by serotonin syndrome.

Effects Documented in Nonhuman Animals

Cats

In laboratory studies, clonazepam is substantially less toxic to cats than chlordiazepoxide, diazepam, or flurazepam (Table 3.4).

Other

Clonazepam has been shown to have a taming effect on aggressive primates, with concurrent muscle weakness and hypnosis.

IV. Clorazepate Dipotassium

Chemical Compound: Potassium 7-chloro-2,3,-dihydro-2-oxo-5-phenyl-1H-1,4 benzodiazepine-3-carboxylate

DEA Classification: Class IV non-narcotic agent

Table 3.4   Dose at which muscle relaxation is achieved and lethal dose of some benzodiazepines when given orally to cats

Benzodiazepine	Muscle relaxation mg/kg PO	Lethal dose mg/kg PO
Chlordiazepoxide hydrochloride	2	200
Clonazepam	0.05	>1,000
Diazepam	0.2	500
Flurazepam	2	400

Note: The lethal dose for clonazepam is listed as >1000 mg/kg because this dose was not fatal, and higher doses were not given. The data are based on only two cats per benzodiazepine, and individual variation in metabolism would be expected to produce a wider range of doses than given in this table. However, the data show the relative differences between drugs in these effects.
Source: Randall and Kappell 1973.

Preparations: Generally available as 3.75-, 7.5-, 11.25-, 15-, 22.5-mg tablets and 3.75-, 7.5-, 15-mg capsules

Clinical Pharmacology

Clorazepate is metabolized in the liver and excreted in the urine. In the acidity of the digestive tract, it is rapidly decarboxylated to form nordiazepam, also called desmethyldiazepam, which is the active metabolite (Troupin et al. 1979; Greenblatt et al. 1988). Plasma levels of nordiazepam will be proportionate to clorazepate dose. Nordiazepam is further metabolized by hydroxylation to conjugated oxazepam (3-hydroxynordiazepam) and *p*-hydroxynordiazepam (Abbott Laboratories 2004).

Nordiazepam is also an active metabolite of diazepam. Clorazepate provides higher concentrations of nordiazepam over a longer period of time than does diazepam and has less sedative effect (Lane and Bunch 1990).

After administration of a 50-mg dose of clorazepate to humans, 62–67% of the radioactivity was excreted in the urine and 15–19% was excreted in the feces within 10 days (Abbott Laboratories 2004).

As with other benzodiazepines, dogs metabolize clorazepate more rapidly than do humans. After administrations of oral clorazepate, humans have been reported to have a half-life elimination of nordiazepam of 40.8 ± 10.0 hours (Wilensky et al. 1978) or over 80 hours (Boxenbaum 1980). In contrast, the half-life of nordiazepam in dogs is about 9 hours (Brown and Forrester 1991).

In humans, Tranxene SD (sustained delivery) has longer efficacy than does the regular-release product, Tranxene. In dogs, there is no difference in either time of peak plasma concentration or serum concentrations 2 hours after administration. However, 12 hours after administration of a single 2.5–3.8 mg/kg-dose serum concentration of regular release was 24 ± 77.9 ng/ml of nordiazepam, while serum concentration of nordiazepam with sustained delivery was 215 ± 66.1 ng/ml (Brown and Forrester 1991). There was no gender effect on disposition of the drug, although this study only involved four males and three females and so cannot be considered conclusive on this issue. Peak nordiazepam concentrations were 372–1140 ng/ml with the regular release. Peak nordiazepam concentrations were 450–1150 with sustained delivery. Overall, the bioavailabilities of the two products were not different.

In healthy adult dogs given a single dose of clorazepate orally at a dose of 2 mg/kg maximum nordiazepam concentrations at 59–180 minutes after administration range from 446 to 1542 ng/ml. After multiple such doses given q12h, maximum nordiazepam concentration is reached at 153 ± 58 minutes and range from 927 to 1460 ng/ml. The mean elimination half-life after a single dose is 284 minutes, while the mean elimination half-life after multiple doses is 355 minutes. After multiple doses of clorazepate, there are significant decreases in serum chemical values of albumin, total protein, and calcium, while there are significantly increased concentrations of urea nitrogen and glucose. There are also significant increases in total white blood cell count, segmented neutrophils, lymphocytes, and eosinophils. Urine pH decreases significantly. Also, serum alkaline phosphatase activity increases while alanine transaminase (ALT) values decrease. Despite these changes, all values remain within normal reference ranges after 21 days on 2 mg/kg b.i.d. (Forrester et al. 1990).

Concurrent administration of clorazepate and phenobarbital in dogs results in significantly lower concentrations of nordiazepam, necessitating higher doses in dogs that are on phenobarbital because of epilepsy (Forrester et al. 1993).

Uses in Humans

Clorazepate is used for management of anxiety disorders and short-term relief of anxiety.

Contraindications

Clorazepate is contraindicated in patients with a history of adverse reactions to clorazepate and in patients with acute narrow-angle glaucoma. Since clorazepate has depressant effects on the CNS, avoid concurrent use with other CNS depressants.

Side Effects

As with all benzodiazepines, sedation, ataxia, muscle relaxation, increased appetite, paradoxical excitation, increased friendliness, anxiety, and a variety of other side effects may occur. Transient sedation and ataxia was observed in one of eight healthy adult dogs given a single dose of 2 mg/kg of clorazepate (Forrester et al. 1990).

Potential mutagenic effects of clorazepate have not been studied sufficiently to come to any conclusions. However, other minor tranquilizers, for example, diazepam, have been associated with an increased risk of fetal abnormalities if given during the first trimester of pregnancy. Nordiazepam is excreted in milk. Therefore, use of clorazepate in pregnant and nursing females should be avoided.

Dependence

As with all benzodiazepines, continuous administrations of clorazepate can result in dependence. In humans, the severity of withdrawal symptoms has been shown to be related to the dose that has been taken. Dogs and rabbits have exhibited seizures when clorazepate was abruptly withdrawn after dependence was established (Abbott Laboratories 2004). In all cases, it is recommended that if a patient has received clorazepate regularly over a period of several weeks, the dose be decreased gradually.

Overdose

In case of overdose, immediate gastric lavage and supportive measures should be conducted. Administer intravenous fluids and maintain an open airway. Flumazenil, a benzodiazepine receptor antagonist, can be used to completely or partially reverse the effects of an overdose. Treatment with flumazenil may result in seizures, especially in patients that have frequently been given clorazepate for a long period of time.

Doses in Nonhuman Animals

For nonhuman animals initiate treatment at the lowest dose. If no undesirable side effects occur, titrate the dose up to the desired effect.

Effects Documented in Nonhuman Animals

Clorazepate is used in dogs when a long duration of action is desired, for example, in cases of separation anxiety in which a serotonin reuptake inhibitor has not had time to take effect and the shorter-acting anxiolytics are not sufficient to keep the dog calm while the owner is gone for a full day.

V. Diazepam

Chemical Compound: 7-Chloro-1,3-dihydro-1-methyl-5-phenyl-2H-1,4-benzodiazepin-2-one

DEA Classification: Class IV non-narcotic agent

Preparations: Generally available as 2-, 5-, and 10-mg tablets. Also available as a 1 mg/ml and 5 mg/ml suspension for oral administration and a 5 mg/ml injectable solution. Rectal gels are available in 2.5-, 5-, 10-, 15-, and 20-mg sizes.

Clinical Pharmacology

Diazepam has a CNS depressant effect, specifically on the limbic system, thalamus, and hypothalamus, which results in anxiolytic, calming, sedative, skeletal muscle relaxation, and anticonvulsant effects. It does not have any peripheral autonomic blocking action or produce extra-pyramidal side effects. It acts by activation of the γ-aminobutyric acid system at the $GABA_A$ receptor complex. This results in decreased neural transmission throughout the CNS (Roche 2000).

Following oral administration, the usual route in treating behavior cases, diazepam is rapidly absorbed, with peak plasma levels occurring 0.5–2 hours after administration in humans and 1 hour after administration to rats (Schwartz et al. 1965; see Table 3.5). Diazepam readily crosses the blood–brain barrier, is highly bound to plasma proteins, is highly lipid soluble, and is widely distributed through the body. Blood concentrations are proportional to the dose given. In horses, 87% of diazepam is bound to

Table 3.5 Half-life of diazepam, in hours, and some of its metabolites in the dog, cat, and horse

Benzodiazepine	Dog	Cat	Horse
Diazepam	2.5–3.2	5.5	7–22
Nordiazepam	3.6–10	21.3	12
Oxazepam	3.5–5.7		18–28

Source: Löscher and Frey 1981; Norman et al. 1997; Shini et al. 1997; Plumb 2002.

plasma protein when the serum concentration is 75 ng/ml. This is a lower percentage than for humans (Plumb 2002).

Diazepam undergoes extensive first-pass hepatic metabolism when given orally. In the liver, diazepam is changed into multiple metabolites, including desmethyl-diazepam (nordiazepam), temazepam, and oxazepam. In dogs given an intravenous injection of 1 mg/kg of diazepam, about 61% of it is excreted in the urine while about 34% is excreted in the feces, either as diazepam or, predominantly, as a metabolite. In humans only about 10% of diazepam is excreted in the feces, again predominantly as a metabolite. In contrast to dogs and humans, diazepam given to rats is excreted predominantly through the feces, whether it is given intraperitoneally or orally (Schwartz et al. 1965). Thus, the exact metabolism of diazepam varies between species. This variation happens at many levels and may account for much of the variation in clinical response.

In the cat, the half-life of diazepam is approximately 5.5 hours, and the half-life of nordiazepam is 21.3 hours (Plumb 2002). There is an initial rapid increase in levels of nordiazepam for 2 hours after intravenous injection of diazepam, with about 54% of diazepam being biotransformed to nordiazepam (Cotler and Gustafson 1978; Cotler et al. 1984). After this, nordiazepam levels are maintained within 50% of peak nordiazepam levels for 24–48 hours. Approximately 70% of diazepam given by intravenous injection is excreted in the urine, 50% as known metabolites. Approximately 20% is excreted in the feces, 50% of that as nordiazepam (Cotler and Gustafson 1978). Diazepam is fatal to cats within one day when given at a dose of 500 mg/kg PO (Randall and Kappell 1973).

Diazepam is rapidly metabolized in dogs, with a half-life of 2.5–3.2 hours while the half-life of nordiazepam is 3.6–10 hours (Vree et al. 1979; Löscher and Frey 1981). The metabolite oxazepam reaches maximal plasma concentration in about 2 hours, then declines with a half-life of about 3–5.7 hours (Vree et al. 1979; Löscher and Frey 1981). When dogs were given 25 mg/kg of diazepam per day for 10 days, no diazepam was subsequently found in urine extracts. In these dogs, the main pathway of metabolism of diazepam was *N*-demethylation and hydroxylation, followed by excretion as oxazepam glucuronide. While oxazepam can be conjugated with glucuronic acid, diazepam has to first be hydroxylated in order to produce a compound that can subsequently be excreted as a glucuronide (Ruelius et al. 1965). Dogs chronically administered doses of 0.56, 4.5, 9, or 36 mg/kg daily of diazepam exhibit a linear relationship between total plasma levels and brain levels of diazepam, nordiazepam, and oxazepam, and the chronic dose of diazepam. At higher doses there is more free nordiazepam and oxazepam, and less free diazepam in the plasma, cerebrospinal fluid, and brain (Wala et al. 1995).

The half-life of diazepam is 7–22 hours in the horse. The half-life of nordiazepam is 18–28 hours while the half-life of oxazepam, another active metabolite, is 12 hours (Norman et al. 1997; Shini et al. 1997; Plumb 2002). Peak levels of diazepam occur in the serum 40 minutes after an intramuscular injection of a dose of 10 mg per horse. Diazepam is not detected in horse serum more than 6 hours after administration. Nordiazepam levels in the serum peak 3 hours after administration of diazepam. The metabolites oxazepam and temazepam can be found in the urine up to 121 and 79 hours, respectively, after injection of diazepam, but are not found in the serum after administration by assays that do not detect levels below 1.1 ng/ml. Overall, diazepam is excreted in the urine mainly as oxazepam (37%), temazepam (33%), and nordiazepam (29%), with <0.2% being excreted as diazepam (Marland et al. 1999). Measurements of various cardiopulmonary parameters in horses given clinically usual doses of diazepam intravenously have identified few significant changes. Doses greater than 0.2 mg/kg IV are likely to induce recumbency in this species due to muscle relaxant properties (Muir et al. 1982; Matthews et al. 1991; Kerr et al. 1996).

In rabbits, there are multiple metabolites with the primary metabolite being oxazepam (Jommi et al. 1964; Sawada et al. 1976).

Comparison of research on guinea pigs, rats, rabbits, and mice demonstrates the existence of substantial interspecies variation in metabolism. Rat liver predominantly hydroxylates diazepam in the C_3 position and only slightly causes N-demethylation; mouse liver predominantly N-demethylates, but does hydroxylate, whereas in the guinea pig only N-demethylation occurs. Rabbits, like mice, predominantly demethylate but hydroxylate to some degree. The major metabolite of diazepam in blood, brain, and adipose tissue of guinea pigs is N-demethyldiazepam. Oxazepam is not a significant metabolite in this species, but it is in the mouse (Jommi et al. 1964; Marcucci et al. 1969; Marcucci et al. 1970a, 1970b; Marcucci et al. 1971; Mussini et al. 1971).

Bergamottin, a furanocoumarin that occurs in grapefruit juice, reduces the activity of the P450 enzymes CYP3A12 and CYP1A1/2, concurrently causing an increase in plasma levels of diazepam in dogs, but not in Wistar rats (Sahi et al. 2002).

Uses in Humans

Diazepam is used in humans for the relief of symptoms of anxiety and management of anxiety disorders. It is also used in the treatment of convulsive disorders, for relief of skeletal muscle spasms, and for symptomatic relief of acute alcohol withdrawal.

Contraindications

Diazepam is contraindicated when there is a known hypersensitivity of the patient to the drug, in patients with glaucoma, and in cats that have been exposed to the insecticide chlorpyrifos, because diazepam may potentiate organophosphate toxicity (Plumb 2002). Lower doses should be used in patients with compromised liver or renal function and in geriatric or debilitated patients. Diazepam may cause loss of inhibitions and result in increased aggression in aggressive patients. Its use should be avoided in working animals, for example, drug detection dogs, because their ability to perform their working tasks may be compromised. Extreme caution should be used in giving riding and driving horses diazepam since the muscle fasciculations, ataxia, and sedative properties may be dangerous.

Diazepam crosses the placental barrier and enters the milk. There is an increased risk of congenital malformations when diazepam is given during the first trimester of pregnancy. Therefore, its use should be avoided in pregnant and lactating females (Roche 2000).

Side Effects

Side effects include ataxia, sedation, increased appetite, paradoxical excitation, transient cardiovascular depression, muscle relaxation, increased friendliness, anxiety, apparent hallucinations, muscle spasticity, insomnia, and idiopathic hepatic necrosis in cats. Idiopathic hepatic necrosis in cats is discussed further below. There have been occasional reports of neutropenia and jaundice in humans. Muscle fasciculations may occur in horses given diazepam.

The rate of metabolism may be decreased if diazepam is given concurrently with other medications that compete with it for the P450 isoenzyme system by which it is metabolized, including the selective serotonin reuptake inhibitors.

Reproduction studies on rats given 1, 10, 80, and 100 mg/kg daily of diazepam during pregnancy resulted in lowered pregnancy rates and surviving offspring in rats given 100 mg/kg. There were no teratological effects, lowered pregnancy rates, or reduced survival of offspring given up to 80 mg/kg (Beall 1972). In humans, however, research has suggested a risk of congenital malformations when diazepam is used during the first trimester. Because diazepam crosses the placenta and enters the milk, its use should be avoided in pregnant and lactating females of all species.

The oral LD_{50} in rats is 1240 mg/kg and in mice is 720 mg/kg (Roche 2000). The oral LD_{50} in rabbits is 328 mg/kg (Randall et al. 1965).

Overdose

Immediate gastric lavage and supportive measures should be conducted. Administer intravenous fluids and maintain an open airway. Flumazenil, a benzodiazepine receptor antagonist, can be used to completely or partially reverse the effects of an overdose. Treatment with flumazenil may result in seizures, especially in patients that have frequently been given diazepam for a long period of time.

Doses in Nonhuman Animals

Initiate treatment for nonhuman animals at the lowest dose. If no undesirable side effects occur, titrate dose up to the desired effect. There is a wide range of clinically effective doses for diazepam in veterinary populations. As discussed above under clinical guidelines for benzodiazepines, an initial test dose of the lowest usual dose for the species should be given when the owners will be home to observe the pet for sensitivity to the medication. This guideline is mentioned because diazepam is often used to treat anxiety problems for which symptoms may be exhibited primarily or entirely when the owners are absent. If the pet does not exhibit untoward side effects, this dose can then be used in the context of the situation for which the medication is being used, for example, storms or being alone. If humans will not be present, as is the case with separation anxiety, a video camera should be positioned to evaluate whether or not this dose of medication is effective in treating the behavioral signs. If the dose is insufficient, the dose can gradually be increased over a period of days until a clinically effective dose is identified or undesirable side effects occur. If the anxiety is effectively controlled before significant side effects occur, the dose that accomplishes this result can then be used. If significant side effects occur before effective treatment is accomplished, then the use of this particular medication in the patient must be reevaluated.

Discontinuation

Patients that have been treated with diazepam on a daily basis for several weeks should be gradually withdrawn. Diazepam is more addicting than some of the other benzodiazepines, such as lorazepam and oxazepam.

Other

Diazepam appears to interfere with the acquisition of new learning, but not with the recall of material already learned (e.g., Ghoneim et al. 1984).

Diazepam is commonly used in the treatment of seizure disorders in various species. A detailed discussion of this use is beyond the subject of this book.

Effects Documented in Nonhuman Animals

Cats

A single oral dose of diazepam has no prominent behavioral effects at a dose of 0.2 mg/kg. A mixture of ataxia, muscle relaxation, increased playfulness, and exploratory behavior occurs at a single oral dose of 1 mg/kg. Interestingly, the higher of these two doses produces increased wakefulness and decreased REM sleep during the one- to four-hour period after administration, while the lower dose produces no change in wakefulness when compared with placebo (Hashimoto et al. 1992).

Captive feral cats injected with 1 mg/kg of diazepam exhibit decreased defensive aggression, but have no change in flight behavior (Langfeldt and Ursin 1971).

Spraying is a common behavior problem in cats, affecting about 10% of prepubertally castrated males and about 5% of prepubertally neutered females (Hart and Cooper 1984). While the causes and function of spraying are poorly understood, the behavior often decreases or ceases if an anxiolytic is administered. Marder (1991) gave 19 castrated male cats and 4 spayed female cats with problems of spraying behavior 1 mg q12h. If spraying did not cease after three days, the dose was increased to 2 mg q12h. Treatment was continued for 1 month, at which point the dose was halved. Subsequently medication was gradually reduced at weekly intervals until the cats were off medication 1 month after beginning to decrease the dose. Success was defined as at least a 75% reduction and owner satisfaction at a 1- to 10-month follow-up. Sixteen out of the 19 castrated males exhibited reduced spraying, while one out of the four females exhibited reduced spraying. Eleven of the cats had previously been treated with synthetic progestins. All of those cats responded to diazepam. However, 75% of the cats that had responded well relapsed at a later date. Side effects observed by Marder were increased affection, lethargy, increased appetite, and ataxia.

Cooper and Hart (1992) also evaluated the effect of diazepam on spraying. Their subjects were 14 castrated males and 6 spayed females. Diazepam was given at 1–2 mg/cat q12h for 2 weeks. If spraying was eliminated or reduced to the client's satisfaction, this dose was continued for an additional 6–8 weeks. If the cat still sprayed, however, the dose was increased 50% for an additional 2 weeks. If the cat responded favorably at the higher dose, treatment was continued for another 6–8 weeks. If the cat still sprayed at the higher dose, it was weaned off medication over a 2-week period. For the cats that responded to the 1- or 2-mg q12h doses, treatment continued for 8 to 12 weeks, after which the cat was weaned off medication. If, during weaning, a cat resumed spraying, dosage was increased back to the previously effective dose. Some cats were treated for four years. Eleven out of 20 cats responded by complete cessation or decrease to a level that was acceptable to the owner. However, 10 of those 11 resumed spraying when treatment was discontinued. Eleven of the initial 20 cats had previously been treated ineffectively with progestins. Five of these responded to diazepam. Side effects observed in this study included sedation, ataxia, increased appetite, weight gain, reduced aggression, and a calmer and more affectionate temperament. Treatment with buspirone has subsequently been found to result in a lower recidivism rate than treatment with diazepam. See the discussion of buspirone in chapter 6, azapirones.

Overall (1994a) treated a spraying cat with diazepam 1 mg q12h PO with initial success. However, the cat could not be weaned off of medication without recurrence of the problem, and the spraying gradually recurred over a one-year period. An increase to 2 mg q12h was likewise initially successful, for three months, but was again followed by relapse. This cat was later treated with buspirone with greater success, although the cat could not be weaned off of medication (Overall 1994a).

In the cat, about 50% of diazepam is transformed into nordiazepam. Several clinicians have documented acute onset of hepatic necrosis in cats given diazepam (Levy et al. 1994; Levy 1994; Center et al. 1996; Hughes et al. 1996). Onset was usually eight to nine days after daily medication with diazepam was initiated. Initial signs include anorexia, vomiting, dehydration, lethargy, hypothermia, jaundice, and coma (Center et al. 1996). Most affected cats have died, usually within 24 hours, even with vigorous supportive therapy, but some have survived (Levy et al. 1994). The exact cause is unknown. Speculations have included (1) a toxic intermediate metabolite produced by some cats and (2) a toxic substance incorporated into the pill during manufacture. The latter hypothesis is questionable due to the hepatic necrosis having occurred with multiple different brands of diazepam (Center et al. 1996). Hughes et al. (1996) reviewed the premedication health status of six cats that developed hepatic necrosis subsequent to medication with diazepam. In all cases, the cat had prior cardiac, pancreatic, or renal disease. Current recommendations for the use of diazepam in cats are to do a baseline physical exam, complete blood count (CBC), and blood chemistries to confirm that the cat is in good health. Repeat the blood chemistries at three to five days. If there is elevated ALT or aspartate transferase (AST), discontinue the medication (Center et al. 1996). While hepatic necrosis in response to treatment with diazepam is usually fatal, the problem itself is rare. Some clients who have cats for which diazepam is otherwise a good choice, and for whom cost is a significant issue, may wish to try diazepam without monitoring of liver function. In all cases, however, the client should be informed of the rare, but present, potential for a fatal consequence with this inexpensive drug.

Dogs

Dogs medicated with increasing doses of diazepam until they started losing weight did so at doses of 20–36 mg/kg/day after 11–29 days on the increasing dose regimen (Martin et al. 1990; Sloan et al. 1991). Acute withdrawal of these dogs, precipitated by administering flumazenil, results in tremors, twitches, jerks, and seizures (Martin et al. 1990; Sloan et al. 1991). Dogs given 0.05625, 0.225, 0.5625, 4.5, 9, or 36 mg/kg/day of diazepam exhibited dose-dependent variation in both the quantity and quality of symptoms that occurred when acute withdrawal was precipitated by administration of flumazenil. At the two lowest doses, only minimal signs were precipitated. Seizure activity occurs only with dogs at the two highest doses of 9 and 36 mg/kg/day, both of which are well above routinely used clinical doses (Sloan et al. 1993).

All four of four laboratory beagles treated for abnormal withdrawn and depressed behavior resolved on 2.5 mg/kg of diazepam (Iorio et al. 1983).

Diazepam has been reported to be more effective than chlorpromazine in reducing signs of fear in dogs (Hart 1985).

Horses

Sexual behavior in stallions can be inhibited both by a novel environment and by classical conditioning. Sexual behavior has been shown to be normalized by slow intravenous injection of 0.05 mg/kg of diazepam (McDonnell et al. 1986, 1987; McDonnell 1999).

Performance horses are sometimes given diazepam as an anxiolytic and muscle relaxant, a practice which is generally illegal (Jaussaud and Courtot 1990). Medication of a horse with diazepam can be detected at least 38 days later using gas chromatography-high resolution mass spectrometry (Jouvel et al. 2000).

Parrots

Diazepam has been suggested as a treatment for feather-picking at a starting dose of two drops of the 5 mg/ml solution per ounce of drinking water, with subsequent increases in dose until feather-picking discontinues or the bird becomes excessively sedated. However, no data on results are presented (Galvin 1983).

Rabbits

Diazepam given to rabbits at a dose of 0.05–0.1 mg/kg decreases behavioral arousal as measured by electroencephalogram (Goldberg et al. 1974). When given at doses of 0.6 mg/kg/day PO for 30 days, it has no effect on blood sugar levels (Dixit et al. 2001).

Other Species

Diazepam decreases fear in the marmoset (*Callithrix penicillata*) when exposed to a potential predator. Doses of 1 mg/kg IM produce only a small reduction in behaviors considered indicative of fear. Doses of 2 mg/kg IM produce a much stronger anxiolytic effect without a significant sedative effect. Doses of 3 mg/kg IM produce a sufficient sedative effect that overall activity levels are compromised (Barros et al. 2000).

Diazepam has been used to tame monkeys at a dose of 1 mg/kg (Zbinden and Randall 1967). Within social colonies of rhesus monkeys, diazepam (2.5–5 mg/kg by mouth daily) produces dose-dependent increases in social grooming, approach, contact, self grooming, feeding, and resting with the eyes open. There is also decreased vigilance and aggression (Kumar et al. 1999).

VI. Flurazepam Hydrochloride

Chemical Compound: 7-Chloro-1-[2-(diethylamino)ethyl]-5-(*o*-fluorophenyl)-1,3-dihydro-2 *H*-1,4-benzodiazepin-2-one-dihydrochloride

DEA Classification: Schedule IV drug

Preparations: Generally available as 15- and 30-mg capsules

Clinical Pharmacology

Flurazepam is rapidly absorbed from the gastrointestinal (GI) tract, rapidly metabolized, and excreted primarily through the urine. In humans, peak flurazepam plasma concentrations occur 30 to 60 minutes after a single oral dose. The half-life in humans is 2.3 hours. In humans, its major metabolite is N_1–desalkyl-flurazepam with a half-life of 47–100 hours. The long half-life of this metabolite may be responsible for the clinical observation that flurazepam is increasingly effective on the second and third nights of consecutive use and that efficacy continues for one to two nights after discontinuation (Roche Laboratories 1994).

In humans, older men have a longer elimination half-life of desalkyl-flurazepam than younger men, after both single dose and multiple dose treatment. There is no difference between older women and younger women (Roche Laboratories 1994). Whether this age/gender interaction exists in nonhuman patients has not been tested.

When dogs are given ^{14}C-labeled flurazepam at a dose of 2 mg/kg PO or IV, fecal excretion predominates, and over 80% is eliminated by either route within nine days (Schwartz and Postma 1970).

Flurazepam is fatal to cats within one hour when given at a dose of 400 mg/kg PO (Randall and Kappell 1973).

Uses in Humans

Flurazepam is used to treat insomnia.

Contraindications

Flurazepam is contraindicated in patients with known hypersensitivity to this drug or other benzodiazepines.

Flurazepam crosses the placenta and also enters milk. Its use should therefore be avoided in pregnant and lactating females.

Side Effects

Side effects are similar to those reported for other benzodiazepines and include sedation and ataxia. Flurazepam has not been as extensively used in nonhuman patients as some of the other benzodiazepines. Therefore, it is likely that some probable side effects have not yet been reported.

Rare cases of leucopenia, granulocytopenia, elevated AST/ALT, elevated total/direct bilirubin, elevated alkaline phosphatase, and skin rashes have been reported in humans. Two cases of cholestatic jaundice secondary to treatment with flurazepam have been reported in humans (Fang et al. 1978; Reynolds et al. 1981). Blurred vision has been reported in humans (Roche Laboratories 1994). While subtle changes in vision are difficult to detect in nonhuman patients, this should be kept in mind if significant difficulty navigating the environment occurs after administration of flurazepam.

Rebound insomnia can occur with discontinuation. However, it is less likely to occur than with shorter-acting benzodiazepines such as triazolam (Rickels 1983).

Overdose

In case of overdose, conduct gastric lavage and provide supportive measures, including intravenous fluids. Flumazenil, a benzodiazepine receptor antagonist, is indicated for the complete or partial reversal of flurazepam toxicity.

Doses in Nonhuman Animals

Initiate treatment at the lowest dose. If no undesirable side effects occur, titrate the dose up to the desired effect.

Effects Documented in Nonhuman Animals

Flurazepam may be a preferred benzodiazepine for pets that wake during the night due to its long half-life (Landsberg et al. 2003). There are no reports of clinical studies on the use of flurazepam in the treatment of pets.

VII. Lorazepam

Chemical Compound: 7-Chloro-5-(*o*-chlorophenyl)-1,3-dihydro-3-hydroxy-2H-1,4-benzodiazepine-2-one
DEA Classification: Schedule IV drug
Preparations: Generally available in 0.5-, 1-, and 2-mg tablets and 2 mg/ml oral solution

Clinical Pharmacology

Lorazepam is identical to oxazepam except that it has a chlorine atom on the phenyl ring (Elliott 1976). Absorption of lorazepam is fairly rapid, except in the cat (Ruelius 1978). In humans, peak concentrations in the plasma occur in approximately 2 hours. The time to peak plasma levels of lorazepam in the cat, dog, pig, and rat is given in Table 3.6. In humans, the mean half-life for lorazepam is about 12 hours, while the half-life for its major metabolite, lorazepam glucuronide, is about 18 hours. In African green monkeys, the mean half-life of lorazepam is 1.7 hours (Friedman et al. 1991; Wyeth Laboratories 1999b).

Lorazepam glucuronidate is the primary metabolite in the dog, cat, human, and pig, but not in the rat (Schillings et al. 1971). Lorazepam glucuronidate has no significant CNS activity (Gluckman and Stein 1978). Peak plasma levels of unchanged lorazepam are almost identical in humans and dogs when dogs are given a dose about 30 times higher than a human on a per kilogram basis. This is because formation of lorazepam glucuronide is much faster in dogs than in humans (Ruelius 1978). Cats do glucuronidate lorazepam, but not as rapidly or extensively as dogs. However, the finding that cats form the glucuronide is unexpected, because they often conjugate exogenous molecules with glucuronic acid poorly or not at all (Ruelius 1978).

When cats are given a single dose of 1 mg/kg PO, plasma levels of unconjugated lorazepam peak at 12 hours and then begin declining, with a half-life of 17 hours. Plasma levels of conjugated lorazepam run at about one-third to one-half the levels of unconjugated lorazepam in this species (Schillings et al. 1975).

Table 3.6 Peak plasma levels and percentage of lorazepam eliminated in the urine and feces of cats, dogs, rats, and pigs

Species	Dose	Time to peak plasma concentration	Peak plasma concentration (ng/ml)	Eliminated in the urine (%)	Eliminated in the feces (%)
Cat	20 mg/kg PO	12	9310	47.3	54
Dog	1 mg/kg PO	0.5	28	66.4	22
Pig	0.04 mg/kg PO	3	1.2	87.8	7.9
Rat	1 mg/kg IG	0.5	108	21.7	68.9

Source: Ruelius 1978.

Dogs and pigs excrete lorazepam primarily in the urine, rats predominantly in the feces, and cats excrete it roughly equally in urine and feces (Ruelius 1978). Six days after a single dose of 1 mg/kg lorazepam PO, cats will have excreted about 47% in the urine and about 54% in the feces (Schillings et al. 1975). Within a species, no gender effect has been identified in the qualitative urinary excretion pattern (Schillings et al. 1971; Schillings et al. 1975). No changes in urinary excretion patterns have been identified in dogs, pigs, rats, and humans treated with lorazepam for periods of five to eight weeks (Schillings et al. 1971).

In rats, about three times as much lorazepam occurs in the brain as in plasma for about 0.5–12 hours after dosing (Ruelius 1978).

Both lorazepam and lorazepam glucuronide are transferred by the placenta (Wyeth Laboratories 1999b).

There is good separation between anxiety-reducing doses and sedative-hypnotic doses (Gluckman and Stein 1978).

Uses in Humans

Lorazepam is used for the short-term relief of symptoms of anxiety and for management of anxiety disorders in humans.

Contraindications

Lorazepam is contraindicated in patients with a history of sensitivity to lorazepam or other benzodiazepines and in patients with acute narrow angle glaucoma. It should be used with extreme caution in aggressive animals because it may cause disinhibition and in pregnant or nursing females because it may cause fetal malformations and loss, and is probably transmitted through the milk.

Side Effects

As with all benzodiazepines, sedation, ataxia, muscle relaxation, increased appetite, paradoxical excitation, increased friendliness, anxiety, and a variety of other side effects may occur. When they occur, side effects are usually observed early in therapy and disappear with continued treatment or a decreased dose.

No evidence of carcinogenesis has been identified. In rabbits used to study effects on reproduction, random anomalies of various sorts occurred at all doses. At doses of 40 mg/kg fetal resorption and increased fetal loss occur in rabbits (Wyeth Laboratories 1999b).

Overdose

Induce vomiting and/or conduct gastric lavage. Provide supportive therapy as needed. Flumazenil may be used to partially or fully reverse the effect of lorazepam.

Doses in Nonhuman Animals

Initiate treatment at the lowest dose. If no undesirable side effects occur, titrate dose up to effect. While variation between individuals and species makes exact comparison impossible, 1 mg/kg of lorazepam is about equivalent to 5 mg/kg of diazepam (Gluckman and Stein 1978).

Discontinuation

As with all the benzodiazepines, withdrawal of a patient that has been on lorazepam should be accomplished gradually. Dogs that have been addicted to lorazepam by chronic administration of 100 mg/kg/day and acutely withdrawn by administration of flumazenil exhibit tremor, rigidity, and decreased food intake (McNicholas et al. 1983).

Effects Documented in Nonhuman Animals

Dogs

Dogs given an increasing dose of lorazepam until they reached a dose of 140 mg/kg/day at 16 days of treatment, and subsequently for another 52 days, did not lose weight but did become physically addicted to lorazepam. However, in dogs, physical dependence to lorazepam was found to be less intense than was physical dependence to some other benzodiazepines such as diazepam (Martin et al. 1990).

Primates

Lorazepam reduces anxiety and conflict behavior in squirrel monkeys (Stein and Berger 1971; Gluckman and Stein 1978).

Within social colonies of rhesus monkeys, lorazepam (0.5–1.0 mg/kg PO daily) produces dose-dependent increases in social grooming, approach, contact, self-grooming, feeding, and resting with the eyes open. There is also decreased vigilance and aggression (Kumar et al. 1999).

Rats and Mice

Lorazepam reduces conflict behavior in rats. In mice, it suppresses foot shock-induced fighting behavior (Gluckman and Stein 1978). Rats treated with lorazepam at 1.25 mg/kg/day for over a year have shown no adverse effects. However, rats treated at 6 mg/kg/day for the same period of time developed esophageal dilation. The esophageal dilation reversed if medication was withdrawn within two months of detection.

VIII. Oxazepam

Chemical Compound: 7-Chloro-1,3-dihydro-3-hydroxy-5-phenyl-2*H*-1,4-benzodiazepin-2-one

DEA Classification: Schedule IV controlled substance

Preparations: Generally available as 10-, 15-, and 30-mg capsules and as 15- and 30-mg tablets

Clinical Pharmacology

Oxazepam has no active intermediate metabolites and therefore may be safer for patients with liver disease, obese patients, and geriatric patients than some of the other benzodiazepines. An inactive glucuronide conjugation of oxazepam is the primary metabolite, accounting for over 95% of urinary metabolites in pigs and humans and likewise being the primary metabolite in rabbits (Sisenwine et al. 1972; Sawada et al. 1976). There are at least six other minor metabolites that account for <5% of the urinary metabolites in these species. In the rat, conjugated oxazepam is a minor metabolite, and conversion to inactive metabolites that are minor in humans and pigs is conversely greater (Sisenwine et al. 1972).

In human studies absorption has been identified as equivalent when oxazepam is given as a tablet, capsule, or suspension. Mean elimination half-life is approximately 8.2 hours, while peak plasma levels occur at about 3 hours after oral dosing in humans (Wyeth Laboratories 1999a).

In dogs given 5–10 mg/kg PO of C^{14}-labeled oxazepam, peak plasma levels occur in 4–6 hours, with some drug, or a metabolite, remaining in the system for at least 120 hours. Twenty-four hours after administration, about three-fourths of the total dose is excreted. At 96 hours (four days) after administration, urinary excretion has accounted for about 68% of the C^{14}, while fecal excretion has accounted for about 35% of the C^{14} (Walkenstein et al. 1964).

Oxazepam exerts an anticonvulsant effect in 50% of mice given a dose of 0.6 mg/kg orally, while ataxia is observed in 50% of mice given a dose of 5 mg/kg orally. Thus, there is a wide separation of effective doses and doses that induce side effects. There is also a significant dose separation between effective antianxiety levels in rats subjected to shock and the doses required to produce motor incoordination.

Oxazepam has a larger spread than either chlordiazepoxide or diazepam between the minimal effective dose and the dose that causes side effects. It causes better anxiolytic effects with less depressant effects as well (Gluckman 1965).

The acute oral LD_{50} in mice is more than 5000 mg/kg.

Uses in Humans

Oxazepam is used for the management of anxiety disorders and for the short-term amelioration of anxiety symptoms that occur with or without depression. It is considered to be especially useful in the treatment of anxiety, tension, agitation, and irritability in geriatric patients.

Contraindications

Oxazepam is contraindicated in patients with a history of hypersensitivity to this or other benzodiazepines. Because it crosses the placental barrier and enters the milk, it should not be used in pregnant or lactating females.

Side Effects

As with all benzodiazepines, sedation, ataxia, and temperament changes due to loss of inhibition may occur.

Rarely, leucopenia and hepatic dysfunction have been reported in humans treated with oxazepam. Fetal abnormalities have not been observed in rats subjected to breeding studies of the oxazepam.

Rats given oxazepam as 0.5% of their diet for six weeks exhibit fatty metamorphosis of the liver without necrosis or fibrosis.

Mice given 35 or 100 times the human dose of oxazepam for nine months exhibit dose-related increases in liver adenomas (Fox and Lahcen 1974). Rats given 30 times the human maximum dose over two years showed an increase in benign thyroid follicular cell tumors, testicular interstitial cell adenomas, and prostatic adenomas. There is no evidence that clinical use of oxazepam is carcinogenic.

Overdose

In case of an overdose, induce vomiting and/or conduct gastric lavage. Provide supportive treatment. Flumazenil can be used to partially or fully reverse the effect of oxazepam.

Doses in Nonhuman Animals

Initiate treatment at the lowest dose for nonhuman animals. If no undesirable side effects occur, titrate the dose up to the desired effect.

Discontinuation

As with all benzodiazepines, dose reduction should be done gradually for patients that have been medicated daily for several weeks. However, oxazepam is less addicting than some other benzodiazepines, such as diazepam.

Other Information

Some research in humans has suggested that oxazepam may be more effective than chlordiazepoxide in treating aggression (Gardos et al. 1968; Kochansky et al. 1975).

Effects Documented in Nonhuman Animals

Cats

Oxazepam is used as an appetite stimulant in cats, with a longer duration of action than diazepam (Landsberg et al. 2003).

Dogs

Dogs given increasing doses of oxazepam to 270 mg/kg by day 72 of treatment, and subsequently given this dose for an additional 30 days, did not lose weight. While chronic administration of oxazepam at such a high dose did produce physical dependence, the dependence was not as intense as with some other benzodiazepines such as diazepam (Martin et al. 1990).

Dogs given 480 mg/kg daily for 4 weeks showed no specific changes. Two of eight dogs given 960 mg/kg died with evidence of circulatory collapse. In chronic toxicity studies dogs given 120 mg/kg/day for 52 weeks exhibited no toxic effects. Thus, there is a wide margin of safety.

IX. Triazolam

Chemical Compound: 8-Chloro-6-(*o*-chlorophenyl)-1-methyl-4H-s-tria-zolo-[4,3-α][1,4] benzodiazepine

DEA Classification: DEA Schedule IV controlled drug

Preparations: Generally available 0.125-, 0.25-, and 0.5-mg tablet

Clinical Pharmacology

Triazolam has a short plasma half-life, 1.5–5.5 hours in humans. The initial step in metabolism is hydroxylation, which is catalyzed by cytochrome P450 3A (CYP 34A). The primary metabolites are conjugated glucuronides, which are presumably inactive. Both triazolam and its metabolites are excreted primarily in the urine (Pharmacia and Upjohn 1999).

When triazolam is administered orally to pregnant mice, it is uniformly distributed in the fetus. The fetal brain develops approximately the same concentration in the brain as does the mother (Pharmacia and Upjohn 1999).

Initially, triazolam decreases latency to sleep and number of nocturnal awakenings and increases the duration of sleep. However, after two weeks of consecutive nightly doses, its efficacy decreases. On the first and/or second night after discontinuation from two weeks of continuous use, a rebound effect occurs, with the total time asleep becoming less than at baseline (Pharmacia and Upjohn 1999).

Uses in Humans

Triazolam is used for the short-term (7–10 days) treatment of insomnia in humans.

Contraindications

Triazolam is contraindicated in any patient with a history of sensitivity to this or other benzodiazepines. Triazolam should not be given concurrently with any medications that substantially impair metabolism mediated by cytochrome P450 3A, including ketoconazole, itraconazole, and nefazodone (Pharmacia and Upjohn 1999).

Side Effects

Interdose withdrawal sometimes produces daytime anxiety in human patients after as little as 10 days' treatment with triazolam (Pharmacia and Upjohn 1999). Increased anxiety should be considered as a potential side effect in nonhuman patients for which this short-acting benzodiazepine is being used to treat nighttime restlessness or anxiety.

Otherwise, side effects common to the benzodiazepines, including sedation, ataxia, and temperament changes due to loss of inhibition, may occur.

In a 24-month study of carcinogenesis that was conducted on mice given up to 4000 times the recommended human dose, no evidence of carcinogenesis was identified (Pharmacia and Upjohn 1999).

Overdose

Triazolam is a very potent benzodiazepine. Therefore, signs of overdosage may occur at moderate overdoses, for example, four times the maximum recommended therapeutic dose in humans.

In case of overdose, conduct immediate gastric lavage and provide supportive treatment. Flumazenil can be used for the complete or partial reversal of triazolam.

Doses in Nonhuman Animals

Initiate treatment at the lowest dose. If no undesirable side effects occur, titrate the dose up to the desired effect.

Effects Documented in Nonhuman Animals

Rabbits

Triazolam, at doses of 0.01 or 0.1 mg/kg IV or PO given to rabbits, reduces wakefulness during the subsequent six hours and, in most cases, significantly increases non-REM sleep (except that at 0.01 mg/kg PO it significantly increases REM, rather than non-REM, sleep) (Scherschlicht and Marias 1983).

Important Information for Owners of Pets Being Placed on Any Benzodiazepine

The following should be considered when placing an animal on a benzodiazepine.

1. Benzodiazepines are fast-acting, but only last a few hours.
2. Some pets become unsteady, sleepy, or excited when on a benzodiazepine. The first dose should be given when the owner is home and can observe the pet.
3. There is wide variation between individuals regarding the optimal dose to use to treat a particular problem. Also, some pets respond well to one benzodiazepine but not to another. Pet owners should work closely with their veterinarian until the best drug and dose for their pet is identified.
4. If the owner's pet is medicated with a benzodiazepine for several weeks, withdrawal needs to be gradual.
5. Benzodiazepines are DEA Schedule IV drugs. Therefore, special restrictions apply to their prescription and use.

Clinical Examples

See also Case 1 discussed in the tricyclic antidepressants section.

Case 1

Signalment
Tobler was a 13-year-old female spayed chocolate Labrador retriever weighing 35.5 kg.

Presenting Complaint
Tobler presented with fear of storms.

History
Upon presentation, Tobler was being treated with thyroxin for hypothyroidism and carprofen (Rimadyl) for arthritis. She had a small elevation in alkaline phosphatase (311: normal range 13–122), a small liver, and a urinary tract infection. She was also obese and had multiple subcutaneous masses that were identified as lipomas upon aspiration. Otherwise, results of the physical exam, CBC, blood chemistries, and urinalysis were normal. Her Georgia Storm Phobia Assessment score (SPA) upon presentation was 29 (Crowell-Davis et al. 2003). Her primary behaviors during storms were whining, hiding, pacing, and panting. Otherwise Tobler had no behavior problems, and cognitive function was good.

Diagnosis
The diagnosis was storm phobia.

Treatment Plan
The owners were instructed in behavior modification, including desensitization and counterconditioning to storm sounds that Tobler reacted to in the clinic. Because of

Tobler's age, the multiple medical problems, and the elevated alkaline phosphatase, initial medication treatment was restricted to 1–2 mg of alprazolam (0.03–0.06 mg/kg) to be given 30–60 minutes prior to storms.

Follow-up

Three months later, Tobler's storm phobia had improved and her SPA score had decreased to 19. The owners reported that they had found timing to be critical, that is, Tobler's response was significantly improved if they managed to medicate her early enough. The score of 19 applied to storms in which they did not manage to medicate her until after the storm had started and she was already showing fear. Her alkaline phosphatase had declined to 162. The dose of alprazolam was increased to 2–3 mg (0.06–0.09 mg/kg) to be given prior to storms, but long-acting medications were not added to her treatment protocol.

Tobler continued to be improved on this treatment. After 18 months on treatment, that is, continuing behavior modification and 2–3 mg of alprazolam prior to storms, the owners considered her to be substantially improved. Her SPA score at this point was still 19, but that was affected by the severity of storms she had recently been exposed to. Her 18-month recheck occurred in the wake of the summer of 2004, when four hurricanes hit Florida, three of which made it into Georgia as tropical storms. Many very severe storms and tornadoes occurred during the three months prior to this recheck, and, under the circumstances, the owners considered to her behavioral responses to be good.

Comments

In addition to being an example of the importance of evaluating concurrent medical problems when making medication decisions, this case demonstrates the importance of evaluating context when assessing a patient's improvement.

References

Abbott Laboratories 2004. Tranxene product information. *Physicians desk reference,* Medical Economics Company, Montvale, New Jersey.

Al-Tahan F, Löscher W and H-H Frey 1984. Pharmacokinetics of clonazepam in the dog. *Archives Internationales de Pharmacodynamie et de Therapie* 268(2): 180–193.

Angel C, DeLuca DC, Newton JE and Reese WG 1982. Assessment of pointer dog behavior. Drug effects and neurochemical correlates. *The Pavlovian Journal of Biological Science* 17(2): 84–88.

Barnhill JG, Greenblatt DJ, Miller LG, Gaver A, Harmatz JS and Shader RI 1990. Kinetic and dynamic components of increased benzodiazepine sensitivity in aging animals. *The Journal of Pharmacology and Experimental Therapeutics* 253(3): 1153–1161.

Barros M, Boere V, Huston JP and Tomaz C 2000. Measuring fear and anxiety in the marmoset (*Callithrix penicillata*) with a novel predator confrontation model: Effects of diazepam. *Behavioural Brain Research* 108: 205–211.

Bauen A and Possanza GJ 1970. The mink as a psychopharmacological model. *Archives Internationales de Pharmacodynamie et de Therapie* 186(1): 133–136.

Beall JR 1972. Study of the teratogenic potential of diazepam and SCH 12041. *Canadian Medical Association Journal* 106: 1061.

Bertini S, Buronfosse F, Pineau X, Berny P and Lorgue G 1995. Benzodiazepine poisoning in companion animals. *Veterinary and Human Toxicology* 37: 559–562.

Boissier JR, Simon P and Aron C 1968. A new method for rapid screening of minor tranquilizers in mice. *European Journal of Pharmacology* 4: 145–151.

Boxenbaum H 1980. Interspecies variations in liver weight, hepatic blood flow, and antipyrine intrinsic clearance: extrapolation of data to benzodiazepines and phenytoin. *Journal of Pharmacokinetics and Biopharmaceutics* 8: 165–176.

Boyle D and Tobin JM 1961. Pharmaceutical management of behavior disorders: chlordiazepoxide in covert and overt expressions of aggression. *Journal of the Medical Society of New Jersey* 58: 427–429.

Braestrup C and Squires RF 1977. Specific benzodiazepine receptors in rats characterized by high affinity [3H]-diazepam binding. *Proceedings of the National Academy of Science USA* 74(9): 3805–3809.

Brennan CH and Littleton JM 1991. Chronic exposure to anxiolytic drugs, working by different mechanisms causes up-regulation of dihydropyridine binding sites on cultured bovine adrenal chromaffin cells. *Neuropharmacology* 30(2): 199–205.

Brown SA and Forrester SD. 1991. Serum disposition of oral clorazepate from regular-release and sustained-delivery tablets in dogs. *Journal of Veterinary Pharmacology and Therapeutics* 14 (4): 426–429.

Center SA, Elston TH, Rowland PH, Rosen DK, Reitz, BL, Brunt JE, Rodan I, House J, Bank S, Lynch LR, Dring LA and Levy JK, 1996. Fulminant hepatic failure associated with oral administration of diazepam in 11 cats. *Journal of the American Veterinary Medical Association* 209: 618–625.

Charney DS, Woods SW, Goodman WK, Rifkin B, Kinch M, Aiken B, Quadrino LM and Heninger GR 1986. Drug treatment of panic disorder: The comparative efficacy of imipramine, alprazolam, and trazodone. *Journal of Clinical Psychiatry* 47(12): 580–586.

Christmas AJ and Maxwell DR 1970. A comparison of the effects of some benzodiazepines and other drugs on aggressive and exploratory behaviour in mice and cats. *Neuropharmacology* 9: 17–29.

Cole HF and Wolf HH 1970. Laboratory evaluation of aggressive behavior of the grasshopper mouse (*Onychomys*). *Journal of Pharmaceutical Sciences* 59: 969–971.

Cooper L and Hart BL 1992. Comparison of diazepam with progestin for effectiveness in suppression of urine spraying behavior in cats. *Journal of the American Veterinary Medical Association* 200(6): 797–801.

Cotler S and Gustafson JH 1978. The fate of diazepam in the cat. *Proceedings of the Academy of Pharmaceutical Sciences*, 25th APS National Meeting, Hollywood, Florida, November 12–16, p.98.

Cotler S, Gustafson JH and Colburn WA 1984. Pharmacokinetics of diazepam and nordiazepam in the cat. *Journal of Pharmaceutical Sciences* 73: 348–351.

Crowell-Davis SL 1986. Maternal behavior. *The Veterinary Clinics of North America, Equine Practice* 2(3): 557–571.

Crowell-Davis SL, Seibert LM, Sung W, Parthasarathy V and Curtis TM 2003. Use of clomipramine, alprazolam and behavior modification for treatment of stormphobia in dogs. *Journal of the American Veterinary Medical Association* 222(6): 744–748.

Danneberg P and Weber KH 1983. Chemical structure and biological activity of the diazepines. *British Journal of Clinical Pharmacology* 16: 231S–243S.

DiMascio A 1973. The effects of benzodiazepines on aggression: reduced or increased? In *The benzodiazepines,* pp.433–440, edited by S Garattini, E Mussini and LO Randall, Raven Press, New York.

Dixit RK, Puri JN, Sharma MK, Jain IP, Singh S, Ansari NA and Singh SP 2001. Effect of anxiolytics on blood sugar level in rabbits. *Indian Journal of Experimental Biology* 39: 378–380.

Dodman NH and Shuster L 1994. Pharmacologic approaches to managing behavior problems in small animals. *Veterinary Medicine* 89(10): 960–969.

Elliott HW 1976. Metabolism of lorazepam. *British Journal of Anaesthesia* 48(10): 1017–1023.

Fairchild MD, Jenden DJ, Mickey MR and Yale C 1980. The quantitative measurement of changes in EEG frequency spectra produced in the cat by sedative-hypnotics and neuroleptics. *Electroencephalography and Clinical Neurophysiology* 49: 382–390.

Fang MH, Ginsberg AL and Dobbins WO 1978. Cholestatic jaundice associated with flurazepam hydrochloride. *Annals of Internal Medicine* 89(3): 363–364.

Forrester SD, Wilcke JR, Jacobson JD and Dyer KR 1993. Effects of a 44-day administration of phenobarbital on disposition of chlorazepate in dogs. *American Journal of Veterinary Research* 54(7): 1136–1138.

Forrester SD, Brown SA, Lees GE and Hartsfield SM 1990. Disposition of clorazepate in dogs after single- and multiple-dose oral administration. *American Journal of Veterinary Research* 51(12): 2001–2005.

Fox KA and Lahcen RB 1974. Liver-cell adenomas and peliosis hepatis in mice associated with oxazepam. *Research Communications in Chemical Pathology and Pharmacology* 8: 481–488.

Fox KA and Snyder RL 1969. Effect of sustained low doses of diazepam on aggression and mortality in grouped male mice. *Journal of Comparative and Physiological Psychology* 69: 663–666.

Fox KA, Tockosh JR and Wilcox AH 1970. Increased aggression among grouped male mice fed chlordiazepoxide. *European Journal of Pharmacology* 11(1): 119–121.

Friedman H, Redmond DE and Greenblatt DJ 1991. Comparative pharmacokinetics of alprazolam and lorazepam in humans and in African green monkeys. *Psychopharmacology* 104: 103–105.

Galvin C 1983. The feather picking bird. In *Current veterinary therapy VIII*, pp. 646–651, edited by RW Kirk, W.B. Saunders, Philadelphia, Pennsylvania.

Gao B and Cutler MG 1993. Buspirone increases social investigation in pair-housed male mice, comparison with the effects of chloridazepoxide. *Neuropharmacology* 32 (5): 429–437.

Gardos G, DiMascio A, Salzman C and Shader RI 1968. Differential actions of chlordiazepoxide and oxazepam on hostility. *Archives of General Psychiatry* 18: 757–760.

Ghoneim MM, Hinrichs JV and Mewaldt SP 1984. Dose-response analysis of the behavioral effects of diazepam: I. Learning and memory. *Psychopharmacology* 82: 291–295.

Gluckman MI 1965. Pharmacology of oxazepam (Serax), a new antianxiety agent. *Current Therapeutic Research* 7(11): 721–740.

Gluckman MI and Stein L 1978. Pharmacology of lorazepam. *The Journal of Clinical Psychiatry* 39(10) Sec. 2: 3–10.

Goldberg H, Horvath TB and Meares RA 1974. Visual evoked potentials as a measure of drug effects on arousal in the rabbit. *Clinical and Experimental Pharmacology & Physiology.* 1(2): 147–154.

Goldberg ME, Manian AA and Efron DH. 1967. A comparative study of certain pharmacologic responses following acute and chronic administrations of chlordiazepoxide. *Life Sciences* 6(5): 481–491.

Gorman JM 2003. Treating generalized anxiety disorder. *Journal of Clinical Psychiatry* 64: 24–29.

Greenblatt DJ, Divoll MK, Soong MH, Boxenbaum HG, Harmatz JS and Shader RI 1988. Desmethyldiazepam pharmacokinetics: studies following intravenous and oral desmethyl-diazepam, oral clorazepate and intravenous diazepam. *Journal of Clinical Pharmacology* 28: 853–859.

Guaitani A, Marcucci F and Garattini S 1971. Increased aggression and toxicity in grouped male mice treated with tranquilizing benzodiazepines. *Psychopharmacologia* (Berlin) 19: 241–245.

Harris T 1960. Methaminodiazepoxide. *Journal of the American Medical Association* 172: 1162–1163.

Hart BL 1985. Behavioral indications for phenothazine and benzodiazepine tranquilizer in dogs. *Journal of the American Veterinary Medical Association* 186: 1192–1193.

Hart BL and Cooper L 1984. Factors relating to urine spraying and fighting in prepubertally gonadectomized cats. *Journal of the American Veterinary Medical Association* 184: 1255–1258.

Hashimoto T, Hamada C, Wada T and Fukada N 1992. Comparative study on the behavioral and EEG changes induced by diazepam, buspirone and a novel anxioselective anxiolytic, DN-2327, in the cat. *Neuropsychobiology* 26: 89–99.

Heise GA and Boff E 1961. Taming action of chlordiazepoxide. *Proceedings of the 45th* annual meeting of American Societies for Experimental Biology 20: 393.

Heuschele WP 1961. Chlordiazepoxide for calming zoo animals. *Journal of the American Veterinary Medical Association* 139: 996–998.

Hodges H and Green S 1987. Are the effects of benzodiazepines on discrimination and punishment dissociable? *Physiology & Behavior* 41: 257–264.

Hoffmeister F and Wuttke W. 1969. On the actions of psychotropic drugs on the attack—and aggressive-defensive behavior of mice and cats. In *Aggressive behavior*, pp. 273–280, edited by S. Garattini and B. Sigg, Wiley & Sons, New York.

Horowitz ZP, Furgiuele AR, Brannick LJ, Burke JC and Craver BN 1963. A new chemical structure with specific depressant effects on the amygdale and on the hyperirritability of the "septal rat". *Nature* 200: 369–370.

Hughes D, Moreau RE, Overall KL and van Winkle TJ 1996. Acute hepatic necrosis and liver failure associated with benzodiazepine therapy in six cats, 1986–1995. *Journal of Veterinary Emergency and Critical Care* 6: 13–20.

ICN Pharmaceuticals 1996. Librium product information. In *2002 Physicians desk reference*, pp. 1736–1737, Montvale, New Jersey.

Iorio LC, Eisenstein N, Brody PE and Barnett A 1983. Effects of selected drugs on spontaneously occurring abnormal behavior in beagles. *Pharmacology Biochemistry & Behavior* 18: 379–382.

Iwahara S and Sugimura T 1970. Effects of chlordiazepoxide on black-white discrimination acquisition and reversal in white rats. (In Japanese with an English abstract) *The Japanese Journal of Psychology* 41(3): 142–150.

Iwasaki T, Ezawa K and Iwahara S 1976. Differential effects of chlordiazepoxide on simultaneous and successive brightness discrimination learning in rats. *Psychopharmacology (Berlin)* 48 (1): 75–78.

Jaussaud P and Courtot D 1990. Diazepam et dopage du cheval. *Revue de Médecine Vétérinaire* 141(3): 171–175.

Jommi G, Manitto P and Silanos MA 1964. Metabolism of diazepam in rabbits. *Archives of Biochemistry and Biophysics* 108: 334–340.

Jouvel C, Maciejewski P, Garcia P, Bonnaire Y, Horning S and Popot M 2000. Detection of diazepam in horse hair samples by mass spectrometric methods. *Analyst* 125(10): 1765–1769.

Kaplan SA, Lewis M, Schwartz MA, Postma E, Cotler S, Abruzzo CW, Lee TL and Weinfeld RE 1970. Pharmacokinetic model for chlordiazepoxide HCl in the dog. *Journal of Pharmaceutical Sciences* 59(11): 1569–1574.

Kerr CL, McDonnell WN and Young SS 1996. A comparison of romifidine and xylazine when used with diazepam/ketamine for short duration anesthesia in the horse. *Canadian Veterinary Journal* 37(10): 601–609.

Kimmel HB and Walkenstein SS 1967. Oxazepam excretion by Chlordiazepoxide-^{14}C-dosed dogs. *Journal of Pharmaceutical Sciences* 56(4): 538–539.

Kochansky GE, Salzman C, Shader RI, Harmatz JS and Ogeltree AM 1975. The differential effects of chlordiazepoxide and oxazepam on hostility in a small group setting. *American Journal of Psychiatry* 132(8): 861–863.

Koechlin BA and D'Arconte L 1963. Determination of chlordiazepoxide (Librium) and of a metabolite of lactam character in plasma of humans, dogs, and rats by a specific spectrofluorometric micro method. *Analytical Biochemistry* 5: 195–207.

Koechlin BA, Schwartz MA, Krol G and Oberhansli W 1965. The metabolic fate of C^{14}-labelled chlordiazepoxide in man, in the dog, and in the rat. *The Journal of Pharmacology and Experimental Therapeutics* 148(3): 399–411.

Kumar R, Palit G, Singh JR and Dhawan BN 1999. Comparative behavioural effects of benzodiazepine and non-benzodiazepine anxiolytics in rhesus monkeys. *Pharmacological Research* 39(6): 437–444.

Landsberg G, Hunthausen W and Ackerman L 2003. *Handbook of behavior problems of the dog and cat*, W.B. Saunders.

Lane SB and Bunch SE. 1990. Medical management of recurrent seizures in dogs and cats. *Journal of Veterinary Internal Medicine* 4: 26–39.

Langfeldt T and Ursin H 1971. Differential action of diazepam on flight and defense behavior in the cat. *Psychopharmacologia* (Berlin) 19: 61–66.

Levy JK 1994. Letters to the editor. *Journal of the American Veterinary Medical Association* 205(7): 966.

Levy JK, Cullen JM, Bunch SE, Weston HL, Bristol SM and Elston TH 1994. Adverse reaction to diazepam in cats. *Journal of the American Veterinary Medical Association* 205(2): 156–157.

Löscher W and Frey H-H 1981. Pharmacokinetics of diazepam in the dog. *Archives Internationales de Pharmacodynamie et de Therapie* 254: 180–195.

Marcucci F, Fanelli R, Mussini E and Garattini S 1969. The metabolism of diazepam by liver microsomal enzymes of rats and mice. *European Journal of Pharmacology* 7: 307–313.

Marcucci F, Fanelli R, Mussini E and Garattini S 1970a. Further studies on species difference in diazepam metabolism. *European Journal of Pharmacology* 9: 253–256.

Marcucci F, Mussini E, Fanelli R and Garattini S 1970b. Species differences in diazepam metabolism. I. Metabolism of diazepam metabolites. *Biochemical Pharmacology* 19(5): 1847–1851.

Marcucci F, Guaitani A, Fanelli R, Mussini E and Garattini S 1971. Metabolism and anticonvulsant activity of diazepam in guinea pigs. *Biochemical Pharmacology* 20(7): 1711–1713.

Marder A 1991. Psychotropic drugs and behavioral therapy. In *The veterinary clinics of North America: Small animal practice, advances in companion animal behavior*, pp. 329–342, edited by Marder and Voith, W.B. Saunders, Philadelphia, Pennsylvania.

Marland A, Sarkar P and Leavitt R 1999. The urinary elimination profiles of diazepam and its metabolites, nordiazepam, temazepam, and oxazepam, in the equine after a 10-mg intramuscular dose. *Journal of Analytical Toxicology* 23: 29–34.

Margules DL and Stein L 1968. Increase of "antianxiety" activity and tolerance of behavioral depression during chronic administration of oxazepam. *Psychopharmacologia* (Berlin) 13: 74–80.

Martin WR, Sloan JW and Wala E 1990. Precipitated abstinence in orally dosed benzodiazepine-dependent dogs. *The Journal of Pharmacology and Experimental Therapeutics* 255(1): 744–755.

Matthews NS, Hartsfield SM, Cornick JL, Williams JD and Beasley A 1991. A comparison of injectable anesthetic combinations in horses. *Veterinary Surgery* 20: 268–273.

McDonnell SM 1999. Libido, erection, and ejaculatory dysfunction in stallions. *Compendium on Continuing Education for the Practicing Veterinarian* 21(1): 263–266.

McDonnell SM, Kenney RM, Meckley PE and Garcia MC 1986. Novel environment suppression of stallion sexual behavior and effects of diazepam. *Physiology & Behavior* 37: 503–505.

McDonnell SM, Garcia MC and Kenney RM 1987. Pharmacological manipulation of sexual behaviour in stallions. *Journal of Reproduction and Fertility* (suppl. 35): 45–49.

McNicholas LF, Martin WR and Cherian S 1983. Physical dependence on diazepam and lorazepam in the dog. *The Journal of Pharmacology and Experimental Therapeutics* 226(3): 783–789.

Miczek KA 1974. Intraspecies aggression in rats: effects of d-amphetamine and chlordiazepoxide. *Psychopharmacologia* 39(4): 275–301.

Miczek KA and O'Donnell JM 1980. Alcohol and chlordiazepoxide increase suppressed aggression in mice. *Psychopharmacology* 69: 39–44.

Miczek KA, Weerts EM, Vivian JA and HM Barros 1995. Aggression, anxiety and vocalizations in animals: GAB$_A$ and 5-HT anxiolytics. *Psychopharmacology* 121: 38–56.

Möhler H and Okada T 1977. Benzodiazepine receptor: Demonstration in the central nervous system. *Science* 198: 849–851.

Mos J and Olivier B 1989. Ultrasonic vocalizations by rat pups as an animal model for anxiolytic activity: effects of serotonergic drugs. In *Behavioural pharmacology of 5-HT*, pp. 361–366, edited by P Bevan, AR Cools and T Archer, Lawrence Erlbaum, Hillsdale.

Mos J, Olivier B and Van der Poel AM 1987. Modulatory actions of benzodiazepine receptor ligands on agonistic behaviour. *Physiology and Behavior* 41: 265–278.

Muir WW, Sams RA, Huffman RH, and Noonan BA 1982. Pharmacodynamic and pharmacokinetic properties of diazepam in horses. *American Journal of Veterinary Research* 43(10): 1756–1762.

Mussini E, Marcucci R, Fanelli R and Garattini S 1971. Metabolism of diazepam and its metabolites by guinea pig liver microsomes. *Biochemical Pharmacology* 20(9): 2529–2531.

Norman WM, Court MH and Greenblatt DJ 1997. Age-related changes in the pharmacokinetic disposition of diazepam in foals. *American Journal of Veterinary Research* 58(8): 878–880.

Olivier B, Mos J and Miczek KA 1991. Ethopharmacological studies of anxiolytics and aggression. *European Neuropsychopharmacolgy* 1: 97–100.

Overall K 1994a. Behavior case of the month. *Journal of the American Veterinary Medical Association* 205(5): 694–696.

Overall K 1994b. State of the art: Advances in pharmacological therapy for behavioral disorders. *Proceedings of the North American Veterinary Conference* 8: 43–51.

Overall K 1997. *Clinical behavioral medicine for small animals*, Mosby, St. Louis, Missouri.

Overall K 2004. Paradigms for pharmacologic use as a treatment component in feline behavioral medicine. *Journal of Feline Medicine and Surgery* 6: 29–42.

Pecknold JC, Swinson RP, Kuch K and Lewis CP. 1988. Alprazolam in panic disorder and agoraphobia: Results from a multicenter trial. *Archives of General Psychiatry* 45(5): 429–436.

Pharmacia & Upjohn 1999. Halcion® product information. *2002 Physicians desk reference*, Montvale, New Jersey.

Pharmacia & Upjohn 2001. Xanax® product information. In 2003 *Physicians desk reference*, pp.2794–2798, Montvale, New Jersey.

Plumb DC 2002. *Veterinary drug handbook*. Iowa State University Press, Ames, Iowa.

Randall LO 1960. Pharmacology of methaminodiazepoxide. *Diseases of the nervous system* 21(suppl.): 7–10.

Randall LO. 1961. Pharmacology of chlordiazepoxide (Librium). *Diseases of the Nervous System* 20(suppl.): 7–15.

Randall LO and Kappell B 1973. Pharmacological activity of some benzodiazepines and their metabolites. In *The benzodiazepines*, pp. 27–51, edited by S Garattini, E Mussini and LO Randall, Raven Press, New York.

Randall LO, Schallek W, Heise GA, Keith EF and Bagdon RE 1960. The psychosedative properties of methaminodiazepoxide. *Journal of Pharmacology and Experimental Therapeutics* 129: 163–171.

Randall LO, Scheckel CL and Banziger RF 1965. Pharmacology of the metabolites of chlordiazepoxide and diazepam. *Current Therapeutic Research* 7(9): 590–606.

Reynolds R, Lloyd DA and Slinger RP 1981. Cholestatic jaundice induced by flurazepam hydrochloride. *Canadian Medical Association Journal* 124(7): 893–894.

Rickels K 1983. Clinical trials of hypnotics. *Journal of Clinical Psychopharmacology* 3: 133–139.

Roche Laboratories. 2000. Valium® product information. In *2003 Physicians desk reference*, pp. 2964–2965, Montvale, New Jersey.

Roche Laboratories 2001. Klonopin® product information. In *2003 Physicians desk reference*, pp.2905–2908, Montvale, New Jersey.

Roche Laboratories 1994. Dalmane® product information. In *1998 Physicians desk reference*, pp. 2520–2521, Montvale, New Jersey.

Rodgers RJ and Waters AJ 1985. Benzodiazepines and their antagonists: A pharmacoethological analysis with particular reference to effects on "aggression". *Neuroscience and Biobehavioral Reviews* 9:21–35.

Ruelius HW 1978. Comparative metabolism of lorazepam in man and four animal species. *The Journal of Clinical Psychiatry* 39(10): 11–15.

Ruelius HW, Lee JM and Alburn HE 1965. Metabolism of diazepam in dogs: Transformation to oxazepam. *Archives of Biochemistry and Biophysics* 111: 376–380.

Ryan TP 1985. Feather picking in caged birds. *Modern Veterinary Practice* 66(3): 187–189.

Sahi J, Reyner EL, Bauman J, Gueneva-Boucheva K, Burleigh JE and Thomas VH 2002. The effect of bergamottin on diazepam plasma levels and P450 enzymes in beagle dogs. *Drug Metabolism and Disposition* 30: 135–139.

Salzman C, Kochansky GE, Shader RI, Porrino LJ, Harmatz JS and Swett CP 1974. Chlordiazepoxide-induced hostility in a small group setting. *Archives of General Psychiatry* 31 (3): 401–405.

Sawada H, Hara A, Asano S and Matsumoto Y 1976. Isolation and identification of benzodiazepine drugs and their metabolites in urine by use of amberlite XAD-2 resin and thin-layer chromatography. *Clinical Chemistry* 22(10): 1596–1603.

Scheckel CL and Boff E 1966. Effects of drugs on aggressive behavior in monkeys. *Proceedings of the Fifth International Congress of the Collegium Internationale Neuro-psycho-pharmacologium*. Washington, DC, 28–31 March, 1966.

Scherkl R, Scheuler W and Frey H-H 1985. Anticonvulsant effect of clonazepam in the dog: Development of tolerance and physical dependence. *Archives Internationales de Pharacodynamie et de Therapie* 278(2): 249–260.

Scherschlicht R and Marias J 1983. Effects of oral and intravenous midazolam, triazolam and flunitrazepam on the sleep-wakefulness cycle of rabbits. *British Journal of Clinical Pharmacology* 16: 29S–35S.

Schillings RT, Shrader SR and Ruelius HW 1971. Urinary metabolites of 7-chloro-5-(o-chlorophenyl)-1,3-dihydro-3-hydroxy-2H-1,4-benzodiazepin-2-one (lorazepam) in humans and four animal species. *Arzneimittel Forschung* 21: 1059–1065.

Schillings RT, Sisenwine SF, Schwartz MH and Ruelius HW 1975. Lorazepam: Glucuronide formation in the cat. *Drug Metabolism and Disposition* 3(2): 85–88.

Schwartz MA, Koechlin BA, Postma E, Palmer S and Krol G 1965. Metabolism of diazepam in rat, dog, and man. *The Journal of Pharmacology and Experimental Therapeutics* 149(3): 423–435.

Schwartz MA and Postma E 1966. Metabolic N-demethylation of chlordiazepoxide. *Journal of Pharmaceutical Sciences* 55(12): 1358–1362.

Schwartz MA and Postma E 1970. Metabolism of flurazepam, a benzodiazepine, in man and dog. *Journal of Pharmaceutical Sciences* 59(12): 1800–1806.

Schwartz MA, Postma E and Kolis SJ 1971. Metabolism of demoxepam, a chlordiazepoxide metabolite, in the dog. *Journal of Pharmaceutical Sciences* 60(3): 438–444.

Shini S, Klaus AM and Hapke HJ 1997. Eliminationskinetik von diazepam nach intravenöser applikation beim Pferd (Kinetics of elimination of diazepam after intravenous injection in horses. *Deutsche tierärztliche Wochenschrift* 104(1): 22–25.

Simpson BS 2002. Psychopharmacology primer. *Proceedings of the North American Veterinary Conference*, pp. 73–74, 3.

Simpson BS and Simpson DM 1996. Behavioral pharmacotherapy II. Anxiolytics and mood stabilizers. *Compendium on Continuing Education for the Practicing Veterinarian* 18(11): 1203–1213.

Sisenwine SF, Tio CO, Shrader SR and Ruelius HW 1972. The biotransformation of oxazepam (7-chloro-1,3-dihydro-3-hydroxy-5-phenyl-2H-1,4-benzodiazepin-2-one) in man, miniature swine and rat. *Arzneimittel Forschung (Drug research)* 22(4): 682–687.

Sloan JW, Martin WR and Wala EP 1990. Dependence-producing properties of alprazolam in the dog. *Pharmacology Biochemistry & Behavior* 35: 651–657.

Sloan JW, Martin WR and Wala E 1993. Effect of the chronic dose of diazepam on the intensity and characteristics of the precipitated abstinence syndrome in the dog. *The Journal of Pharmacology and Experimental Therapeutics* 265(3): 1152–1162.

Sloan JW, Martin WR, Wala E and Dickey KM 1991. Chronic administration of and dependence on halazepam, diazepam, and nordiazepam in the dog. *Drug and Alcohol Dependence* 28: 249–264.

Sofia RD 1969. Effects of centrally active drugs on four models of experimentally-induced aggression in rodents. *Life Sciences* 8(1): 705–716.

Stein L and Berger BD 1971. Psychopharmacology of 7-chloro-5-(—chlorophenyl)-1,3-dihydro-3-hydroxy-2H-1,4-benzodiazepin-2-one (Lorazepam) in squirrel monkey and rat. *Arzneimittel Forschung (Drug Research)* 21(7): 1075–1078.

Sternbach Leo H 1973. Chemistry of 1,4-benzodiazepines and some aspects of the structure-activity relationship. In *The benzodiazepines*, pp. 1–26, edited by S Garattini, E Mussini and LO Randall, Raven Press, New York.

Thiébot M-H, Le Bihan C, Soubiré P and Simon P 1985. Benzodiazepines reduce the tolerance to reward delay in rats. *Psychopharmacology* 81(1–2): 147–152.

Tornatzky W and Miczek KA 1995. Alcohol, anxiolytics and social stress in rats. *Psychopharmacology* 121: 135–144.

Troupin AS, Friel P, Wilensky AJ, Morettiojemann L, Levy RH and Feigl P 1979. Evaluation of clorazepate (tranxene) as an anticonvulsant—a pilot study. *Neurology* 29:458–466.

Löcher W and Frey HH 1981. Pharmacokinetics of diazepam in the dog. *Archives Internationales de Pharmacodynamie et de Therapie.* 254: 180–195.

Vachon L, Kitsikis A and Roberge AG 1984. Chlordiazepoxide, Go-Nogo successive discrimination and brain biogenic amines in cats. *Pharmacology Biochemistry and Behavior* 20: 9–22.

Valzelli L, Giacalone E and Garattini S. 1967. Pharmacological control of aggressive behavior in mice. *European Journal of Pharmacology* 2: 144–146.

Vree TB, Baars AM, Hekster YA, van der Kleijn E and O'Reilly WJ 1979. Simultaneous determination of diazepam and its metabolites N-desmethyldiazepam, oxydiazepam and oxazepam in plasma and urine of man and dog by means of high-performance liquid chromatography. *Journal of Chromatography* 162: 605–614.

Wala EP, Martin WR and Sloan JW 1995. Brain-plasma distribution of free and total benzodiazepines in dogs physically dependent on different doses of diazepam. *Pharmacology Biochemistry and Behavior* 52(4): 707–713.

Walkenstein SS, Wiser R, Gudmundsen CH, Kimmel HB and Corradino RA 1964. Absorption, metabolism, and excretion of oxazepam and its succinate half-ester. *Journal of Pharmaceutical Sciences* 53(10): 1181–1186.

Wilensky AJ, Levy RH, Troupin AS, Moretti-Ojemann L and Friel P 1978. Clorazepate kinetics in treated epileptics. *Clinical Pharmacology and Therapeutics* 24: 22–30.

Wismer TA 2002. Accidental ingestion of alprazolam in 415 dogs. *Veterinary and Human Toxicology* 44: 22–23.

Wyeth Laboratories Inc. 1999a. Serax product information. In *1999 Physicians desk reference*, pp. 3383–3384, Montvale, New Jersey.

Wyeth Laboratories Inc. 1999b. Ativan product information. In *2002 Physicians desk reference*, pp. 3482–3483, Montvale, New Jersey.

Zbinden G and Randall LO 1967. Pharmacology of benzodiazepines: Laboratory and clinical correlations. *Advances in Pharmacology* 5: 213–291.

Chapter Four
Biogenic Amine Neurotransmitters: Serotonin

Introduction

Psychopharmacology had its beginnings as recently as the early 1950s, but it has since has grown rapidly into one of the major areas of pharmacology and psychiatry. Before the advent of these psychoactive drugs, various central nervous system (CNS) agents, such as the narcotics, barbiturates, and stimulants, were known, but none of these represented important psychotherapeutic agents; the psychiatrist had an extremely limited chemotherapeutic armamentarium. The initial breakthrough came when the drugs chlorpromazine and reserpine proved to be effective antipsychotic and antischizophrenic agents.

Soon after the development of the antipsychotic (or neuroleptic) drugs, the antidepressant action of iproniazid was discovered, and this therapeutic effect became correlated with inhibition of monoamine oxidase (MAO) and a consequent rise in brain biogenic amines. A great deal of research has been carried out on a diverse array of psychoactive drugs in an attempt to understand the nature of their action. From all of this research one striking common denominator emerges, namely, that many of these agents appear to involve in some way the biogenic amines found in the CNS. Almost all of the psychoactive drugs, ranging from lysergic acid diethylamide (LSD) and other hallucinogens to the antipsychotics and antidepressants, as well as other centrally acting agents, such as medetomidine, clomipramine, and L-deprenyl, are now associated with biogenic amine mechanisms.

The Biogenic Amines

The term *biogenic amines*, as used in psychopharmacology, includes the two catecholamines, dopamine (DA) and norepinephrine (NE), and the indoleamine, 5-hydroxytryptamine (5-HT, serotonin), the structures of which are indicated in Figure 4.1. Norepinephrine has been known for many years as the transmitter in peripheral sympathetic neurons, and much is now known regarding its biosynthesis, storage, uptake, release, and degradation mechanisms. Serotonin has also been extensively investigated; and while its distribution is less ubiquitous, it also regulates critical functions in the CNS. Dopamine, which until the early 1960s was considered primarily as a precursor of NE, is now established as a CNS transmitter in its own right. Its presence in the neostriatum and limbic system in high concentrations initially led to speculation of its possible role in CNS function. These observations and other related studies have demonstrated that degeneration of DA neurons is involved in Parkinson's disease. In

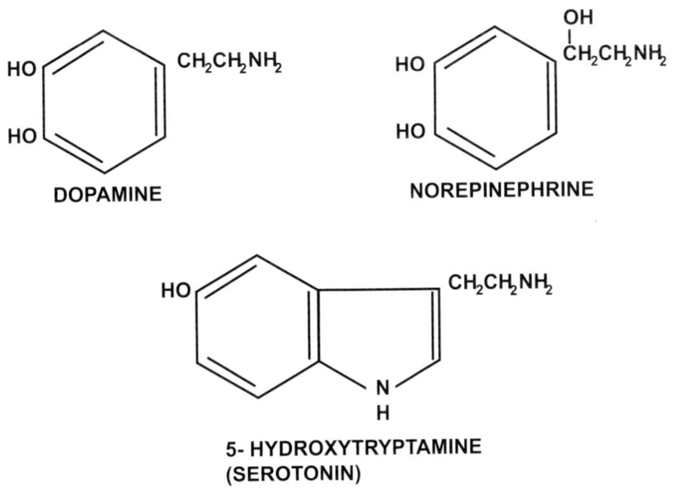

Figure 4.1 Structures of biogenic amine (catecholamine and indoleamine) neurotransmitters dopamine, norepinephrine, and serotonin.

fact, the use of its precursor, L-DOPA, in the treatment of this disease is based on that concept. The development of histochemical fluorescence techniques for the visualization of the biogenic amines within the nerve cell bodies and terminals has permitted the mapping of the biogenic amine pathways throughout the various parts of the CNS. From such investigations it is now known that NE and 5-HT neurons, whose cell bodies are found largely in the locus coeruleus and midbrain raphe, respectively, terminate more or less in the same regions of the CNS. DA cell bodies originate largely in the substantia nigra, the ventral tegmental area, and in the arcuate nucleus of the hypothalamus, and their neurons terminate in the neostriatum, the limbic structures, and the median eminence and pituitary, respectively.

Serotonin

Serotonin was first chemically identified in the 1940s, although its existence in the gastrointestinal tract was previously known. Its presence in blood serum and platelets, and the fact that it exerted vasoconstrictor activity, led to the derivation of the name *serotonin*. It was, however, only its discovery in mammalian brain that initiated the extensive neurochemical and pharmacologic investigations that have led to our current understanding of serotonin as a central neurotransmitter.

Early interest in serotonin functions in the brain intensified with the recognition that many hallucinogenic drugs (LSD) were structurally related to the serotonin molecule. Because these hallucinogens act like serotonin, it was postulated that the hallucinogenic activity of LSD is related to its serotonergic agonist activity. Thus, the compound bufotenin, or *N,N*-dimethylserotonin, a very close analog of serotonin, is a potent hallucinogen when administered centrally. Several other compounds, such as the substances psilocybin and psilocin, the indoleamines found in the "magic" mushrooms of Mexico, and other drugs of abuse, such as the dimethyl- and diethyl- analogs of tryptamine, have the basic indole ethylamine structure. The final mechanism of hallucinogenic activity of these compounds has yet to be determined, but a serotonin-like action on specific subtypes of serotonin receptors is likely involved.

Inasmuch as serotonin is found in many cells that are not neurons, only about 1–2% of the whole body serotonin content is found in the brain. Serotonergic neurons synthesize this transmitter beginning with the conversion of dietary tryptophan to 5-hydroxytryptophan. Plasma tryptophan varies as a function of diet, and elimination of dietary tryptophan can dramatically lower levels of serotonin in the brain. Following the production of 5-hydroxytryptophan by hydroxylation of tryptophan in serotonergic neurons, the 5-hydroxytryptophan is rapidly decarboxylated to produce serotonin (5-hydroxytryptamine). The serotonin precursor, 5-hydroxytryptophan, is sold as an over-the-counter dietary supplement (sometimes termed Griffonia seed extract) for its claimed ability to treat conditions such as depression, headaches, obesity, and insomnia in humans. The oral administration of 5-hydroxytryptophan results in rapid absorption from the gastrointestinal tract and, in turn, readily crosses the blood–brain barrier (Gwaltney-Brant et al. 2000). This 5-hydroxytryptophan can be rapidly converted to serotonin in the brain and spinal cord. Excessive stimulation of serotonin receptors due to dramatic elevations of 5-HT causes a "serotonin syndrome" that may be associated with muscle rigidity, myoclonus, salivation, agitation, and hyperthermia in animals and humans. The most common cause of this syndrome is an interaction between a monoamine oxidase inhibitor and a selective serotonin reuptake inhibitor. The accidental ingestion of 5-hydroxytryptophan by dogs, however, has recently been documented to result in a life-threatening syndrome resembling a serotonin syndrome (Gwaltney-Brant et al. 2000). A review of 21 cases of accidental 5-hydroxytryptophan by dogs indicated that ingestion of a single 500-mg capsule of these dietary supplements would be sufficient to produce adverse sequelae in dogs.

In the mammalian brain serotonergic neurons are localized to clusters of cell bodies of the pons and brain stem termed the *raphe nuclei* (Figure 4.2). These groups of 5-HT neurons project in both ascending and descending pathways to the forebrain and spinal cord, respectively. Forebrain structures receiving 5-HT innervation include the cerebral cortex, striatum, and hippocampus. These ascending projections to the cerebral cortex and limbic regions emanate from rostral raphe nuclei axons, while the caudal raphe nuclei in the brain stem give rise to the descending projections terminating in the medulla and spinal cord.

Serotonergic terminals are the sites of vesicular release of the transmitter at synapses in the projection field (e.g., cerebral cortex, limbic structures). Following the release of 5-HT in the synapse, the action of the transmitter is terminated through a high-affinity reuptake into the presynaptic terminal. This reuptake is mediated by specific transporter proteins that have evolved to recognize and transport serotonin. These serotonin transporters are members of a gene family of Na^+- and Cl^--dependent transport proteins. The serotonin transporters are expressed in the brain in presynaptic and somatodendritic membranes of serotonin neurons. These 5-HT transporters also exist in other tissues such as platelets, placenta, and lung. Given the critical role of serotonin transporters in the regulation of the synaptic actions of 5-HT, they have been an important target for drug development. As a consequence, a number of 5-HT reuptake blockers have been developed, such as fluoxetine, sertraline, paroxetine, and clomipramine for use in the treatment of depression, anxiety, panic attack, and

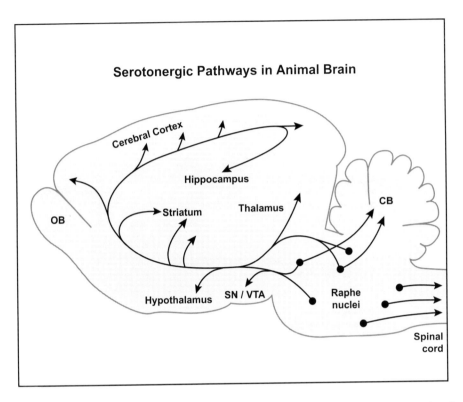

Figure 4.2 Schematic diagram of the serotonergic pathways in animal brain. Serotonergic cell bodies are localized to clusters of cells in the pons and rostral brain stem referred to as the Raphe nuclei. CB, cerebellum; OB, olfactory bulb; SN, substantia nigra; VTA, ventral tegmental area.

obsessive-compulsive disorder (OCD) in humans. Clomipramine has been approved for the treatment of separation anxiety in dogs. These reuptake inhibitors act as indirect serotoninmimetics by increasing the half-life of serotonin in the synapse resulting in prolonged activation of multiple serotonin receptor subtypes. The localization of the serotonin transporter (SERT) on the presynaptic terminal of serotonergic neurons is depicted in Figure 4.3.

The function of serotonin is exerted upon its interaction with specific receptors. Presently, 14 distinct 5-HT receptor subtypes have been identified, and all can be found postsynaptically in various brain areas. All 5-HT receptors except the 5-HT$_3$ receptor are G protein-coupled receptors. Those serotonin receptors that have been cloned include the 5-HT$_1$, 5-HT$_2$, 5-HT$_3$, 5-HT$_4$, 5-HT$_5$, 5-HT$_6$, and 5-HT$_7$ types. Within the 5-HT$_1$ group there are subtypes: 5-HT$_{1A}$, 5-HT$_{1B}$, 5-HT$_{1D}$, 5-HT$_{1E}$, and 5-HT$_{1F}$. There are three 5-HT$_2$ subtypes, 5-HT$_{2A}$, 5-HT$_{2B}$, and 5-HT$_{2C}$, as well as two 5-HT$_5$ subtypes, 5-HT$_{5A}$ and 5-HT$_{5B}$. Most of these receptors are coupled to G proteins that affect the activities of either adenylate cyclase or phospholipase Cγ. The 5-HT$_3$ class of receptors are ion channels. Some serotonin receptors are presynaptic and others postsynaptic. The 5-HT$_{2A}$ receptors mediate platelet aggregation and smooth muscle contractions. The 5-HT$_{2C}$ receptors are suspected in control of food intake because mice lacking this gene become obese from increased food intake and are also

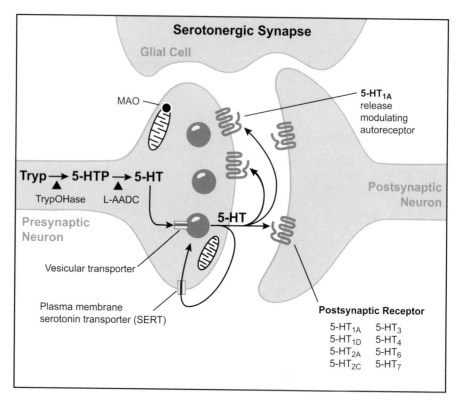

Figure 4.3 Schematic representation of a serotonergic synapse. Tryptophan is the dietary precursor for 5-HT synthesis and is converted to 5-hydroxytryptophan (5-HTP) by the enzyme tryptophan hydroxylase (TrypOHase). The 5-HTP is converted to 5-HT by the enzyme L-aromatic amino acid decarboxylase (L-AADC). The 5-HT is stored in and released from vesicles, and synaptic 5-HT activates both pre- and postsynaptic receptors. Synaptic 5-HT action is terminated by the reuptake of the transmitter into the presynaptic terminal. This reuptake is mediated by the plasma membrane SERT. Cytoplasmic 5-HT can be degraded by the mitochondrial enzyme MAO.

subject to lethal seizures. The 5-HT$_3$ receptors are present in the gastrointestinal tract and chemoreceptor trigger zone in area postrema and are related to vomiting. Also present in the gastrointestinal tract are 5-HT$_4$ receptors that function in secretion and peristalsis. The 5-HT$_6$ and 5-HT$_7$ receptors are distributed throughout the limbic system in the brain, and 5-HT$_6$ receptors are unique in that they display high affinity for both typical (chlorpromazine) and atypical (clozapine) antipsychotic drugs.

Serotonergic drugs such as fenfluramine have a different mechanism of action from the reuptake inhibitors; fenfluramine interacts with the 5-HT transporter to promote the release of serotonin via reverse transport through SERT. Fenfluramine is also a direct acting agonist at 5-HT$_{2B}$ receptors. Until recently, fenfluramine was used in human medicine as an anorectic agent in combination with phenteramine (Fen-Phen). An association between fenfluramine use and valvular heart disease and pulmonary hypertension, however, led to the removal of this preparation from the market. The 5-HT$_{2B}$ receptor is enriched in human cardiac valves and appears to be the target for fenfluramine-induced cardiac valve abnormalities.

Serotonergic neurons possess two functional types of autoreceptors. One autoreceptor is the 5-HT_{1B} receptor that is expressed primarily on serotonergic neuron terminals and functions as a regulator of 5-HT release. Activation of the 5-HT_{1B} receptor inhibits serotonin release from axon terminals and therefore functions as a local negative feedback regulator of serotonin levels in the synapse. These 5-HT_{1B} autoreceptors have been suggested to play a role in depression, anxiety states, aggression, migraine, and locomotor activity. Serotonergic involvement in aggression was indicated in studies with transgenic mice lacking the 5-HT_{1B} receptor; these 5-HT_{1B} knockout mice are more aggressive than the normal 5-HT_{1B} receptor-expressing mice (Sari 2004). A second functional autoreceptor is the 5-HT_{1A} receptor that is found on serotonergic cell bodies and dendrites (somatodendritic), as well as on postsynaptic neurons receiving input from 5-HT pathways (Figure 4.4). Activation of 5-HT_{1A} somatodendritic autoreceptors inhibits 5-HT neuron firing, 5-HT synthesis, and 5-HT release from axon terminals. Direct application of 5-HT onto 5-HT neurons in the dorsal raphe produces an inhibitory effect on serotonergic neuron-firing activity. The 5-HT_{1A} autoreceptors on the cell bodies of serotonergic neurons in the raphe nuclei presumably respond to extracellular 5-HT released from soma and dendrites of these neurons. These 5-HT autoreceptors function in the feedback inhibition of raphe neurons to maintain a regular firing pattern of serotonin neurons.

One of the primary postulated mechanisms of action of selective serotonin reuptake inhibitors (SSRI) is the desensitization of somatodendritic 5-HT_{1A} autoreceptors after chronic administration. This 5-HT_{1A} receptor desensitization after chronic SSRI administration leads to an enhancement of 5-HT synaptic transmission in the terminal field due to increased 5-HT neuronal firing (Blier et al. 1998). The temporal pattern of SSRI-induced desensitization of 5-HT_{1A} receptors parallels the delayed onset of action of the relief of depressive symptomatology in humans that takes two to three weeks to fully manifest. The desensitization of somatodendritics 5-HT_{1A} autoreceptors allows 5-HT neuron-firing rates to increase in forebrain terminal fields where 5-HT_{1A} postsynaptic receptors do not desensitize and may be involved in the therapeutic response to SSRIs (Blier et al. 1998). Recent studies in animals have shown that the somatodendritic 5-HT_{1A} receptor desensitization may be related to the ability of SSRIs to trigger the internalization of these receptors into cytoplasmic compartments (Riad et al. 2004).

A role for limbic serotonergic neurotransmission being involved in anxiety-related behavioral traits has recently emerged from human studies of genetic differences in serotonin transporter function. These studies demonstrated that 5-HT transporter gene polymorphism was associated with SERT functional differences and increased amygdala response to fearful stimuli (Hariri et al. 2002). The link between serotonergic neurotransmission and affective disorders was further established through studies of gene–environment interaction. Individuals with a particular allele of the 5-HT transporter gene appeared to be more vulnerable to stressful events in that they were more likely to become clinically depressed (Caspi et al. 2003). These important studies indicate that rather than cause disease, genes may interact with the environment to control susceptibility to affective disorders such as depression.

Serotonin pathways have also been shown to be involved in obsessive-compulsive disorder (OCD). Clomipramine, a tricyclic antidepressant with some selectivity for the serotonin transporter, was first shown to have efficacy in the treatment of OCD in 1980.

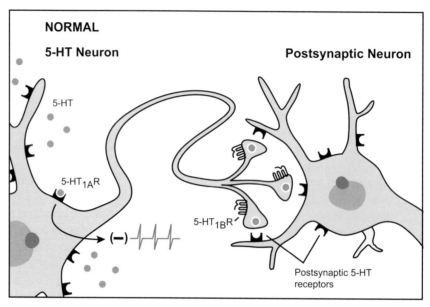

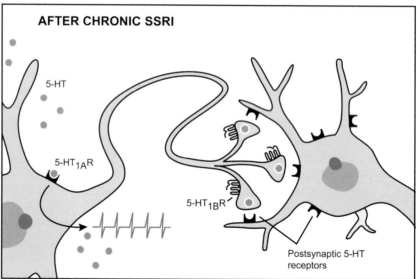

Figure 4.4 Diagram depicting the regulation of the firing activity of 5-HT neurons by 5-HT_{1A} autoreceptors localized on soma and dendrites (somatodendritic). Endogenous 5-HT released from dendrites of serotonergic neurons activates 5-HT_{1A} autoreceptors and decreases neuronal firing activity. After chronic treatment with an SSRI, the 5-HT_{1A} autoreceptors desensitize, and firing activity is restored or enhanced in the presence of the SSRI. This adaptive change in 5-HT neuronal control may be obligatory for an antidepressant response to manifest.

In the 1990s this clinical effectiveness was extended to SSRIs, such as fluoxetine, sertraline, and paroxetine. The therapeutic response of clomipramine and SSRIs in treating OCD in humans and acral lick dermatitis in dogs may be mediated by increased activation of 5-HT_{2C} receptors through elevated synaptic levels of serotonin in forebrain structures such as the orbitofrontal cerebral cortex. The efficacy of SSRIs in treating OCD to some extent generalizes to 5-HT$_{1A}$ receptor agonists; these direct activators of a serotonin receptor represent a group of structurally related compounds, the aza-pirones, best exemplified by buspirone. The azapirones possess significant affinity and selectivity for 5-HT$_{1A}$ receptors, where they exert partial agonist activity. Acute treatment with buspirone produces a transient reduction in the firing rate of 5-HT neurons similar to that seen initially with SSRIs. This response is presumed to reflect the consequences of direct activation of 5-HT$_{1A}$ somatodendritic autoreceptors by buspirone. Chronic administration with azapirones does, however, lead to a gradual increase in 5-HT neuron firing due to the progressive desensitization of 5-HT$_{1A}$ autoreceptors. In addition to the activation of 5-HT$_{1A}$ autoreceptors, buspirone acts as a partial agonist at postsynaptic 5-HT$_{1A}$ receptors in forebrain structures. This pharmacologic profile for azapirones differs from that of SSRIs, tricyclic antidepressants, and monoamine oxidase inhibitors (MAOI) in that these latter drug classes produce an indiscriminate activation of all serotonin receptor subtypes (Blier and Ward 2003). This generalized activation of multiple 5-HT receptor subtypes is consequently associated with a number of adverse effects of SSRIs, MAOIs, and tricyclics, such as nausea, vomiting, sleep disturbance, and sexual dysfunction. The most common side effects of azapirones are limited to headache, dizziness, and nausea. Buspirone and other azapirone agonists are also used in the treatment of generalized anxiety disorder, where they produce less sedation, psychomotor disruption, and cognitive impairment than benzodiazepines. Although in clinical trials buspirone is typically shown to be efficacious in treating anxiety, the patient's response is more delayed than with benzodiazepines; this most likely reflects the requirement for 5-HT$_{1A}$ autoreceptor desensitization to achieve the therapeutic response. The azapirones are therefore an alternative to either SSRIs or benzodiazepines for the treatment of specific behavioral disorders in companion animals.

References

Blier P and Ward NM 2003. Is there a role for 5-HT$_{1A}$ agonists in the treatment of depression? *Biological Psychiatry* 53: 193–203.

Blier P, Pi–eyro G, El Mansari M, Bergeron R and DeMontigny C 1998. Role of somatodendritic 5-HT autoreceptors in modulating 5-HT neurotransmission. *Annals of the New York Academy of Science* 861: 204–216.

Caspi A, Sugden K, Moffitt TE, Tayor A, Craig IW, Harrington H, McClay J, Mill J, Martin J, Braithwaite A and Poulton R 2003. Influence of life stress on depression: moderation by a polymorphism in the 5-HTT gene. *Science* (301): 291–293; 386–389.

Gwaltney-Brant SM, Albretson JC and Khan SA 2000. 5-Hydroxytryptophan toxicosis in dogs: 21 cases (1989–1999). *Journal of the American Veterinary Association* 216: 1937–1940.

Hariri AR, Mattay VS, Tessitore A, Kolachana B, Francesco F, Goldman D, Egan MF and Weinberger DR 2002. Serotonin transporter genetic variation and the response of the human amygdala. *Science* 297: 400–403.

Riad M, Zimmer L, Rbah L, Watkins KC, Hamon M and Descarries L 2004. *Journal of Neuroscience* 24(23): 5420–5426.

Sari Y 2004. Serotonin$_{1B}$ receptors: from protein to physiological function and behavior. *Neuroscience and Biobehavioral Reviews* 28: 565–582.

Chapter Five
Selective Serotonin Reuptake Inhibitors

Action

The selective serotonin reuptake inhibitors (SSRIs) are a class of antidepressant that inhibit the reuptake of serotonin. This results in an increase in serotonergic neurotransmission by allowing serotonin molecules to act for extended periods of time. With prolonged use, there is also down-regulation of serotonin receptors.

Overview of Indications

The SSRIs are classified as antidepressants; however, they have anxiolytic, anticompulsive, and some antiaggressive effects (e.g., Kavoussi et al. 1994; Charney et al. 1990; Coccaro et al. 1990; Sanchez and Hyttel 1994; Stein and Stahl 2000; Walsh and Dinan 2001). It is primarily for these reasons that they are used in veterinary medicine. The onset of all effects is usually slow, and clients of pets that are put on any SSRIs must be informed of this so that they do not have unrealistic expectations. While some response may be observed within a few days of initiation of treatment, improvement commonly does not occur for three to four weeks, or even longer. Thus, if an SSRI is recommended, caution the client that the pet's response to the medication will not be evaluated until it has been on medication daily for at least one month. SSRIs should never be given on an "as needed" basis, because they will generally be ineffective if used this way. They can be used in cases of specific anxieties, such as agoraphobia or storm phobia, and are particularly useful in cases of anxiety that occurs pervasively and frequently, as in the case of generalized anxiety disorder (e.g., Gorman 2002). Pets with generalized anxiety disorder exhibit an almost constant state of low-level anxiety, regardless of their current environment, and are hyperreactive to a variety of fear-inducing environmental stimuli.

Fluoxetine has been used in the treatment of behavior problems in domestic animals more commonly than any other SSRI. As a consequence, there is more information about safety, side effects, and efficacy in various species for this medication than any other. Following fluoxetine, paroxetine (Paxil), and sertraline (Zoloft) have been used the most and are mentioned in various textbooks, even though there is a lack of clinical trials on their use for treatment of animal behavior problems.

Common uses in domestic animals include anxiety, affective aggression, compulsive disorder, and urine marking. They can potentially be used for predatory aggression. However, medication should never be considered a substitute for adequate restraint for patients with this or any other problem of aggression. As discussed in Chapter 1, serotonin is involved in the control of aggression. Reisner et al. (1996)

measured CSF levels of 5-hydroxyindole acetic acid (5-HIAA) in 21 dogs with a diagnosis of dominance aggression and 19 control dogs. The dogs with dominance aggression had significantly lower concentrations of cerebrospinal fluid (CSF) 5-HIAA
than did the 19 controls (Reisner et al. 1996). When used in the treatment of compulsive disorder, response to serotonin reuptake inhibitor (SRIs) varies with the specific
signs of the disorder and the duration of the problem.

All SSRIs are metabolized in the liver and excreted through the kidneys. Therefore,
premedication blood work to assess the function of these organs is recommended.

Contraindications, Side Effects, and Adverse Events

Side effects observed in various species include sedation, tremor, constipation, diarrhea, nausea, anxiety, irritability, agitation, insomnia, decreased appetite, anorexia, aggression, mania, decreased libido, hyponatremia, and seizures. Mild sedation and decreased appetite are the most common side effects observed by the author in dogs. Both
are typically transient. If the appetite decrease is sufficient to cause concern about adequate food intake, temporarily increasing the palatability of the diet and/or hand feeding is usually sufficient to induce adequate food consumption until this phase passes.

Serotonin syndrome is a phenomenon reported in humans. It is a consequence of
taking excessive quantities of medications that increase serotonin levels and/or taking
certain medications that are incompatible with SRIs at the same time as SRIs. Signs
and symptoms can be grossly grouped into mental changes, neuromuscular changes
and autonomic changes. Treatment should include decontamination, anticonvulsants,
thermoregulation, and fluid therapy (Mills 1995; Martin 1996; Brown et al. 1996).
This phenomenon is discussed in further detail in chapter 15, Combinations.

When mothers are given various SRIs (fluoxetine, sertraline, paroxetine or one of
the previous with clonazepam), the neonatal acute pain response is decreased and
parasympathetic cardiac modulation during the recovery period is increased (Oberlander et al. 2002).

Adverse Drug Interactions

SSRIs are competitive inhibitors of a number of cytochrome P450 liver enzymes.
Therefore, if a patient is placed on an SSRI and another medication that is metabolized by the P450 liver enzymes, elevated plasma levels may develop in the medications, potentially resulting in toxic side effects (Albers et al. 2002). To date, there is
minimal data on variation between breeds and species in the P450 enzymes as it re-
lates to metabolism of various psychoactive drugs. Therefore, findings in humans
must be substantially relied upon for the time being. Since there is substantial variation, even within the human population, it is expected that further studies will also reveal substantial variation in veterinary populations (DeVane 1994).

The following are of special note. All of the SSRIs can increase levels of warfarin
due to P450 interactions and due to competition for plasma protein binding sites.
Fluoxetine and fluvoxamine are the strongest inhibitors of CYP1A2 and CYP2C9,
P450 enzymes that metabolize warfarin (Albers et al. 2002).

Fluoxetine, fluvoxamine, sertraline, and paroxetine cause significant inhibition of CYP2D6, which metabolizes amitriptyline, amphetamine, clomipramine, desipramine, haloperidol, imipramine, and nortriptyline (Crewe et al. 1992; Albers et al. 2002).

Fluvoxamine causes the greatest degree of inhibition of CYP3A4, which metabolizes alprazolam, buspirone, clomipramine, clonazepam, and imipramine (Albers et al. 2002).

Fluoxetine and fluvoxamine cause the greatest degree of inhibition of CYP2C19, which metabolizes amitriptyline, clomipramine, diazepam, imipramine, and propranolol (Albers et al. 2002).

Fluvoxamine causes the greatest degree of inhibition of CYP1A2, which metabolizes amitriptyline, caffeine, clomipramine, clozapine, haloperidol, imipramine, and olanzapine, in addition to warfarin (Brøsen et al. 1993; Albers et al. 2002).

In addition, SSRIs should not be given with monoamine oxidase inhibitors (MAOIs), because fatal drug interactions can occur.

Overdose

In case of overdose, conduct gastric lavage, give activated charcoal, give anticonvulsants as needed, and provide supportive therapy.

Clinical Guidelines

SSRIs should generally be given once a day. If large doses are required for efficacy, the total daily dose can be divided to minimize side effects. SSRIs should not be given on a sporadic, as-needed basis. While some response may be observed in a few days, it may require three to four weeks before a response occurs. Efficacy of a given SSRI on a given patient should not be evaluated until the patient has been on medication daily for a full month. If, at one month, some degree of improvement is observed, the medication should be continued at the same dose, or at a higher dose if improvement has been only slight.

SSRIs may alter blood glucose levels. Therefore, while they can be used with diabetic patients, they should be used with caution, and blood glucose levels should be monitored closely. Decreased doses should be used in patients with mild dysfunction of the liver or kidneys. SSRIs should not be used at all in patients with severe dysfunction of the liver or kidneys. There is no relationship between plasma levels of SSRIs and clinical response. Therefore, measuring plasma levels will not be useful (Albers et al. 2002). Animal doses and some cost comparisons are given in Tables 5.1, 5.2, and 5.3.

Specific Medications

I. Citalopram Hydrobromide

Chemical Compound: (±)-1-(3-Dimethylaminopropyl)-1-(4-fluorophenyl)-1,3 dihydroisobenzofuran-5-carbonitrile

DEA Classification: Not a controlled substance

Table 5.1 Doses of various SSRIs for dogs, cats, horses, and parrots

SSRI	Dog	Cat	Parrot	Horse
Citalopram	0.5–1.0 mg/kg			
Fluoxetine	1.0–2.0 mg/kg	0.5–1.5 mg/kg	2.0–5.0 mg/kg	0.25–0.5 mg/kg
Fluvoxamine	1–2 mg/kg	0.25–0.5 mg/kg		
Paroxetine	1.0–1.5 mg/kg	0.5–1.5 mg/kg	2.0 mg/kg q12h	0.5 mg/kg
Sertraline	0.5–4.0 mg/kg	0.5–1.5 mg/kg		

Note: All doses given are orally, once daily, unless otherwise specified. Do not evaluate efficacy until the patient has received the medication daily for at least one full month.

Preparations: Generally available as 10-, 20-, and 40-mg tablets and as a 2-mg/ml peppermint-flavored oral solution

Clinical Pharmacology

Citalopram is a strong inhibitor of serotonin reuptake and has little effect on reuptake of dopamine or norepinephrine. Of the currently available SSRIs, it appears to be the most selective inhibitor of 5-hydroxytryptamine (5-HT) uptake (Pollock 2001). It has very little to no effect on the $5-HT_{1A}$, $5-HT_{2A}$, dopamine D_1 and D_2, α_1, α_2 and β-adrenergic, histamine H_1, γ-aminobutyric acid (GABA), muscarinic cholinergic, and benzodiazepine receptors.

Citalopram is metabolized to demethylcitalopram (DCT), di-demethylcitalopram (DDCT), citalopram-*N*-oxide, and a deaminated propionic acid. At steady state, while the parent compound, citalopram, is the predominant component, DCT and DDCT occur in significant amounts. Citalopram is more effective than its metabolites in preventing serotonin reuptake. Dogs appear to convert more citalopram to metabolites than do humans. Specifically, in dogs, peak DDCT concentrations are approximately equal to peak citalopram concentrations, whereas in humans, steady-state peak DDCT plasma concentrations are less than 10% of citalopram concentrations (Forest Laboratories, Inc. 2002).

In humans, when a single oral dose is given peak blood levels are reached in two to four hours (Pollock 2001). When it is given daily, steady-state plasma concentrations are reached in about 7 days (Forest Laboratories, Inc. 2002). The half-life in humans is about 1.5 days, while the half-life of demethylcitalopram is 2 days and DDCT, 4 days (Pollock 2001).

Citalopram is metabolized by CYP2C19, CYP3A4, and CYP2D6 (Pollock 2001; Forest Laboratories, Inc. 2002). Since citalopram is metabolized by multiple enzyme systems, it is not expected that concurrent medication with drugs that affect only one of these systems would cause clinically significant effects.

In geriatric populations and individuals with reduced hepatic or renal function citalopram clearance time is slower than for younger populations without reduced hepatic or renal function. Citalopram doses should be reduced in these populations (Forest Laboratories, Inc. 2002).

Uses in Humans

Citalopram is used to treat depression. Citalopram has also been shown to be significantly more effective than placebo in treating impulsive aggressive behavior in humans (Reist et al. 2003).

Contraindications

Citalopram is contraindicated in patients taking MAOIs. MAOIs should be discontinued for at least two weeks before beginning treatment with citalopram. Likewise, citalopram should be discontinued for at least two weeks before beginning an MAOI.

Side Effects

In a small number of patients, treatment with citalopram can result in anxiety, changes in appetite, vomiting, diarrhea, changes in urinary frequency, insomnia, sedation, excitement, seizures, hyponatremia, abnormal bleeding, mydriasis, and various other side effects unique to individuals, including anaphylaxis.

In studies of carcinogenesis, mice were given up to 240 mg/kg/day of citalopram for 18 months, and rats were given up to 24 mg/kg/day for 24 months. No increased carcinogenesis occurred in the mice. Rats exhibited an increased incidence of small intestine carcinoma. Albino rats given 80 mg/kg/day for two years exhibited degeneration and atrophy of the retinas. Retinal degeneration did not occur in rats given 24 mg/kg/day, mice treated at doses of up to 240 mg/kg/day for 18 months, or dogs treated for a year with doses of up to 20 mg/kg/day. These doses are greater than what would be used therapeutically in mice and rats. The implication of these findings for other domestic species is not known.

Citalopram has been mutagenic in some bacterial assays. It has not been found to be mutagenic in mammalian assays, however (Forest Laboratories, Inc. 2002).

Citalopram at doses of 16–72 mg/kg/day decreased mating behavior in both male and female rats and decreased fertility at doses $\leq$ 32 mg/kg/day. In rat embryo/fetal development studies, pregnant rats were given citalopram at doses of 32, 56, or 112 mg/kg/day. This resulted in decreased embryo/fetal growth and survival and an increased rate of abnormalities at the high dose of 112 mg/kg/day. Toxicity, with clinical signs, occurred in the pregnant females at this dose. There were no harmful effects on the fetuses at 56 mg/kg/day or lower. In rabbit embryo/fetal development studies, pregnant females were given 15 mg/kg/day with no adverse consequences (Forest Laboratories, Inc. 2002).

Citalopram is excreted in milk. In humans, sedation, decreased feeding, and weight loss have been recorded in the infants of mothers being treated with citalopram. When considering giving citalopram to a pregnant or nursing female, the potential benefits must be weighed against the potential risks to the embryo, fetus, or young animal (Forest Laboratories, Inc. 2002).

Citalopram has a longer half-life in geriatric patients than in younger patients. It is recommended that the lower range of the dose be given in geriatric patients (Forest Laboratories, Inc. 2002).

Five of 10 beagles given citalopram at a dose of 8 mg/kg/day died between days 17 and 31 after initiation of treatment. Some data suggest that dogs convert citalopram to its metabolites more than do humans. The phenomenon of sudden death was not observed in rats given up to 120 mg/kg/day, which produced plasma levels of citalopram and its metabolites similar to those observed in dogs on 8 mg/kg/day. Subsequent intravenous studies showed that DDCT produced prolonged QT intervals. Combined with the fact that dogs metabolize more citalopram to DDCT than do other species studied, this medication should not be considered a first-choice SSRI to use in this species (Forest Laboratories, Inc. 2002).

Overdose

Gastric lavage may be useful if conducted soon after ingestion. Induction of emesis is not recommended. Give activated charcoal and provide supportive therapy. There is no specific antidote.

Other Information

While the peppermint-flavored solution may seem an obvious choice for use in very small animals, taste aversion could be a problem with various species and individuals. Other SSRIs may be better choices for animals under 10 kg.

In humans, citalopram has not been shown to significantly affect the metabolism of digoxin, warfarin, theophylline, or triazolam (Forest Laboratories, Inc. 2002).

Effects Documented in Nonhuman Animals

Dogs

Citalopram has been effectively used to treat canine acral lick dermatitis (ALD) in dogs when given at a dose of 0.5–1.0 mg/kg daily. Specifically, six of nine dogs responded, with the average time to achieving a status of "much improved" or better being 2.6 weeks. Side effects that were observed in this population included sedation, anorexia, and constipation. Long-term follow-up of more than one year was available on three dogs. One was continued on a dose of 0.5 mg/kg and remained lesion free. One relapsed on two occasions when medication was discontinued, but recovered when medication was resumed at a maintenance dose of 0.33 mg/kg; a third relapsed when medication was discontinued. This dog was changed to fluoxetine for economic reasons and responded to that agent, on which it was likewise maintained for more than one year (Stein et al. 1998).

Table 5.2 Comparative cost of some selective serotonin reuptake inhibitors for a one-month supply for a 5-kg cat

Medication	Prescription	Cost for cat
Fluoxetine	10-mg tablets, #8 Give 1/4 tablet daily	$
Paroxetine	10-mg tablets, #8 Give 1/4 tablet daily	$$

Note: See Chapter 1 for a complete explanation.

Table 5.3 Comparative cost of various SSRIs for a one-month supply for a 20-kg dog

Medication	Cost for dog
Citalopram	$$$
Fluoxetine	$$
Fluvoxamine	$$$$
Paroxetine	$$$
Sertraline	$$$$$

Note: See Chapter 1 for a complete explanation.

II. Fluoxetine Hydrochloride

Chemical Compound: (+)-*N*-methyl-3-phenyl-3-($\alpha\alpha\alpha$-trifluoro-p-tolyl) oxypropylamine hydrochloride

DEA Classification: Not a controlled substance

Preparations: Generally available as 10- and 20-mg tablets, 10-, 20-, and 40-mg capsules, a slow release 90-mg tablet, and a mint-flavored solution of 20 mg/5 ml

Clinical Pharmacology

Fluoxetine is a strong inhibitor of serotonin reuptake and a very weak inhibitor of norepinephrine reuptake. Fluoxetine also has very little binding to muscarinic, histaminergic, and α1-adrenergic receptors compared with other antidepressants such as the tricyclic antidepressants.

Fluoxetine is well absorbed after oral administration, although food may delay its absorption by one to two hours. Metabolism is not proportional to dose; that is, when fluoxetine is given repeatedly, it is metabolized more slowly than if it is given as a single dose. In humans, peak plasma concentrations of a single oral dose occur in six to eight hours, while the elimination half-life of fluoxetine is 1–6 days (Altamura et al. 1994; Eli Lilly 2004). It is extensively metabolized in the liver to norfluoxetine, its principle metabolite, which is a less-potent SRI, but which has an elimination half-life of 4–16 days. In animal models, S-norfluoxetine has been found to be comparable to the parent compound in inhibition of serotonin reuptake (Altamura et al. 1994; Eli Lilly 2004). While exact elimination half-lives for veterinary patients have not been determined, clinical responses indicate that, as in humans, the drug may be present in the body for weeks after discontinuation.

Elimination of fluoxetine is primarily by metabolism in the liver and excretion of metabolites via the kidney. The elimination half-life of fluoxetine is substantially delayed in patients with liver disease as compared to patients without liver disease. In contrast, human patients on dialysis had steady-state fluoxetine and norfluoxetine concentrations similar to those of patients with normal kidneys. Thus, while the presence of liver disease should always be considered cause for reducing the dose, patients with renal disease may be able to tolerate a normal dose. Elderly patients have not been observed to have a higher incidence of adverse events than young adult patients (Eli Lilly 2004).

The median lethal dose in rats is 452 mg/kg PO. The median lethal dose in mice is 248 mg/kg. Phospholipids have been shown to increase in the tissues of dogs, mice, and rats chronically medicated with fluoxetine (Eli Lilly 2004).

Uses in Humans

Fluoxetine hydrochloride is used to treat depression, premenstrual dysphoric disorder, obsessive-compulsive disorder (OCD), and bulimia in humans.

Contraindications

The combination of fluoxetine and MAOIs can result in serious and sometimes fatal drug interactions. The two medications should never be given together. Because of the long half-life of fluoxetine, treatment with a MAOI should not be initiated until five weeks have passed since the discontinuation of fluoxetine. Conversely, fluoxetine

treatment should not be initiated until two weeks have passed since the discontinuation of an MAOI. Thioridazine should also not be given with fluoxetine or until at least
five weeks have passed since discontinuation of fluoxetine, because fluoxetine may
result in elevated levels of thioridazine. Rarely, various allergic events may occur in
response to fluoxetine, including anaphylactoid reactions.

Fluoxetine inhibits the liver enzymes cytochrome CYP2C9, CYP2D6, CYP2C19,
and CYP3A4. Therefore, elevated levels of medications that are metabolized by any
of these enzymes may occur when given concurrently, for example, tricyclic antidepressants, benzodiazepines, carbamazepine, and haloperidol. Low doses should be
used when these are combined with fluoxetine.

Co-administration of fluoxetine and tryptophan may lead to adverse events.
Because tryptophan is available over the counter, clients should be cautioned to not
supplement their pet with tryptophan when it is being medicated with fluoxetine or
any other serotonin reuptake inhibitor.

Co-administration with warfarin can result in increased bleeding.

Side Effects

In a small number of patients, treatment with fluoxetine can result in anxiety,
changes in appetite, vomiting, diarrhea, changes in urinary frequency, insomnia, sedation, excitement, seizures, hyponatremia, abnormal bleeding, and decreased sexual motivation. Decreased sexual motivation has been documented to occur in nonhuman animals, as well as humans (Matuszcyk et al. 1998). While this side effect
makes fluoxetine undesirable for use in breeding animals, it makes it potentially
useful for treatment of problems of undesirable sexual behavior in neutered animals
and is irrelevant for animals with behavior problems that are not intended for breeding. Veterinary patients that exhibit increased anxiety with administration of fluoxetine may improve and be subsequently maintained on this medication if the dose is
decreased.

Fluoxetine may alter metabolism of blood glucose. In particular, hyperglycemia
may develop during treatment with fluoxetine, while hypoglycemia may develop upon
withdrawal from fluoxetine. However, in humans, fluoxetine is effectively used to
treat depression in diabetic patients (Lustman et al. 2000). In diabetic patients, insulin
doses may need to be modified when initiating and discontinuing treatment with
fluoxetine.

Fluoxetine is tightly bound to plasma protein. Therefore, concomitant administration with drugs that are also tightly bound to plasma protein (e.g., digitoxin) can produce plasma levels of either (or both) drugs that are high compared with what they are
if given alone, resulting in adverse side effects.

Fluoxetine can alter anticoagulant effects and cause increased bleeding in patients
concurrently given warfarin.

Fluoxetine has not been found to be carcinogenic, mutagenic, or impair fertility.
However, in rats given 7.5 mg/kg daily or 12 mg/kg daily of fluoxetine during pregnancy, there was increased postpartum pup death. Rats given 5 mg/kg daily did not
have increased pup mortality. Also, when ewes in late gestation are given a 70 mg IV
bolus of fluoxetine over a two-minute period, transient decreases in uterine artery
blood flow, fetal PO_2, and oxygen saturation occur within the first 15 minutes. These
values do not return to normal after the passage of 24 hours. In addition, fetal pH de-

creases and fetal PCO_2 increases during the first 4 hours and then they return to normal within 24 hours. There are no differences in uterine artery blood flow, blood gas status, or cardiovascular measures between fluoxetine-treated ewes and control ewes (Morrison et al. 2002).

Because of potential risks to the fetus, fluoxetine should not be given to pregnant females unless the potential benefits clearly outweigh the potential risks to the fetus. Likewise, because fluoxetine is excreted in milk, it is recommended that it not be given to nursing females unless either a clear need outweighs the fact that the offspring are also being medicated or the offspring are fed a milk substitute. While caution is indicated, children of women who took fluoxetine throughout pregnancy did not show any decrement in birth weight, preschool IQ, language development, or behavior (Nulman et al. 2001).

During toxicity testing, rats were given up to 12 mg/kg daily of fluoxetine for two years without any evidence of carcinogenicity.

Overdose

There are no specific antidotes for overdose with fluoxetine. In 87 cases in which humans ingested an acute overdose of fluoxetine without concurrent ingestion of other drugs, the most common symptoms were tachycardia, drowsiness, tremor, vomiting, or nausea. Thirty of the patients (47%) did not develop any symptoms. Asymptomatic patients ingested a mean dose of 341 mg and a maximum dose of 1200 mg (Borys et al. 1992). Gastric lavage may be helpful if done soon after the overdose. Induction of emesis is not recommended. Give activated charcoal and supportive therapy. Give diazepam for seizures.

Doses in Nonhuman Animals

Doses reported for dogs generally range from 1.0–2.0 mg/kg/day, while doses reported for cats run a bit lower, generally ranging from 0.5–1.5 mg/kg/day. Smaller animals and/or species with faster metabolism, such as birds, will need higher doses to obtain clinical efficacy. Doses reported for birds range from 2.0 mg/kg/day to 5 mg/kg/day. Conversely, larger animals are likely to need smaller doses on a per kilogram basis. While there are no clinical reports of the treatment of rats, mice, or rabbits with fluoxetine, these species have tolerated very high doses in laboratory studies of toxicity. Horses may be effectively treated with 100–200 mg daily, or approximately 0.25–0.50 mg/kg.

Discontinuation of Fluoxetine

For patients that have been on fluoxetine for several weeks or months, it is recommended that discontinuation be done gradually rather than abruptly. In practice, if fluoxetine is effective in the treatment of the target behavior problem, continue medication for another one to three months, depending on the severity of the primary problem. Once it is confirmed that the problem has achieved long-term remediation with medication, fluoxetine is decreased at a rate not to exceed 25% of the maintenance dose per week. Some patients experience relapses at given decreases. If this happens, go back up to the lowest effective dose and continue for another one to three months, and then attempt to decrease the dose again.

Other Information

Fluoxetine has been more extensively used in the treatment of behavior problems in domestic animals than any other SSRI. Cats exhibit a strong distaste for the mint-flavored solution designed for humans. Rather than attempt to give this orally, it is recommended that a compounding pharmacist prepare a solution in a tuna or chicken flavored liquid.

While fluoxetine is not approved for use in the treatment of aggression in humans, several small studies have supported the hypothesis that it is effective in treating aggression in some patients (see, for example, Charney et al. 1990; Coccaro et al. 1990; Cornelius et al. 1991; Markowitz 1992; Kavoussi et al. 1994). In addition, a meta-analysis of 3992 patients treated with fluoxetine or placebo during clinical trials revealed that aggressive events were four times less likely to occur in fluoxetine-treated patients than in placebo-treated patients (Heiligenstein et al. 1993). Fluoxetine has been shown to suppress aggression in various laboratory animal species, for example, golden hamsters (*Mesocricetus auratus*) and lizards (*Anolis carolinensis*) (Deckel 1996; Deckel and Jevitts 1997; Ferris et al. 1997).

Effects Documented in Nonhuman Animals

Cats

Fluoxetine in a 15% pluronic lecithin organogel (PLO gel) formulation can be absorbed through the skin of cats into the systemic circulation. However, bioavailability of transdermally administered fluoxetine is only 10% that of the oral route. When concentrations are increased to achieve clinically effective levels, dermatitis results. Thus, transdermal administration of fluoxetine is not recommended (Ciribassi et al. 2003).

Hartmann (1995), in a letter to the *American Journal of Psychiatry*, reported on a cat with ALD that had not responded to more conventional treatments, including hypoallergenic diets, diphenhydramine, and diazepam, but the condition resolved when given fluoxetine, 0.25–0.38 mg/kg daily. The only side effect observed was some mild sedation.

Romatowski (1998) described two clinical cases of cats that responded to fluoxetine. One was a 16-month-old, 3-kg, spayed female Siamese cat that was presented with symmetrical, self-induced alopecia on the forelimbs. The cat was also a nervous and hyperactive pet. There were no cutaneous lesions other than the hair loss, and the cat had no fleas or flea manure. Treatment with methylprednisolone, phenobarbital, a commercial lamb and rice diet, and finally, megestrol acetate, all failed to resolve the problem. In fact, during these treatments, the hair loss became more extensive and eventually involved the abdomen, flanks, and thighs in a symmetrical pattern. Finally, treatment with fluoxetine, 0.66 mg/kg (2 mg daily) was attempted. The cat discontinued the excessive licking and after five months had grown a full hair coat. The owner also reported that the cat was more relaxed and was, therefore, a more pleasant pet.

The second case described by Romatowski involved two 5-year-old, spayed female, domestic shorthair littermates. The two cats had gotten along well until they were moved to a new home approximately one year prior to presentation. Before the move, the cats had been entirely indoors. After the move, they were allowed access to the backyard. One cat began rejecting the other, hissing whenever she approached. The rejected cat began intermittently urinating in various places in the house on a variety of substrates, for example, countertops, plastic or paper bags, the sleeping place of the cat that was rejecting her, and the owner's clothes. Urinalysis of the cat with the elimination behavior problem was unremarkable. Treatment with buspirone, 5 mg two times a day (b.i.d) for 30 days, was ineffective, as was treatment with diazepam, 1 mg b.i.d. Both cats were then placed on 2 mg fluoxetine daily. This treatment resulted in a discontinuation of the hissing behavior. The cats resumed sleeping together and grooming each other, behavior that had not occurred since the move. Inappropriate elimination was decreased 50%.

Pryor et al. (2001) treated 17 neutered urine spraying cats, all over 1 year of age, with fluoxetine or a fish-flavored liquid placebo in a randomized, double-blind, placebo-controlled trial. The initial dose was 1 mg/kg PO given once daily. If the patient did not achieve a 70% reduction in urine spraying by the fifth week, the dose was increased to 1.5 mg/kg. To maintain blinding, any cat that did not show improvements, including those on placebo, were given a 50% increased dose of their compounded medication. Treatment was carried out for eight weeks, followed by an additional four weeks of monitoring the cats after they had discontinued medication.

Standardized environmental management was as follows: (1) the owners were provided with an enzymatic cleaner that they were to use on all soiled areas; (2) the owners were instructed to provide as many litter boxes as cats in the household, plus one more; (3) the owners were instructed to clean all feces and urine from the litter boxes once a day and to completely change the litter material and wash the litter boxes once per week; and (4) the owners were instructed to refrain from physically or verbally punishing the cats.

Cats on the treatment showed a significant decrease in spraying behavior, compared with baseline premedication measures after two weeks of treatment. Their spraying rate continued to decrease throughout treatment. In contrast, the mean weekly spraying rate of cats on placebo decreased slightly during the first week and did not decrease further thereafter. This slight decrease was probably a response to the environmental management and increased regular supervision that was necessarily occurring because of the research. By the end of the trial, all cats on treatment had demonstrated a 90% reduction in the number of urine marks each week. Total cessation of spraying occurred in 66% of the cats on treatment by the eighth week. For weeks two through eight, there was a significant difference in response for the cats on placebo versus the cats on treatment. The most common side effect reported was decreased food intake; however, this was reported in four of the nine cats on treatment and three of the seven cats on placebo. The decreased food intake was never to such a degree that it was cause for concern or considered clinically significant. Vomiting occurred in one cat on treatment and two cats on placebo. Lethargy occurred in three cats on treatment and two cats on placebo.

After medication was discontinued, two of the nine cats that had been treated did not resume spraying. However, the other seven cats resumed some degree of marking. There was a linear correlation between the rate of marking during baseline and the rate of marking four weeks after treatment. Because of this finding, it is recommended that most cats, particularly those with higher rates of urine marking prior to treatment, that is, four or more marks per week, should be treated for a period of time longer than eight weeks.

S-norfluoxetine, at doses of 3–10 mg/kg, causes small but significant increases in bladder capacity (Katofiasc et al. 2002).

Dogs

Six laboratory dogs overdosed with fluoxetine given orally developed grand mal seizures that were controlled with intravenous boluses of diazepam. In another study, the electrocardiogram (ECGs) of dogs given high doses of fluoxetine were evaluated. Tachycardia and increased blood pressure occurred. However, no changes occurred in the PR, QRS, or QT intervals (Eli Lilly 2004).

In 1995, Overall described a case of a dog with dominance-related interdog aggression, dominance aggression to the dog's owner, fear of strangers, and stereotypic circling. Initial treatment with behavior modification alone resulted in resolution of the dominance aggression toward the owner, but did not resolve the interdog aggression or fear of strangers. Therefore, medication treatment was initiated. After an initial period of treatment with fluoxetine alone, then buspirone, then buspirone with fluoxetine, and finally fluoxetine alone, the dog was maintained on fluoxetine at a dose of 0.54 mg/kg daily for a period of 28 months. During this time, there was only one incident of interdog aggression, and there was no owner-directed dominance aggression. Side effects included constant mydriasis after the initiation of treatment with fluoxetine. Renal and hepatic function were not compromised while on the long-term fluoxetine treatment.

In a later study, Dodman et al. (1996) conducted a single-blind crossover trial of the treatment of owner-directed dominance aggression in nine dogs. Diagnosis was based entirely on context and frequency of aggression and did not include signaling behavior. Therefore, patients with what the author considers to be other forms of affective aggression may have been included in this study's population. Patients were treated with fluoxetine at a dose of 1 mg/kg PO q24h, and one week of a placebo. The fluoxetine and placebo were placed into gelatin capsules so that they were visually indistinguishable. While owners were not told which week their dog would be getting the placebo, all dogs received the placebo during the first week of the trial to avoid a carryover effect from the fluoxetine, since it has a long half-life. No behavior modification or training was carried out during the five-week study.

A significant reduction in owner-directed incidents of aggression was observed by the end of treatment. While on medication, some dogs exhibited changes in level of activity, changes in food or water intake, increased alertness, shaking, barking, and reclusion. While it is not recommended that medication be used alone in the treatment of canine affective aggression, it is clear from this report that SSRI medications such as fluoxetine can be useful adjuncts to treatment with behavior modification. Fluoxetine has also been used to treat interdog dominance-motivated aggression (Dodman 2000).

Rapoport et al. (1992) compared fluoxetine to fenfluramine in 14 dogs with ALD in an 11-week crossover treatment trial. Dogs were treated for 5 weeks with up to 0.96 ± 0.29 mg/kg daily of fluoxetine and for another 5 weeks with up to 0.92 ± 0.24 mg/kg daily of fenfluramine. Owners used a 10-point scale to rate their dogs' licking with 0 being no licking at all and 10 being the worst licking ever observed. There was no order effect, so ratings were combined across both orders. Dogs on fluoxetine exhibited, on average, a 39% decrease from baseline scores. By 5 weeks, improvement on fluoxetine was significantly greater than improvement on fenfluramine, which was slight. Concurrent studies were carried out on an additional 13 dogs that were treated with clomipramine or desipramine and another 10 dogs that were treated with sertraline or placebo in a similar crossover trial. Comparisons in response across trials showed that fluoxetine was more effective than desipramine, fenfluramine, and sertraline in reducing licking. Four of the 14 dogs treated with fluoxetine showed lethargy, 1 showed loss of appetite, and 1 showed hyperactivity. Two of the dogs treated with fluoxetine showed complete remission of excessive licking, while 4 showed a 50% reduction in licking.

Stein et al. (1992) likewise used fluoxetine, 1–2 mg/kg daily for an eight-week open trial on five dogs with ALD. One dog almost entirely discontinued self-injurious behavior, but developed polyuria and polydipsia. Two others showed substantial improvement with no side effects. One dog was removed from the study at two weeks when there was no response, while another was removed from the study because it exhibited sedation. Subsequent use of fluoxetine in cases of OCD manifested as canine acral lick have been reported as having about a 50% success rate (Karel 1994). In the author's experience, improvement may not be exhibited for four weeks or more. Sedation, when it occurs, is often transient, and dogs usually return to normal levels of activity after a couple of weeks.

Wynchank and Berk (1998) subsequently conducted a double-blind, randomized, placebo-controlled trial of the use of fluoxetine in the treatment of ALD in dogs. All dogs on treatment were dosed at 20 mg/day, regardless of size, for six weeks. The smallest dog was 5 kg. Thus, this dog was dosed at 4 mg/kg. For a dog to qualify for the study, a veterinarian must have diagnosed the dog with ALD at least six months before the beginning of the trial. Other causes of licking behavior must have been ruled out, as well.

Fifty-eight dogs, ranging in age from 1 to 13 years, completed the trial. For dogs that were on the treatment, owner rating of the licking behavior and appearance of the lesion decreased significantly over the course of treatment. The placebo group did not exhibit a significant decline. There was a significant difference between treatment and placebo groups in both change in appearance of the lesion and general condition of the dog by the end of the study. Veterinarians who were blinded as to whether or not the photographs were before or after treatment evaluated photographs of the lesions. Changes in the scores for lesion severity were significantly better for the treatment group than for the placebo group. No adverse events were reported.

Interdog dominance aggression in a Welsh terrier has been successfully treated with fluoxetine, 1.1 mg/kg PO daily, in combination with behavior modification (Dodman 2000).

Of 40 dogs treated for generalized anxiety disorder with fluoxetine at 0.37–1.2 mg/kg, 27 (67%) improved, 9 showed no significant behavior change, and 4 got worse while on this treatment (Reisner 2003).

Parrots

Mertens (1997) reported that 12 of 14 birds treated with fluoxetine for feather-picking (2.3 mg/kg daily for at least four weeks) exhibited initial improvement but subsequently relapsed. An increased dose up to as high as 3 mg/kg b.i.d. again resulted in improvement with a subsequent relapse. Side effects observed included frequent sneezing (2 birds) one week after initiation of treatment, temporary ataxia, and lethargy about one hour after medication (2 birds). Additionally, 1 bird that had an extensive vocabulary, including songs and poems, forgot word sequences and exhibited a reduced vocabulary. All problems disappeared after treatment was discontinued. All birds were kept in good housing conditions, with provision of intra- and interspecific social contact, good dietary management, and exercise.

Seibert (2004) treated a 3.5-year-old white female cockatiel (*Nymphicus hollandicus*) (1 mg/kg of fluoxetine PO, q24h) with a compulsive disorder that was specifically manifested as chewing the third digit of the right foot. The bird responded two weeks after initiation of treatment. After three months of treatment, the dosage was decreased. By five months treatment was successfully discontinued.

Primates

Vervet monkeys with various stereotypic behaviors, for example, saluting, somersaulting, weaving, and head tossing, were treated with fluoxetine (1 mg/kg daily for six weeks) or placebo. Results of assessment by a rater blind to treatment status identified a significant difference between fluoxetine-treated and placebo-treated monkeys by the end of the trial (Hugo et al. 2003).

III. Fluvoxamine

Chemical Compound: 5-Methoxy-4′-(trifluoromethyl)valerophenone-(E)-*O*-(2-aminoethyl)oxime maleate
DEA Classification: Not a controlled substance
Preparations: Generally available as 25-, 50-, and 100-mg tablets

Clinical Pharmacology

Fluvoxamine specifically inhibits reuptake of serotonin in both blood platelets and brain synaptosomes (Claasen et al. 1977). It has a weak affinity for histaminergic, α- or β-adrenergic, muscarinic, or dopaminergic receptors. Absorption is not affected by food intake. In humans, steady-state plasma concentrations are achieved in about 10 days. Once people have achieved steady state, peak plasma concentrations occur in three to eight hours. The pharmacokinetics of fluvoxamine are nonlinear. Specifically, higher doses of fluvoxamine produce proportionally higher concentrations in the plasma than do lower doses.

Fluvoxamine is metabolized by the liver, primarily via oxidative demethylation and deamination. Nine metabolites have been identified. The major human metabolites are fluvoxamine acid, the *N*-acetyl analog of fluvoxamine acid, and fluvoxethanol, all of which have little to no serotonin reuptake prevention activity. Humans excrete only about 2% of fluvoxamine as the parent compound. The remaining 98% is excreted as various metabolites (Solvay Pharmaceuticals 2002).

Excretion occurs primarily via the kidneys. In healthy humans, an average of 94% of the medication is excreted in the urine within 71 hours of dosing. Geriatric patients clear fluvoxamine more slowly than do young adults. Patients with liver disease clear fluvoxamine more slowly than do healthy patients. However, patients with renal disease have not been found to clear fluvoxamine any more slowly than do persons without renal disease (Solvay Pharmaceuticals 2002).

Uses in Humans

Fluvoxamine is used to treat OCD in humans.

Contraindications

Fluvoxamine should not be administered with terfenadine or cisapride. These are metabolized by the P450 isozyme 3A4. While there is no definitive proof that fluvoxamine is a 3A4 inhibitor, there is strong evidence that it is. Thus, co-administration could result in elevated terfenadine or cisapride levels, which could result in QT prolongation, ventricular tachycardia, and other cardiac symptoms (Solvay Pharmaceuticals 2002).

Fluvoxamine should not be administered at the same time as MAOIs. It should not be used in patients that have previously received an MAOI until the patient has been off the MAOI for at least two weeks. Conversely, MAOIs should not be given until a patient has been off of fluvoxamine for at least two weeks.

The metabolism of benzodiazepines metabolized by hepatic oxidation, including alprazolam, midazolam, and triazolam (see Chapter 3) can be reduced by combined use with fluvoxamine. Benzodiazepines metabolized by glucuronidation, including lorazepam, oxazepam, and temazepam, are not likely to be affected by co-administration with fluvoxamine (Solvay Pharmaceuticals 2002).

Fluvoxamine can alter the efficacy and activity of warfarin, propanaolol, tricyclic antidepressants, and theophylline, as well as other drugs metabolized by the P450 enzyme system. Tryptophan may increase the serotonergic activity of fluvoxamine and should be used in combination with caution (Solvay Pharmaceuticals 2002).

Side Effects

In a small number of patients, treatment with fluvoxamine can result in anxiety, changes in appetite, vomiting, diarrhea, changes in urinary frequency, insomnia, sedation, excitement, seizures, hyponatremia, abnormal bleeding, mydriasis, decreased libido, and various other side effects unique to individuals, including anaphylaxis.

Studies of the potential for carcinogenicity, mutagenicity, and impairment of fertility by fluvoxamine have not revealed any such effects. Rats were treated with doses of up to 240 mg/kg/day for 30 months, and hamsters were treated with doses of up to 240 mg/kg day for up to 20 months, with no carcinogenic effect. In fertility studies, male and female rats were given up to 80 mg/kg/day PO of fluvoxamine, with no deleterious effects on mating, duration of gestation, or pregnancy (Solvay Pharmaceuticals 2002).

In teratology studies in which pregnant rats were given up to 80 mg/kg/day PO and pregnant rabbits were given up to 40 mg/kg/day PO, there were no fetal malformations. In other studies in which pregnant rats were dosed through weaning with 5, 20, 80, and 160 mg/kg/day PO there was an increase in pup mortality at birth in rats that were dosed at 80 mg/kg and higher, decreased neonatal pup weights at 160 mg/kg, and decreased long-term survival of the pups at all doses. Results of a cross-fostering study suggested that some of the postnatal deficits in survival were due to maternal toxicity; that is, the mothers being chronically medicated at such high doses were not as competent mothers as were unmedicated rats. However, there may have been some direct drug effect on the offspring.

Fluvoxamine is excreted in the milk. In deciding whether to medicate pregnant or lactating females, potential risks to the offspring must be weighed against the potential benefits to the mother (Solvay Pharmaceuticals 2002).

In human studies, the side-effect profile for pediatric patients has been found to be similar to the side-effect profile for adult patients (Solvay Pharmaceuticals 2002).

Overdose

Gastric lavage may be useful if it is conducted soon after ingestion of an overdose. Give activated charcoal, and provide supportive therapy. There is no specific antidote.

Other Information

Comparisons of humans treated with either placebo or fluvoxamine showed no significant effect of fluvoxamine on various vital sign indicators, serum chemistries, hematology, urinalysis, or ECG changes. Fluvoxamine has not been found to significantly effect the pharmacokinetics of digoxin (Solvay Pharmaceuticals 2002).

Effects Documented in Nonhuman Animals

Fluvoxamine has a specific antiaggressive effect on maternal aggression, because it results in decreased aggression at doses that do not cause concurrent nonspecific decreases in activity (Olivier and Mos 1992).

IV. Paroxetine Hydrochloride

Chemical Compound: (-)-Trans-4R-(4'-fluorophenyl)-3S-[(3',4'-methylene-dioxyphenoxyl)methyl]piperidine hydrochloride hemihydrate

DEA Classification: Not a controlled substance

Preparations: Generally available as 10-, 20-, 30-, and 40-mg tablets and a 2-mg/ml orange-flavored suspension. Controlled-release tablets are available in 12.5-, 25-, and 37.5-mg sizes.

Clinical Pharmacology

Paroxetine has weak effects on neuronal reuptake of norepinephrine and dopamine, but is primarily a highly selective inhibitor of serotonin reuptake. It has little affinity for muscarinic, α_1-, α_2-, β-adrenergic, dopamine (D_2)-, 5-HT_1-, 5-HT_2-, or histamine (H_1)receptors. Thus, there are fewer anticholinergic, sedative, and cardiovascular side effects than some other serotonin reuptake inhibitors, such as amitriptyline, that also have substantial effects on muscarinic, histaminergic and α_1-adrenergic receptors. Paroxetine has multiple metabolites, each about 1/50th as potent as the parent compound. Thus, clinical efficacy of paroxetine is essentially from the parent compound, and there are no significant contributions from metabolites (SmithKline Beecham Pharmaceuticals 2004).

Paroxetine is completely absorbed when given orally and can be given with or without food. In humans, the half-life is about 10 days, with 64% being excreted in the urine, 2% as paroxetine, and the remainder as metabolites of paroxetine. The remaining 36% is excreted in the feces, <1% as paroxetine, and the remainder as metabolites. With chronic daily dosing, steady-state plasma concentrations are achieved in about 10 days. Paroxetine is distributed throughout the body, including the central nervous system, with about 95% being bound to plasma protein (SmithKline Beecham Pharmaceuticals 2004).

The presence of renal or hepatic disease produces increased concentrations of paroxetine in the plasma. Therefore, patients with mild renal or hepatic impairment should be started on a very low dose and the dose titrated upward over time. Plasma levels in older patients are also elevated. Therefore, the starting dose should be low in all geriatric patients and subsequently titrated upward as necessary (SmithKline Beecham Pharmaceuticals 2004).

Paxil CR tablets are formulated so that dissolution occurs gradually over a period of several hours. There is also an enteric coat that prevents release of the active ingredient until after the tablet has left the stomach. The consumption of food does not significantly affect release or absorption. For the slower release to occur, the tablet cannot be cut, broken, or chewed (SmithKline Beecham Pharmaceuticals 2004). This limits its potential usefulness in animals weighing less than approximately 10 kg. Even in animals large enough to theoretically be given the controlled release tablets, it is important to remember that these tablets are designed for the human digestive system and dissolve and are absorbed at substantially slower or faster rates in various other species.

Uses in Humans

Paroxetine is used to treat depression, OCD, panic disorder, social anxiety disorder, generalized anxiety disorder, and posttraumatic stress disorder (PTSD).

Contraindications

Do not use paroxetine in combination with any MAOI or with thioridazine, because serious and sometimes fatal drug interactions can result. Patients should not be given paroxetine for at least two weeks before initiating medication with either of these drugs. Patients should not have been given MAOIs for at least two weeks before initiation of paroxetine (SmithKline Beecham Pharmaceuticals 2004).

Paroxetine inhibits the liver enzyme CYP2D6 but otherwise causes less inhibition of liver enzymes than do other SSRIs such as fluoxetine and fluvoxamine. Nevertheless, there are a large number of medications that are metabolized by this enzyme, including amitriptyline, clomipramine, dextromethorphan, imipramine, propranolol, and thioridazine. Thus, lower doses should be used in patients concurrently receiving any drug that is metabolized by this enzyme (SmithKline Beecham Pharmaceuticals 2004).

Do not use in patients with narrow angle glaucoma.

Concurrent use of paroxetine and tryptophan can result in adverse events. Because tryptophan is available over the counter, clients should be advised of this (SmithKline Beecham Pharmaceuticals 2004).

Paroxetine may interact with warfarin, altering its effect on bleeding. Paroxetine is strongly bound to plasma protein, resulting in a greater plasma concentration of any drug administered concurrently that is likewise strongly bound to plasma protein (SmithKline Beecham Pharmaceuticals 2004).

Side Effects

In a small number of patients, treatment with paroxetine can result in anxiety, changes in appetite, vomiting, diarrhea, changes in urinary frequency, insomnia, sedation, excitement, seizures, hyponatremia, abnormal bleeding, mydriasis, decreased libido, and various other side effects unique to individuals, including anaphylaxis (SmithKline Beecham Pharmaceuticals 2004). Studies conducted in humans have shown that the incidence of many side effects is dose dependent, that is, the higher the dose, the more likely it is that side effects will occur. Withdrawal reactions occur at a higher rate for paroxetine than for fluoxetine, fluvoxamine, or sertraline in the human population (Price et al. 1996). In case of decreased libido, while this side effect makes paroxetine undesirable for use in breeding animals, it makes it potentially useful for treatment of animals with undesirable sexual behavior. In cats, constipation has been reported to be a common side effect of paroxetine.

Carcinogenicity studies were conducted in mice and rats on paroxetine for two years. Mice were given 1, 5, or 25 mg/kg daily, and rats were given 1, 5, or 20 mg/kg daily. The male rats in the high-dose group had significantly more sarcomas than did the male rats in the low- or medium-dose group or on placebo. There was no carcinogenic effect identified in mice or female rats. The implications of these findings for other domestic animals are unknown (SmithKline Beecham Pharmaceuticals 2004). Since the dose that induced cancer in male rats was greater than what would be used as a therapeutic dose for the treatment of behavior problems in pet rats, the findings are probably not of concern in treating this group. Nevertheless, owners should be cautioned.

Studies of potential mutagenicity of paroxetine have not identified any mutagenic effects of this medication.

Female rats experienced a reduced pregnancy rate when given 15 mg/kg daily of paroxetine. Male rats given 25 mg/kg daily had atrophic changes in the seminiferous tubules and aspermatogenesis. Male rats given 50 mg/kg/day had vacuolation of the epididymal tubular epithelium (SmithKline Beecham Pharmaceuticals 2004).

In studies of teratogenic effects, pregnant rabbits were given 6 mg/kg daily, and pregnant rats were given 50 mg/kg daily during organogenesis. There were no terato-genic effects in either species and no increased postnatal pup deaths in rabbits. However, in rats there was increased pup mortality when paroxetine was continued during the last trimester and lactation. The cause of this mortality has not been iden-tified. The implications of these findings for other domestic animals are not known. However, because of these findings and the fact that paroxetine is secreted in milk, it should be used in pregnant and lactating females only when the potential benefits clearly outweigh the risks (SmithKline Beecham Pharmaceuticals 2004).

Geriatric patients have decreased clearance time as compared with younger pa-tients. Therefore, lower dosing is recommended in geriatric patients (SmithKline Beecham Pharmaceuticals 2004).

Overdose

Gastric lavage may be useful if conducted soon after ingestion. Induction of emesis is not recommended. Give activated charcoal, and provide supportive therapy. There is no specific antidote.

Discontinuation of Paroxetine

For patients that have been on paroxetine for several weeks, it is recommended that discontinuation be done gradually rather than abruptly. While abrupt discontinuation of a variety of SSRI treatments can cause withdrawal symptoms, this phenomenon has been most frequently reported with paroxetine in the human literature (Price et al. 1996; Michelson et al. 1998). In practice, if paroxetine is effective in the treatment of the target behavior problem, continue medication for another one to three months, de-pending on the severity of the primary problem. Once it is confirmed that the problem has achieved long-term remediation with medication, paroxetine is decreased at a rate not exceeding 25% of the maintenance dose per week. Some patients experience relapses at given decreases. If this happens, go back up to the lowest effective dose and continue for another one to three months, then attempt to decrease the dose again.

Other Information

In double-blind placebo-controlled trials conducted on humans, paroxetine was not found to produce any significant changes in ECGs, heart rate, blood pressure, or liver enzymes.

Paroxetine has an insignificant effect on the liver enzyme CYP2C19. Therefore, there is no need for lower doses of benzodiazepines, which are metabolized by this enzyme, as is the case with fluoxetine and fluvoxamine (SmithKline Beecham Pharmaceuticals 2004).

Effects Documented in Nonhuman Animals

Cats

Paroxetine has been used to treat cats for urine marking and aggression (Pryor 2003).

Dogs

Of 12 dogs treated with paroxetine (0.96–1.75 mg/kg PO q24h), for generalized anxiety disorder, 6 (50%) showed improvement, 4 showed no change, and 1 dog got worse (Reisner 2003). The response of the twelfth dog is not reported.

Horses

A mare with a five-year history of weaving exhibited a 95% decrease in this behavior when given 0.5 mg/kg daily PO. Even when stressed, the mare exhibited a 57% improvement over baseline. Specifically, the frequency of weaving changed from 43.5 per minute with kicking to less than 1 per minute. When the mare was stressed, weaving increased to 18.75 per minute (Nurnberg et al. 1997).

V. Sertraline Hydrochloride

Chemical Compound: (1S-*cis*)-4-(3,4-dichlorophenyl)-(1,2,3,4-tetrahydro-*N*-methyl-1-naphthalenamine hydrochloride

DEA Classification: Not a controlled substance

Preparations: Generally available as 25-, 50-, and 100-mg tablets and a 20-mg/ml liquid

Clinical Pharmacology

Sertraline is a selective inhibitor of neuronal serotonin reuptake. It has very weak effects on reuptake of norepinephrine and dopamine. Sertraline has no substantial affinity for adrenergic (α_1, α_2, and β), cholinergic, GABA, dopaminergic, histaminergic, serotonergic (5-HT$_{1A}$, 5-HT$_{1B}$, 5-HT$_2$), or benzodiazepine receptors. Therefore, the anticholinergic, sedative and cardiovascular effects seen with some other psychoactive drugs, such as the tricyclic antidepressants, are minimal. Chronic administration of sertraline also down-regulates brain norepinephrine receptors. The half-life in humans is about 26 hours. Blood levels reach a steady state after approximately one week of daily dosing in a healthy adult. More time is required to achieve steady state in older patients. Sertraline can be given with or without food (Pfizer Inc. 2004).

Sertraline is metabolized extensively during its first pass through the liver, primarily to *N*-desmethylsertraline, which has a plasma elimination half-life of 62–104 hours. *N*-desmethylsertraline is a less potent serotonin reuptake inhibitor than is the parent compound. In human subjects given a single radiolabeled dose of sertraline, 40–45% of the radioactivity was recovered via the urine within nine days. Another 40–45% was recovered in the feces. The urine contained only metabolites of sertraline, while the feces contained 12–14% of the original sertraline in an unchanged form, the remainder being metabolites produced by oxidative deamination and subsequent reduction, hydroxylation, and glucuronide conjugation (Pfizer Inc. 2004).

In human pediatric studies it was found that children and teenagers (6 to 17 years of age) metabolized sertraline more efficiently than did adults. There was no difference between males and females. In contrast, geriatric patients clear sertraline more slowly than do adults (Pfizer Inc. 2004).

Patients with chronic mild liver impairment clear sertraline more slowly than do age-matched patients with normal liver function. This is not a surprising finding given the significant metabolism of the drug in the liver in normal patients. As discussed above, clearance of unchanged sertraline in the urine is a minor mode of elimination of the parent compound, and almost half of the metabolites are eliminated in the feces. In patients with mild to severe renal impairment the pharmacokinetics of sertraline metabolism and excretion are not significantly different from healthy controls (Pfizer Inc. 2004).

The minimum lethal doses are 350 mg/kg PO in male mice, 300 mg/kg PO in female mice, 1000 mg/kg in male rats, and 750 mg/kg in female rats. Death occurs after one to two days (Pfizer Inc. 2004).

Uses in Humans

Sertraline is used to treat depression, OCD, PTSD, panic disorder, and premenstrual dysphoric disorder in humans.

Contraindications

Do not use sertraline in combination with any MAOI, because serious and sometimes fatal drug interactions can result. Patients should not be given sertraline for at least two weeks before initiating medication with an MAOI. Patients should not have been given monoamine oxidase inhibitors for at least two weeks prior to initiation of paroxetine (Pfizer Inc. 2004).

Side Effects

In a small number of patients, treatment with sertraline can result in anxiety, changes in appetite, vomiting, diarrhea, changes in urinary frequency, insomnia, sedation, excitement, seizures, hyponatremia, abnormal bleeding, mydriasis, decreased libido, and various other side effects unique to individuals, including anaphylaxis. Rarely, patients on sertraline may have altered platelet function and abnormal bleeding (Pfizer Inc. 2004).

Sertraline has some effect of inhibiting the biochemical activity of the liver enzyme CYP2D6. While its effect is not as substantial as paroxetine or fluoxetine (Albers et al. 2002), it should be used with caution with drugs that are metabolized by this enzyme, such as the tricyclic antidepressants dextromethorphan and propranolol.

Lifetime carcinogenicity studies have been conducted on mice and rats given up to 40 mg/kg/day of sertraline. Male mice experienced a dose-related increase in liver adenomas. Female mice did not experience this increase. Female rats experienced an increase in the rate of follicular adenomas of the thyroid gland at 40 mg/kg/day. This change was not accompanied by thyroid hyperplasia. There was an increase in uterine adenocarcinomas in female rats given 10–40 mg/kg/day compared with placebo (Davies and Kluwe 1998; Pfizer Inc. 2004).

In tests of mutagenicity, no mutagenic activity has been identified. Doses of 80 mg/kg/day result in decreased fertility in rats (Davies and Kluwe 1998; Pfizer Inc. 2004).

Pregnant rats have been given sertraline up to 80 mg/kg/day, while pregnant rabbits have been given sertraline up to 40 mg/kg/day. Sertraline was not teratogenic at these doses. When the pregnant rats and rabbits were medicated during the period of organogenesis, delayed ossification occurred in the fetuses when their mothers were on doses of 10 mg/kg/day in rats and 40 mg/kg/day in rabbits. At a dose of 20 mg/kg/day given to rats during the last third of gestation and lactation, there was decreased body weight gain in the pups and increased early postnatal mortality. There was no effect at 10 mg/kg/day. The increased pup mortality was due to the in utero exposure to sertraline at the higher doses (Davies and Kluwe 1998; Pfizer Inc. 2004).

Dogs given ≥ 40 mg/kg PO of sertraline daily orally for two weeks exhibit mydriasis, hindlimb weakness, hyperactivity, and anorexia. Alkaline phosphatase (Alk Ph) activity is increased in dogs given 80 mg/kg/day for two weeks, while serum transaminase activity (ALT) is increased in dogs receiving 160 mg/kg for this period of time. Dogs given ≥ 10 mg/kg daily PO for 3 months or longer exhibit mydriasis. In addition, dogs given ≥ 30 mg/kg daily PO for up to 12 months exhibit transient hyperactivity and restlessness with anorexia and body weight loss or decreased body weight loss. Convulsions may occur at 90 mg/kg. Dogs treated with sertraline for one year exhibit increased Alk Ph activity when dosed at ≥ 10 mg/kg daily PO, increased relative liver weight when dosed at ≥ 30 mg/kg daily PO, and increased ALT when dosed at 90 mg/kg daily PO. Lymphoid depletion may occur in dogs given 15–160 mg/kg for a short period of time, but has not been observed in dogs treated chronically (Davies and Kluwe 1998).

It is unknown whether sertraline is excreted in milk. As with the other SSRIs, medicating pregnant or lactating females with sertraline should be done cautiously, with the potential benefits to the female being weighed against the risks to the fetus and neonate (Pfizer Inc. 2004).

Other Information

While sertraline is not labeled for use in the treatment of aggression in humans, beneficial effects for this problem have been observed (e.g., Kavoussi et al. 1994).

Effects Documented in Nonhuman Animals
Dogs

Rapoport et al. (1992) studied the effects of sertraline versus placebo on dogs with ALD in an 11-week crossover treatment trial, with 5 weeks each on placebo and on sertraline. Sertraline was dosed at up to 3.42 ± 0.52 mg/kg daily. Sertraline was significantly better than placebo, producing a 21% decrease in licking behavior at 5 weeks as compared with baseline. However, sertraline was less effective than fluoxetine, which was being studied in a similar crossover trial with fenfluramine. Fluoxetine produced a 39% decrease by 5 weeks when compared to baseline. No side effects were reported for dogs on sertraline. However, only one dog showed clinically significant (50%) improvement in licking behavior.

Reptiles

Male *Anolis carolinensis* given sertraline at a dose of 10 mg/kg exhibit decreased aggressiveness. In addition, if sertraline is given only to the dominant male of a pair that has established their hierarchical relationship prior to treatment, the dominance order often reverses. In addition, nonaggressive associative behavior increases (Larson and Summers 2001).

Important Information for Owners of Pets Being Placed on Any SSRI

The following should be considered when placing an animal on an SSRI.

1. It is essential that owners inform their veterinarian of all other medication, herbal supplements, and nutritional supplements they are giving their pet, because some of these may interact with the medication.
2. While their pet may respond within a few days, it may be a month before their pet begins responding. They must be patient.
3. If their pet exhibits mild sedation in the beginning, it will probably return to normal levels of activity in two or three weeks as its body adjusts to the medication.
4. If their pet should experience any adverse events such as vomiting, diarrhea or seizures, they should contact their veterinarian immediately.
5. All use of the medication being given is extra-label use. This does not mean that the drug is not indicated for the problem. In fact, there may be an extensive body of scientific and clinical evidence supporting the use of this drug for their pet's problem. It means that the extensive testing required by the FDA for on-label usage of the drug for their particular species of pet and their particular pet's problem has not been conducted or, if in progress, completed. Exceptions to this may occur after the publication of this book if the FDA subsequently approves any of the SSRIs for treatment of various behavior problems in domestic animals.

Clinical Examples

Case 1

Signalment

Sam was an 11-year-old neutered male bichon frise weighing 8.5 kg owned by a couple, both of whom were substantially involved in caring for and interacting with Sam. There were no other pets in the house.

Presenting Complaint

Sam presented with aggression.

History

At the time of his presentation at the age of 10, Sam had been aggressive most of his life. The aggression had become an issue only recently because the couple was expecting their first child in approximately three months. Neutering had resulted in some improvement, but had not cured the problem.

Sam became aggressive if either of the owners picked him up and then moved to put him down, if they were near his toys, if they laughed, if they said "good-bye," if the husband got up during the night and then returned to the bed (Sam slept in the bed), if they moved while in bed, and in a variety of other circumstances. His posture consistently involved erect ears and tail. Sam would solicit "people food" when the couple ate and would persistently bark until they gave him some. If Sam had some food, such as a bagel or some chicken, the owners reported that they couldn't get it back without risk of a serious bite. The owners reported that if they looked him in the eye and used a stern tone of voice he would "bare his fangs," "spit water out of his nose," and adopt an "aggressive posture." Sam never exhibited behaviors indicative of fear or submission; that is, he did not lower his ears or tail, crouch, or avoid. Instead, he had a consistent pattern of moving toward the owners with tail and ears up and staring at them during agonistic encounters. Sam was also aggressive to visitors.

Sam was healthy, except for a urinary tract infection that responded to treatment without complications. Serum chemistry and complete blood count (CBC) results were normal. There was no evidence of cognitive decline.

Diagnosis

Sam was diagnosed with dominance-motivated aggression.

Treatment Plan

The potential dangers that Sam presented, especially to the forthcoming baby, were discussed in depth. The owners were realistic about the dangers, having been previously bitten. While the couple was very concerned about their new baby's safety, they were very attached to Sam, whom they had had since he was six months old. The initial plan was to attempt treatment for two months and then assess Sam's improvement before deciding whether or not to continue treatment or simply make sure that Sam never had access to the baby.

Following is a summary of the initial treatment plan.

1. Fluoxetine, 10 mg (1.2 mg/kg) was given once daily PO.
2. Sam was not to be allowed in bed anymore. This was not difficult to implement since Sam was so small he had to be lifted onto the bed. Sam was also not to be allowed on any of the other furniture. If he got on, he was to be called off for a treat.
3. Sam was to be required to obey a command, for example, "sit" or "down," before he got anything he wanted, including food, going inside, going outside, and being petted.
4. For the short term, Sam was not to be picked up, because this was one of the situations that resulted in aggressive behavior. The owners were also, for the short term, not to attempt to handle Sam's toys or take food away from him. Interactions with visitors were to be restricted. Again, this was to avoid further incidents of aggression.

5. The owners were to practice simple command training, that is, sit-stay and down-stay, with Sam on a daily basis. They were given detailed instructions on how to do this using training techniques that were nonconfrontational and exclusively involved positive reinforcement of desired behaviors.
6. The owners were to frequently give dominance signals that they anticipated Sam would tolerate. Again, the owners were educated in depth about signaling of dominance and submission by dogs.
7. Changes that would occur when the baby arrived were reviewed. The owners were instructed to, as much as possible, make these changes as soon as possible and to expose Sam to the sights, sounds, and smells of a baby in advance. Since Sam was not going to be allowed into the baby's room, which had already been converted into a nursery, the room was to be gated immediately. Sam was never to be allowed in that room. The wife was to get a large baby doll and carry it around the house while maintaining obedience control over Sam. It was anticipated that this would not actually be initiated for about a month, until Sam had been on fluoxetine for four weeks and the wife had gained better obedience control over him without the encumbrance of a baby doll.

Follow-up

After 10 days the owners reported that all rules had been instituted and Sam was taking his medication without difficulty. He experienced no side effects in the first days or later on in the treatment. A sufficient change in Sam's behavior had already occurred such that the husband expressed optimism about the situation. After one month Sam was friendly toward visitors whom he had previously been aggressive toward. A relative who had visited stated that Sam was "a different dog." After two months on medication, Sam was showing clear improvement. He would sit on command without threatening the owner. At three months, the wife reported that when she began carrying the baby doll around him, he barked at it at first, but discontinued after a few days. He had also discontinued showing facial expressions of aggressive threat, which had been common prior to treatment. The couple decided to proceed with treatment.

When the baby was born, the husband brought various items home from the hospital for Sam to smell before the baby's arrival, thus helping him to become familiar with the baby's scent. When the baby was brought home, the couple greeted Sam and brought him a toy. Sam was curious about the baby and displayed no aggression. There were numerous visitors at the house during the first days after the baby's arrival. Sam was well behaved except for one incident when he growled at a relative who was staying for several days to assist. She stared at him and Sam looked away instead of staring back.

Six months after the initial visit, the owners reported that Sam was doing very well with them, the baby, and visitors. They described his progress as "really terrific." They had let Sam back on the bed after he had been kept off for several months. He was no longer aggressive to the couple in this context.

They had also had him in the bed simultaneously with the baby. While they were cautioned about the potential risks of this, Sam's behavior was so much improved that they were comfortable doing so. Sam had been introduced to the baby through a gradual process begun on the floor with mother, Sam, and the baby together during which

Sam was very well behaved and exhibited friendly curiosity and greeting behavior. Sam was only allowed around the baby under close supervision.

A year after the initial visit the owners reported no hostility toward the baby or defense of toys. There had been one biting incident that was inconsistent with the earlier history. Sam's leg became trapped, and he couldn't free himself. As the female owner was maneuvering his leg to free him, he bit her. This isolated incident was probably a pain- and/or fear-elicited bite that can occur with any dog.

As of this writing, Sam has been on fluoxetine for 21 months and continues to be well behaved. In fact, he interacts regularly and well with the baby, who is now a toddler, and the owners have many pictures of the two playing together. Repeated physical exams, blood chemistries, CBCs, urinalyses, and screenings for cognitive decline have been negative. The potential for unknown side effects arising with long-term use has been discussed with the owners. Given his participation in family activities and his interactions with the baby, combined with his dramatically different behavior since he has been on fluoxetine, they wish to continue medicating Sam indefinitely rather than take the risk that, as he is weaned off of medication, he might suddenly become aggressive again.

Case 2

Signalment

Frances was a one-year-old intact female rat, weighing 302 grams, who lived with a single female owner and another rat, Elsie. Two cats were in the household but were kept separate from the rats.

Presenting Complaint

Frances barbered her own forelimbs, one hindlimb, and, to a small degree, barbered Elsie under the chin; that is, she chewed fur until the skin was bare. While the barbered areas were hairless, there was no mutilation, although the owner reported that sometimes the skin appeared a little "raw." The skin on both of Frances' forelimbs was bare for a distance of 2–3 cm. By owner report, she spent about 10% of the day engaged in what appeared to be a combination of normal grooming and quick biting at her fur.

History

Frances had been obtained from a local humane society three months previously. Frances had spent most of the first nine months of her life at the society where, by owner report, cats were able to sit outside her cage and stare at her. She had been left at the humane society as part of an unwanted litter.

At her current home, Frances lived in a four-story ferret cage with Elsie. She had numerous toys, a wheel, a wooden box to hide in, a hammock, and PVC pipe available. The owner regularly offered new toys, such as a toilet paper roll with blueberries stuffed in the middle. The litter box had recycled paper bedding, and numerous rags were available for the rats to manipulate. Overall, management and care were of high quality, and both rats lived in an enriched environment.

The owner had previously had several pet rats and reported that Frances was less active than she had observed in other rats and was less willing to exit her cage to come out into the room for play time that was an option at least one hour a day. At this time, the owner would remove both rats from the cage and place them on her bed. Frances would try to run from the owner when the owner did this. While other rats, including Elsie, would commonly explore their environment in this situation, Frances would either hide under a pillow or run back to her cage and hide.

At the time of presentation Frances was on doxycycline for a probable mycoplasma infection.

Diagnosis

Frances was diagnosed with compulsive disorder.

Treatment

Frances was placed on paroxetine at 1 mg (1/2 ml; 3.3 mg/kg) per day. Paroxetine was selected in part because it is available in an orange-flavored suspension that the owner anticipated Frances would readily take, given her history of food preferences. If Frances had rejected the orange-flavored suspension, creating suspensions in other flavors would have been attempted.

While the owner already provided a high-quality environment, she was encouraged to make time outside the cage more interesting for Frances while providing her with opportunities to feel safe away from the main cage, for example, by setting up upside-down cardboard boxes with small entryways cut in the sides and food placed inside. She was to continue keeping the cats out of the section of the house where the rats were housed, because the sight and smell of cats may have been a stressor contributing to Frances's problem.

Frances also had a history of following Elsie's lead in exploring new objects. Therefore, the owner was instructed to continue social interactions with Elsie and introduce Elsie to new environmental situations, while allowing Frances to follow along.

Follow-up

Getting 1/2 ml of paroxetine solution into Frances proved to be problematic because the owner gave it by soaking a piece of bread with the medicine and offering it to Frances. While Frances readily ate the orange-flavored bread, the quantity necessary to soak up the entire 1/2 ml was high, and there was concern that she wouldn't consume her entire dose every day. Paroxetine was therefore compounded into a 1 mg/0.05 ml solution and Frances was given 0.05 ml daily.

Approximately three to four weeks after beginning medication, Frances had ceased chewing on her limbs and hair was beginning to grow out. She was also less timid, ran from the owner less, and had discontinued hiding under pillows when out of her cage. While she still often ran back to her cage, she would sometimes explore for short periods. The owner was instructed to close the door to Frances' cage when Frances was out, while still providing various "hides" around the room. This was to encourage Frances to continue initiating interactions with her environment.

Frances did well for the next two months. She continued to not barber, to be more investigative, and was also tamer. Five months after beginning treatment, the owner began having difficulty medicating her, possibly due to issues of flavor. While various flavors were tried in attempts to make medication administration easy and consistent,

Frances began showing panic behavior after she had gone 10 days without taking medication. Shortly thereafter, she became seriously ill from a combination of complications due to mycoplasma and the development of cancer, which resulted in her euthanasia.

Case 3

Signalment

Sally was a nine-year-old quarter horse mare.

Presenting Complaint

Sally's problem was aggression directed at people, horses, dogs, and cats. Sally bit, charged, kicked, and struck.

History

Sally had been obtained by her current owner at five years of age and was aggressive at the time of purchase. While she was very aggressive to people on the ground, she was well behaved under saddle and was an excellent show horse in hunter/jumper competition. When under saddle, she kept her ears forward and was consistently cooperative with her rider's requests.

Mistreatment as a young horse and administration of illegal drugs by previous owners was suspected but could not be directly confirmed. Additionally, a full brother of Sally's was known to have similar problems of aggression, but the relative importance of genetics versus management issues could not be evaluated.

At the time of presentation, Sally was consistently aggressive to all people on the ground. At the least, she would lay her ears back, and she would often threaten to bite, even if the people were out of reach. She would bite, kick, and strike if she had the opportunity, but was only handled by professionals and experienced amateurs who knew how to keep themselves as safe as possible and were willing to take the risks involved in handling such an aggressive horse. Four years of gentle handling by experienced horsemen had resulted in improvement in her aggression, in that it was less intense, though still frequent, but Sally had reached a plateau in her improvement.

Sally occasionally spooked at novel objects while being trail-ridden, but there was not a serious problem with this behavior.

Diagnosis

The exact cause of Sally's aggressiveness could not be confirmed. Learning and fear were probably significant contributing factors, because she appeared to have learned to keep people on the ground away from her by threatening them. Genetics and inappropriate medications may have contributed to her aggression.

Treatment

Initially, Sally was too dangerous to attempt any kind of structured behavior modification. Because she was not being shown competitively, the owner could concentrate on treating her problem, and because she was in good health, she was placed on fluoxetine, 80 mg daily. The contents of four 20-mg capsules were mixed into her feed, which she readily consumed.

Follow-up

After one month, Sally's aggressiveness had decreased to the point that she could be handled more safely. She exhibited mild sedation at first, in that she was slightly less active overall than she had been before, but there were no problems riding her. There were no other side effects. After two months on fluoxetine, the dose was increased to 100 mg daily, and systematic desensitization and counterconditioning was initiated. The owner could reliably get Sally to raise her ears and show a friendly face, while not making any threats, with the use of peppermints and carrot slivers. Therefore, these were used during behavior modification sessions. Because of the delayed timing of getting peppermints out of wrappers, clicker training was also initiated to allow the owner to have a means of immediately reinforcing any friendly interactions. Approximately 10 weeks after beginning treatment, people were sometimes able to walk past her stall without Sally's laying her ears back at them; that is, she would watch them with her ears pricked forward. It was recommended that the owner place a small basket of treats outside her stall so that passers-by could reinforce any expressions of friendly, rather than aggressive, behavior.

After five months on fluoxetine, two months at 80 mg/day and three months at 100 mg/day, Sally continues to make steady progress with her behavior modification. Aggression is becoming less intense and of shorter duration, as well as less frequent, but has not entirely resolved. She has not experienced any side effects beyond the initial mild sedation.

References

Albers LJ, Hahn RK and Reist C 2002. *Handbook of psychiatric drugs*, Current Clinical Strategies Publishing, Laguna Hills, California.

Altamura AC, Moro AR and Percudani M 1994. Clinical pharmacokinetics of fluoxetine. *Clinical Pharmacokinetics* 26(3): 201–214.

Borys DJ, Setzer SC, Ling LJ, Reisdorf JJ, Day LC and Krenzelok EP. 1992. Acute fluoxetine overdose: A report of 234 cases. *The American Journal of Emergency Medicine* 10(2): 115–120.

Brøsen K, Skjelbo E, Rasmussen BB, Poulsen HE and Loft S 1993. Fluvoxamine is a potent inhibitor of cytochrome P4501A2. *Biochemical Pharmacology* 45:1211–1214.

Brown TM, Skop BP and Mareth TR 1996. Pathophysiology and management of the serotonin syndrome. *The Annals of Pharmacotherapy* 30: 527–533.

Charney DS, Krystal JH, Delgado PL and Heninger GR 1990. Serotonin-specific drugs for anxiety and depressive disorders. *Annual Review of Medicine* 41: 437–446.

Ciribassi J, Luescher A, Pasloske S, Robertson-Plouch C, Zimmerman A and Kaloostian-Whittymore L 2003. Comparative bioavailability of fluoxetine after transdermal and oral administration to healthy cats. *American Journal of Veterinary Research* 64(8): 994–998.

Claassen V 1983. Review of the animal pharmacology and pharmacokinetics of fluvoxamine. *British Journal of Clinical Pharmacology* 15: 349S–355S.

Claassen V, Davies JE, Hertting G and Placheta P 1977. Fluvoxamine, a specific 5-hydroxytryptamine uptake inhibitor. *British Journal of Pharmacology* 60: 505–516.

Coccaro EF, Astill JL, Herbert JL and Schut AG 1990. Fluoxetine treatment of impulsive aggression in DSM-III-R personality disorder patients. *Journal of Clinical Psychopharmacology* 10(5): 373–375.

Cornelius JR, Soloff PH, Perel JM and Ulrich RF 1991. A preliminary trial of fluoxetine in refractory borderline patients. *Journal of Clinical Psychopharmacology* 11(2): 116–120.

Crewe HK, Lennard MS, Tucker GT, Woods FR and Haddock RE 1992. The effect of selective serotonin reuptake inhibitors on cytochrome P4502D6 (CYP2D6) activity in human liver microsomes. *British Journal of Clinical Pharmacology* 34: 262–265.

Davies TS and Kluwe WM 1998. Preclinical toxicological evaluation of sertraline hydrochloride. *Drug and Chemical Toxicology* 21(4): 521–537.

Deckel AW 1996. Behavioral changes in *Anolis carolinensis* following injection with fluoxetine. *Behavioural Brain Research* 78: 175–182.

Deckel AW and Jevitts E 1997. Left vs. right-hemisphere regulation of aggressive behaviors in *Anolis carolinensis*: Effects of eye-patching and fluoxetine administration. *The Journal of Experimental Zoology* 278: 9–21.

DeVane CL 1994. Pharmacogenetics and drug metabolism of newer antidepressant agents. *Journal of Clinical Psychiatry* 55(12) (suppl.): 38–47.

Dodman NH 2000. Behavior case of the month. *Journal of the American Veterinary Medical Association* 217(10): 1468–1472.

Dodman NH, Donnelly R, Shuster L, Mertens P, Rand W and Miczek K 1996. Use of Fluoxetine to treat dominance aggression in dogs. *Journal of the American Veterinary Medical Association* 209: 1585–632.

Eli Lilly 2004. Prozac® product information. *Physicians' desk reference,* pp. 1840–1846, Montvale PDR, Montvale, New Jersey.

Ferris CF, Melloni RH, Koppel G, Perry KW, Fuller RW and Delville Y 1997. Vasopressin/serotonin interactions in the anterior hypothalamus control aggressive behavior in golden hamsters. *The Journal of Neuroscience* 17(11): 4331–4340.

Forest Laboratories 2002. Celexa Product Information 2004 *Physicians desk reference,* pp. 1292–1296, Thomson PDR, Montvale, New Jersey.

Gorman JM 2002. Treatment of generalized anxiety disorder. *Journal of Clinical Psychiatry* 63(suppl. 8): 17–23.

Hartmann L 1995. Cats as possible obsessive-compulsive disorder and medication models. *American Journal of Psychiatry* 152: 1236.

Heiligenstein JH, Beasley CM Jr. and Potvin JH 1993. Fluoxetine not associated with increased aggression in controlled clinical trials. *International Clinical Psychopharmacology* 8: 277–280.

Hugo C, Seier J, Mdhluli C, Daniels W, Harvey BH, Du Toit D, Wolfe-Coote S, Nel D and Stein DJ 2003. Fluoxetine decreases stereotypic behavior in primates. *Progress in Neuro-Psychopharmacology & Biological Psychiatry* 27(4): 639–643.

Karel R 1994. Fluoxetine use in dogs provides animal model for human mental disorders. *Psychiatric News* 29: 12.

Katofiasc MA, Nissen J, Audia JE and Thor KB 2002. Comparison of the effects of serotonin selective, norepinephrine selective, and dual serotonin and norepinephrine reuptake inhibitors on lower urinary tract function in cats. *Life Sciences* 71: 1227–1236.

Kavoussi RJ, Liu J, and Coccaro EF 1994. An open trial of sertraline in personality disordered patients with impulsive aggression. *Journal of Clinical Psychiatry* 55(4): 137–141.

Larson ET and Summers CH 2001. Serotonin reverses dominant social status. *Behavioural Brain Research* 121: 95–102.

Lustman PJ, Freedland KE, Griffith LS and Clouse RE 2000. Fluoxetine for depression in diabetes—A randomized double-blind placebo-controlled trial. *Diabetes Care* 23(5): 618–623.

Markowitz PI 1992. Effect of fluoxetine on self-injurious behavior in the developmentally disabled: A preliminary study. *Journal of Clinical Psychopharmacology* 12: 27–31.

Matuszcyk JV, Larsson K and Eriksson E 1998. The selective serotonin reuptake inhibitor fluoxetine reduces sexual motivation in male rats. *Pharmacology Biochemistry and Behavior* 60(2): 527–532.

Martin TG 1996. Serotonin syndrome. *Annals of Emergency Medicine* 28(5): 520–526.

Mertens PA 1997. Pharmacological treatment of feather picking in pet birds. *Proceedings of the First International Conference on Veterinary Behavioural Medicine Birmingham,* UK, pp. 209–211.

Michelson D, Tamura R, Tepner R and Potter WZ 1998. Physiological correlates of SSRI withdrawal: Evidence from a controlled, randomized trial of fluoxetine, sertraline, and paroxetine. *Proceedings of the 37th annual meeting of the American College of Neuropsychopharmacology*, Las Croabas, Puerto Rico, p. 314.

Mills KC 1995. Serotonin syndrome. *American Family Physician* 52: 1475–1482.

Morrison JL, Chien C, Riggs KW, Gruber N and Rurak D. 2002. Effect of maternal fluoxetine administration on uterine blood flow, fetal blood gas status, and growth. *Pediatric Research* 51(4): 433–442.

Nulman I, Rovet J, Stewart D, Wolpin J, Loebstein M, Pace AP, Fried S and Koren G 2001. Neurodevelopment of children exposed to maternal antidepressant drugs throughout gestation: A prospective controlled study. *Clinical Pharmacology and Therapeutics* 69: 31.

Nurnberg HG, Keith SJ and Paxton DM 1997. Consideration of the relevance of ethological animal models for human repetitive behavioral spectrum disorders. *Society of Biological Psychiatry* 41: 226–229.

Oberlander TF, Grunau RE, Fitzgerald C, Ellwood A-L, Misri S, Rurak D and Riggs KW 2002. Prolonged prenatal psychotropic medication exposure alters neonatal acute pain response. *Pediatric Research* 51(4): 443–453.

Olivier B and Mos J 1992. Rodent models of aggressive behavior and sertotonergic drugs. *Progress in Neuro-Psychopharmacology & Biological Psychiatry* 16: 847–870.

Overall KL 1995. Animal behavior case of the month. *Journal of the American Veterinary Medical Association* 206(5): 629–632.

Overall K 2004. Paradigms for pharmacologic use as a treatment component in feline behavioral medicine. *Journal of Feline Medicine and Surgery* 6: 29–42.

Pfizer Inc. 2004. Zoloft(r) product information. *Physicians' desk reference*, pp. 2690–2696, Thomson PDR, Montvale, New Jersey.

Pies RW and Popli AP 1995. Self-injurious behavior: Pathophysiology and implications for treatment. *Journal of Clinical Psychiatry* 56(12): 580–588.

Pollock BG 2001. Citalopram: A comprehensive review. *Expert Opinion on Pharmacotherapy* 2(4): 681–698.

Price JS, Waller PC, Wood SM and MacKay AVP 1996. A comparison of the post-marketing safety of four selective serotonin re-uptake inhibitors including the investigation of symptoms occurring on withdrawal. *British Journal of Clinical Pharmacology* 42: 757–763.

Pryor P 2003. Animal behavior case of the month. *Journal of the American Veterinary Medical Association* 223(8): 1117–1119.

Pryor PA, Hart BL, Cliff DC and Bain MJ 2001. Effects of a selective serotonin reuptake inhibitor on urine spraying behavior in cats. *Journal of the American Veterinary Medical Association* 219(11): 1557–1561.

Rapoport JL, Ryland DH and Kriete M 1992. Drug treatment of canine acral lick: An animal model of obsessive-compulsive disorder. *Archives of General Psychiatry* 49: 517–521.

Reisner IR 2003. Diagnosis of canine generalized anxiety disorder and its management with behavioral modification and fluoxetine or paroxetine: A retrospective summary of clinical experience (2001–2003). *Journal of the American Animal Hospital Association* 39: 512.

Reisner IR, Mann JJ, Stanley M, Huang Y, Houpt KA 1996. Comparison of cerebrospinal fluid monoamine metabolite levels in dominant-aggressive and non-aggressive dogs. *Brain Research* 714(1–2): 57–64.

Reist C, Nakamura K, Sagart E, Sokolski KN and Fujimoto KA 2003. Impulsive aggressive behavior: Open-label treatment with citalopram. *Journal of Clinical Psychiatry* 64(1): 81–85.

Romatowski J 1998. Two cases of fluoxetine-responsive behavior disorders in cats. *Feline Practice* 26: 14–15.

Sanchez C and Hyttel J 1994. Isolation-induced aggression in mice: effects of 5-hydroxytryptamine uptake inhibitors and involvement of postsynaptic 5-HT_{1A} receptors. *European Journal of Pharmacology* 264: 241–247.

Seibert LM 2004. Animal behavior case of the month. *Journal of the American Veterinary Medical Association* 224(9): 1433–1435.

SmithKline Beecham Pharmaceuticals 2004. Paroxetine(r) product information. *Physicians desk reference,* pp.1590–1594, Montvale PDR, Montvale, New Jersey.

Solvay Pharmaceuticals 2002. Luvox(r) product information. *Physicians desk reference,* pp. 3256–3261, Montvale PDR, Montvale, New Jersey.

Stein DJ, Mendelsohn I, Potocnik MB, Van Kradenberg J and Wessels C 1998. Use of the selective serotonin reuptake inhibitor citalopram in a possible animal analogue of obsessive-compulsive disorder. *Depression and Anxiety* 8: 39–42.

Stein DJ, Shoulberg N, Helton K and Hollander E 1992. The neuroethological approach to obsessive-compulsive disorder. *Comprehensive Psychiatry* 33: 274–281.

Stein DJ and Stahl S 2000. Serotonin and anxiety: Current models. *International Clinical Psychopharmacology* 15(suppl. 2): S1–S6.

Walsh M-T and Dinan TG 2001. Selective serotonin reuptake inhibitors and violence: A review of the available evidence. *Acta Psychiatrica Scandinavica* 104: 84–91.

Wynchank D and Berk M 1998. Fluoxetine treatment of acral lick dermatitis in dogs: A placebo-controlled randomized double blind trial. *Depression and Anxiety* 8: 21–23.

Chapter Six
Azapirones

Action

Azapirones are serotonin 1A agonists.

Overview of Indications

Azapirones can be used for a variety of anxiety disorders and behaviors that may be affected by chronic anxiety, including general anxiety disorder, marking, separation anxiety, and subordinate or timid cats that are the regular recipients of aggression. Azapirones may be helpful in certain cases of aggression that are triggered by excessively timid behavior by one animal, but should be used cautiously for this problem.

Contraindications, Side Effects, and Adverse Events

Buspirone is the only azapirone that is commercially available in the United States. See the detailed discussion under buspirone below.

Adverse Drug Interactions

Azapirones should not be given in combination with monoamine oxidase inhibitors (MAOIs).

Overdose

See information under buspirone below.

Clinical Guidelines

Buspirone is anxioselective with no substantial sedative effect. While there may be a rapid response, it may require one to four weeks to take effect. The patient should be medicated daily, rather than on an as-needed basis. Doses for dogs, cats, and rabbits are given in Table 6.1.

Table 6.1 Dose and cost of buspirone given orally for various species

Species	Dose	Example	Cost for 30-day supply
Dog	0.5–2.0 mg/kg q8–24h	20-kg dog 30-mg, #30 Give 1/2 q12h	$$$$$$
Cat	2.5–7.5 mg/cat q12h or 0.5–1.0 mg/kg q12h	5-kg cat 5 mg, #30 Give 1/2 q12h	$$
Rabbit	0.25–1.0 mg/kg q12h		

Azapirones are commonly combined with selective serotonin reuptake inhibitors (SSRIs) or tricyclic antidepressants (TCAs) in patients that do not respond to either of those two drugs alone. This topic is discussed in further detail in chapter 15.

Specific Medications

I. Buspirone

Chemical Compound: 8-[4-[4-(2-pyrimidinyl)-1-piperazinyl]butyl]-8-azaspiro[4,5] decane-7,9-dione monohydrochloride
DEA Classification: Not a controlled substance
Preparations: Generally available as 5-, 10-, 15-, and 30-mg tablets. The 15- and 30-mg tablets are scored so that they can readily be split into two or three pieces.

Clinical Pharmacology

Buspirone is a serotonin 1A partial agonist that has been available in the United States since 1987. It is believed to exert its action by blocking presynaptic and postsynaptic serotonin-1A (5-HT$_{1A}$) receptors. It fully antagonizes presynaptic receptors, but only partially antagonizes postsynaptic 5-HT$_{1A}$ receptors. It also down-regulates 5-HT$_2$ receptors (Eison 1989; Cole and Yonkers 2004). It has moderate affinity for D2-dopamine receptors in the brain (Peroutka 1985). It does not have anticonvulsant, muscle relaxant, or sedative effects and is therefore often referred to as anxioselective. The anxiolytic effect appears to be due, at least in part, to action on neurons in the dorsal raphe (Trulson and Trulson 1986).

In humans, buspirone has extensive first-pass metabolism. Food slightly decreases the extent of presystemic clearance of buspirone, but this effect is not known to have any clinical significance. Buspirone is given with or without food (Bristol-Myers Squibb Co. 2000). It reaches maximum concentrations in about 1 hour in humans, with a subsequent elimination half-life of about 2.5 hours.

Buspirone is primarily metabolized by oxidation by the P450 liver enzyme CYP3A4. It has one pharmacologically active metabolite, 1-pyrimidinylpiperazine (1-PP), and several inactive metabolites. In animal tests, there has been found to be about 20 times as much 1-PP as the parent compound in the plasma, but 1-PP is about one-fourth as active (Bristol-Myers Squibb Co. 1999). Urinary excretion of unchanged buspirone accounts for about 0.1% of the initial dose. Thus, it is eliminated almost entirely in a biotransformed state (Caccia et al. 1986).

Buspirone has nonlinear pharmacokinetics so that repeated dosing results in higher blood levels than would be predicted from studies of blood levels after a single dose is given (Bristol-Myers Squibb Co. 1999).

Buspirone does not displace highly protein-bound medications such as phenytoin, warfarin, and propranolol. Thus, concurrent medication with buspirone does not generate the risk of inducing higher plasma levels of such drugs (Bristol-Myers Squibb Co. 1999).

No significant difference has been found between geriatric and younger adult subjects in the pharmacokinetics of buspirone. Both liver and kidney disease result in decreased clearance and higher levels of buspirone (Bristol-Myers Squibb Co. 1999). Buspirone appears to have no significant effect on blood sugar levels (Dixit et al. 2001). In contrast to benzodiazepines, it stimulates rather than depresses respiration (Garner et al. 1989). Buspirone does not appear to have cardiovascular effects at clinical anxiolytic doses (Hanson et al. 1986).

In horses, buspirone and three major metabolite classes can be detected in the urine 1 to 12 hours after administration (Stanley 2000).

Uses in Humans

Buspirone is used to treat general anxiety disorder in humans.

In humans with general anxiety disorder, buspirone is more effective than placebo and similar in efficacy to diazepam and clorazepate, although with a slightly slower onset of action (Goldberg et al. 1979; Rickels et al. 1982, 1988). The benefit of buspirone over the benzodiazepines includes avoidance of excessive sedation and physical dependence. Use of buspirone likewise avoids the sedation and anticholinergic side effects of TCAs, which are also used in general anxiety disorder. It is also more effective than placebo in the treatment of major depression with moderate anxiety (Fabre 1990; Rickels et al. 1990).

Contraindications

Buspirone should be used cautiously with MAOIs (Cole and Yonkers 2004). In humans, co-administration of buspirone and erythromycin results in substantial increases in plasma levels of buspirone with concurrent increases in side effects. The implications of this finding in nonhuman animals are unknown. Nevertheless, if a patient being chronically medicated with buspirone must be given erythromycin, the dose of buspirone should be decreased. Ideally, other antibiotics that do not exhibit this interaction should be selected. Co-administration with itraconazole also results in substantial increases in plasma levels of buspirone (Bristol-Myers Squibb Co. 1999).

Side Effects

Side effects are uncommon, which is one advantage to the use of buspirone. Sedation does not occur in humans, but has been reported in nonhuman animals (e.g., see Hart et al. 1993). In humans, the more common side effects are dizziness, insomnia, nervousness, nausea, headache, and fatigue. One cat placed on buspirone by the author began hiding in the closet. This may have been a behavioral response to increased anxiety, analogous to the nervousness reported in some human patients. Mania has also occasionally been reported in humans (Liegghio and Yeragani 1988; McDaniel et al. 1990; Price and Bielefeld 1989). As with all medications, some individuals may have unique, adverse reactions to buspirone.

Several desirable side effects commonly occur in cats. Many cats on buspirone begin behaving in ways that their owners often summarize as "more affectionate." Specifically, they will stay near the owner more, rub the owner's limbs more, climb in the owner's lap more, and remain in the owner's lap for longer periods of time than before. The end point of this effect appears to be related to the baseline. Thus, cats that were already affectionate become intensely affectionate, whereas cats that were previously not very sociable begin exhibiting some degree of social behavior. While the cat is on medication, it is capable of learning, and the social dynamic between cat and owner changes so that many cats retain increased levels of social behavior even after the medication is discontinued, although it may decrease from peak levels that occur while on buspirone.

Unlike the benzodiazepine anxiolytics, buspirone does not produce dependence, even after several months of treatment (Robinson 1985).

In rats and mice given high doses of buspirone for 24 and 18 months, respectively, there was no evidence of carcinogenicity. Studies of mutagenicity have also revealed no such effect (Bristol-Myers Squibb Co. 1999).

In studies of rats and rabbits given high doses of buspirone during pregnancy, there was no impairment of fertility or damage to the fetuses (Bristol-Myers Squibb 1999).

Buspirone is excreted in milk (Bristol-Myers Squibb Co. 1999).

The LD_{50} (the dose that kills half of the animals tested), given orally, in dogs is approximately 300 mg/kg. Death results from compromised respiratory function (Kadota et al. 1990).

Overdose

Conduct gastric lavage and provide supportive treatment if an overdose is given. There is no specific antidote (Bristol-Myers Squibb Co. 1999).

Dogs given 3 or 10 mg/kg may exhibit emesis. The 10 mg/kg dose produces significantly increased urinary volume and electrolyte excretion (Hanson et al. 1986).

Other Information

Buspirone causes decreased territorial and maternal aggression in rats concurrently with a substantial decrease in social activity and interest, suggesting that the decreased aggression is nonspecific (Olivier and Mos 1992). On the other hand, it causes no significant changes in social or solitary behavior patterns of rhesus monkeys (*Macaca mulatta*) when given at a dose of 5–10 mg/kg daily PO. This is an interesting example of species differences in response because it contrasts with the increased social interaction noted clinically in the domestic cat.

Buspirone has also been observed to decrease territorial aggression in rats but not in mice (Mos et al. 1992; Gao and Cutler 1993).

Effects Documented in Nonhuman Animals
Cats

Absorption of buspirone is poor when administered transdermally as opposed to orally. Therefore, until such time as a transdermal administration technique is developed that is proven to be effective, it is recommended that buspirone always be given orally (Mealey et al. 2004).

At a dose of 5 mg/kg PO buspirone causes increased wakefulness and decreased REM sleep in cats (Hashimoto et al. 1992).

Buspirone, at an average dose of 0.46 mg/kg, blocks motion sickness in cats (Lucot and Crampton 1987). Pet cats susceptible to car sickness and other forms of motion sickness may benefit from a dose of approximately 1.0 mg/kg prior to trips since this will alleviate vomiting and may help with anxiety, although the latter effect may only occur with multiple doses.

Hart et al. (1993) conducted an open trial of the effectiveness of buspirone on spraying and urine marking in cats. The subjects were 47 castrated males and 15 spayed females. Forty-two of the males were from multiple cat households while only five were from single cat households. Thirteen of the females were from multiple cat households while only two were from single cat households. Cats were initially medicated with 2.5 mg/cat q12h PO. If this dose resulted in cessation or substantial reduction by the second week, it was maintained for eight weeks. If the initial dose was not sufficiently effective, the dose was increased to 5 mg/cat q12h PO for an additional two weeks. If the spraying or marking was substantially decreased or ceased at this higher dose, the cats were maintained on buspirone at this dose for eight weeks. Cats that initially stopped spraying on the 5-mg dose, but subsequently resumed spraying during the eight weeks, were increased to 7.5 mg/cat q12h.

After the completion of eight weeks of treatment, the dose of buspirone was gradually decreased over a two-week period. If the cat continued to not spray, medication was discontinued entirely. If the cat resumed spraying at a given lower dose, the cat was then treated for 6–12 months at the lowest effective dose.

Thirty-two of the 62 cats treated with buspirone responded favorably. Thus, about one-half of the cats had a positive response. The majority of cats (81%) were given the 5-mg dose and 12 cats were given the 7.5-mg dose. Twenty-one of the responders exhibited complete cessation of spraying, whereas the remaining 11 responders exhibited a decrease of 75% or more. There was a clear effect of household type. Thirty-two of the 55 cats from multiple cat households responded, whereas none of the 7 cats from single cat households responded. There was no significant effect of sex, although proportionately more females than males responded favorably. Further studies with larger numbers of cats would be required to determine if this trend would become significant with an adequate sample size.

Of the responders, contact was maintained with the owners of 30 cats after treatment. When treatment was discontinued, half of these resumed spraying and half did not resume spraying. When the relapsing cats were placed back on buspirone, 2 failed to respond to the second treatment, while 13 responded.

Owners of 4 of the 62 cats reported sedation. Nine of the cats exhibited increased aggression toward other cats. In at least in some of these cases, the cats that became more aggressive had previously been withdrawn and timid, particularly in their relationship with other cats. While on buspirone, they became more assertive in their social interactions. Five of the cats became agitated. Twelve owners reported increased friendliness toward humans.

Forty of the cats had been previously treated with progesterone. Of these, 30 were nonresponders to progesterone. Fourteen of the 30 that had not responded to progesterone responded to buspirone. Seventeen cats had been previously treated with diazepam, 8 of these being nonresponders. Of the diazepam nonresponders, only 2 responded to buspirone.

While buspirone has approximately the same initial efficacy as diazepam in the treatment of spraying, there is a lower recidivism rate. Specifically, only about 50% of the cats responding to buspirone resume spraying when treatment is discontinued, while over 90% of cats that respond to diazepam relapse when treatment is discontinued (Cooper and Hart 1992). Given the lower incidence of serious side effects and lower rate of recidivism, buspirone is clearly a better choice than diazepam for the treatment of urine spraying and urine marking in cats.

Sawyer et al. (1999) reported on four cats with psychogenic alopecia that were treated with buspirone at 5 mg/cat q12h PO. While the frequency of grooming decreased in one cat, the problem resumed when treatment was discontinued. The problem stopped again when treatment with buspirone was resumed at a dose of 2.5 mg/kg q12h PO. While the cat was on treatment for a second time, the owner moved to a new home. When medication was discontinued for a second time, the problem remained resolved. This result begs the question of whether the second treatment cured the problem or whether the problem was caused by environmental stresses at the original home. The other three cats treated with buspirone did not respond at all. While these poor results suggest that buspirone may not be a good treatment for psychogenic alopecia, the sample size is too small to come to any conclusions other than that buspirone may be effective in some cases.

Dogs

Overall (1995) reported on one case of a dog with multiple behavior problems, including fear of approaches by strangers. As part of the overall treatment program, buspirone was used (10 mg q24h PO, 23-kg dog; 0.4 mg/kg daily) for the fear of strangers. The dog became less fearful and made a clear transition to friendly behavior, jumping up and licking faces, and playing with toys with strangers. This response is similar to the increased friendliness to humans seen in cats.

Marder (1991) has used buspirone in combination with acepromazine or diazepam in intense fear-inducing situations, such as thunderstorms, with no serious side effects, although she does not state the effectiveness of the combination. Acepromazine was also used at a lowered dose. Marder (1991) has also used buspirone in dogs with mild separation anxiety.

Overall (1994) used buspirone at 2.5 mg q12h PO to successfully treat spraying in a low-ranking cat that had previously responded to diazepam, but had stopped responding. The patient had also been socially isolated by its own volition from other cats in the household. While on buspirone, the cat not only stopped spraying, but began venturing into other parts of the house. The cat could not be weaned off buspirone without resumption of the spraying. At the time of publication, the cat had been on buspirone for 16 months with no adverse effects.

Horses

Because buspirone does not have sedative or muscle-relaxant side effects it is a better drug for treating anxiety in horses than the benzodiazepines. Dodman (personal communication, 1996) has treated horses with buspirone at up to 250 mg per day per horse with no adverse side effects. Although it may be useful in the treatment of anxiety disorders, it must not be used in performance horses preparing for competition. A 50-mg dose can be detected in the urine (Stanley 2000).

Rabbits

The rabbit cerebral cortex has 5-HT$_{1A}$ receptors, and the binding rate of buspirone is similar to the binding rate of buspirone in rats and humans (Weber et al. 1997). Rabbits treated with buspirone at 0.05 mg/kg day PO for one month do not exhibit any changes in blood sugar (Dixit et al. 2001). Buspirone may be a useful treatment for timid, anxious rabbits.

References

Bristol-Myers Squibb Company. 2000. Buspar product information. In *Physicians desk reference*, pp. 820–822, Medical Economics Co. Inc., Montvale, NJ.

Caccia S, Conti I, Viganò G and Garattini S. 1986. 1-(2-Pyrimidinyl)-piperazine as active metabolite of buspirone in man and rat. *Pharmacology* 33: 46–51.

Cole KO and Yonkers KA 2004. Nonbenzodiazepine anxiolytics. In *Textbook of psychopharmacology*, pp. 231–244, edited by AF Schatzberg and CB Nemeroff, American Psychiatric Press, Washington, DC.

Cooper LL, and Hart BL. 1992. Comparison of diazepam with progestin for effectiveness in suppression of urine spraying behavior in cats. *Journal of the American Veterinary Medical Association* 200: 797–801.

Dixit RK, Puri JN, Sharma MK, Jain IP, Singh S, Ansari NA and Singh SP. 2001. Effect of anxiolytics on blood sugar level in rabbits. *Indian Journal of Experimental Biology* 39: 378–380.

Eison MS. 1989. Azapirones: Clinical uses of serotonin partial agonists. *Family Practice Recertification* 11(9)(suppl.): 8–16.

Fabre LF. 1990. Buspirone in the management of major depression: A placebo-controlled comparison. *Journal of Clinical Psychiatry* 51 (9)(suppl.): 55–61.

Garner SJ, Eldridge FL, Wagner PG and Dowell RT 1989. Buspirone, an anxiolytic drug that stimulates respiration. *The American Review of Respiratory Disease* 139(4): 946–950.

Gao B and Cutler MG 1993. Buspirone increases social investigation in pair-housed male mice—comparison with the effects of chloridazepoxide. *Neuropharmacology* 32 (5): 429–437.

Goldberg HL and Finnerty RJ 1979. The comparative efficacy of buspirone and diazepam in the treatment of anxiety. *American Journal of Psychiatry* 136: 1184–1187.

Hanson RC, Braselton JP, Hayes DC, Snyder RW, White JB and Deitchman D 1986. Cardiovascular and renal effects of buspirone in several animal models. *General Pharmacology* 17(3): 267–274.

Hart BL, Eckstein RA, Powell KL and Dodman NH 1993. Effectiveness of buspirone on urine spraying and inappropriate urination in cats. *Journal of the American Veterinary Medical Association* 203(2): 254–258.

Hashimoto T, Hamada C, Wada T and Fukuda N 1992. Comparative study on the behavioral and EEG changes induced by diazepam, buspirone and a novel anxioselective anxiolytic, DN-2327, in the cat. *Neuropsychobiology* 26:89–99.

Kadota T, Kawano S, Chikazawa H, Kondoh H, Kuroyanagi K, Ohta S, Ishikawa K, Kai S, Kohmura H, Takahashi N, Funahashi N, Ochiai T, Shimizu K, Mori H, Taniura A and Nakazawa M 1990. Acute toxicity study of buspirone hydrochloride in mice, rats and dogs. *The Journal of Toxicological Sciences* 15: 1–14.

Liegghio NE and Yeragani VK. 1988. Buspirone-induced hypomania: A case report. *Journal of Clinical Psychopharmacology* 8: 226–227.

Lucot JB and Crampton GH 1987. Buspirone blocks motion sickness and xylazine-induced emesis in the cat. *Aviation, Space, and Environmental Medicine* 58: 989–991.

Marder AR 1991. Psychotropic drugs and behavioral therapy. In *Veterinary clinics of North America: Small animal practice*, 21(2), pp. 329–342, edited by AR Marder and V Voith. WB Saunders, Philadelphia.

McDaniel JS, Ninan PT and Magnuson JV 1990. Possible induction of mania by buspirone. *American Journal of Psychiatry* 147: 125–126.

Mealey KL, Peck KE, Bennett BS, Sellon RK, Swinney GR, Melzer K, Gokhale SA and Krone TM 2004. Systemic absorption of amitriptylline and buspirone after oral and transdermal administration to healthy cats. *Journal of Veterinary Internal Medicine* 18(1): 43–46.

Mos J, Olivier B, and Tulp MT 1992. Ethopharmacological studies differentiate the effects of various serotonergic compounds on aggression in rats. *Drug Development Research* 26: 343–360.

Olivier B and Mos J 1992. Rodent models of aggressive behavior and serotonergic drugs. *Progress in Neuro-Psychopharmacology & Biological Psychiatry* 16: 847–870.

Overall KL 1994. Animal behavior case of the month. *Journal of the American Veterinary Medical Association.* 205(5): 694–696.

Overall KL 1995. Animal behavior case of the month. *Journal of the American Veterinary Medical Association* 206(5): 629–632.

Peroutka SJ 1985. Selective interaction of novel anxiolytics with 5-hydroxytryptamine$_{1A}$ receptors. *Biological Psychiatry* 20: 971–979.

Price WA and Bielefeld M 1989. Buspirone-induced mania. *Journal of Clinical Psychopharmacology* 9:150–151.

Rickels K, Weisman K, Norstad N, Singer M, Stoltz D, Brown A and Danton J 1982. Buspirone and diazepam in anxiety: A controlled study. *Journal of Clinical Psychiatry.* 43(12): 81–86.

Rickels K, Schweizer E, Csanalosi I, Case WG and Chung H. 1988. Long-term treatment of anxiety and risk of withdrawal: Prospective comparison of clorazepate and buspirone. *Archives of General Psychiatry* 45: 444–450.

Rickels K, Amsterdam J, Clary C, Hassman J, London J, Puzzuoli G and Schweizer E 1990. Buspirone in depressed outpatients: A controlled study. *Psychopharmacology Bulletin* 26(2): 163–167.

Robinson DS 1985. Buspirone: Long-term therapy. Proceedings of *Anxiety Disorders, an International Update*, April 18–19, Dösseldorf, Germany, pp.93–99, Bristol-Myers, New York, NY.

Sawyer LS, Moon-Fanelli AA and Dodman NH 1999. Psychogenic alopecia in cats: 11 cases (1993–1996). *Journal of the American Veterinary Medical Association* 214: 71–74.

Stanley SMR 2000. Equine metabolism of buspirone studied by high-performance liquid chromatography/mass spectrometry. *Journal of Mass Spectrometry* 35: 402–407.

Trulson ME and Trulson TJ 1986. Buspirone decreases the activity of serotonin-containing neurons in the dorsal raphe in freely-moving cats. *Neuropharmacology* 25(11): 1261–1266.

Weber JT, Hayataka K, O'Connor M-F and Parker KK 1997. Rabbit cerebral cortex 5HT1a receptors. *Comparative Biochemistry and Physiology Part C, Pharmacology, toxicology & endocrinology* 117(1): 19–24.

Chapter Seven
Biogenic Amine Transmitters: Acetylcholine, Norepinephrine, and Dopamine

Acetylcholine

Acetylcholine was the first compound to be identified as a neurotransmitter in the peripheral nervous system; however, knowledge concerning the anatomical organization of cholinergic neurons lagged behind other transmitter substances due to the lack of suitable techniques for mapping cholinergic pathways. These technical obstacles have been surmounted in recent years.

Acetylcholine is synthesized in cholinergic neurons by a reaction catalyzed by the cytosolic enzyme choline acetyltransferase (CAT). This linkage of choline and an acetate group provided by acetyl-coenzyme A (CoA) is not, however, the rate-limiting step in the biosynthesis of acetylcholine; rather, the high-affinity transport of choline from the extracellular medium by a specific transporter protein represents the rate-limiting step. Acetylcholine is stored in vesicles in cholinergic terminals and released into the synaptic cleft by exocytosis (Figure 7.1). The proteins involved in this exocytotic release of acetylcholine are the targets for botulinum toxin; the therapeutic actions of Botox in the treatment of neuromuscular disorders derives from the ability of this toxin to block the release of acetylcholine from cholinergic neuron terminals (Coffield, 2003). Acetylcholine released from neurons into the synaptic cleft is hydrolyzed by the membrane-bound enzyme, acetylcholinesterase, which represents the mechanism for termination of the signal in cholinergic neurotransmission. This distinguishes cholinergic neurons from those of other biogenic amines where the signal is terminated by the high-affinity reuptake of the transmitter. Acetylcholine is the neurotransmitter of all autonomic ganglia, postganglionic parasympathetic synapses, the neuromuscular junction, and cholinergic neurons in the central nervous system.

Cholinergic pathways in the brain have now been identified by histochemical and neurochemical techniques. One important cholinergic system sends projections to the cerebral cortex (corticopetal) from the nucleus basalis of Meynert and the substantia innominata (BMSI) in the basal forebrain (Sarter and Bruno 1999). These projections terminate throughout the cerebral cortex, and their degeneration in senile dementia and Alzheimer's disease has been demonstrated to be correlated with the degree of cognitive decline. The acetylcholine content of the brain in Alzheimer's patients at postmortem is profoundly reduced. These observations have led to the cholinergic hypothesis of cognitive decline in senile dementia that has served as the basis for pharmacological attempts to ameliorate learning and memory deficits by restoration of cholinergic neurotransmission. One pharmacologic strategy for augmenting cholinergic transmission has been the use of inhibitors of acetylcholine esterase (ACHE; see

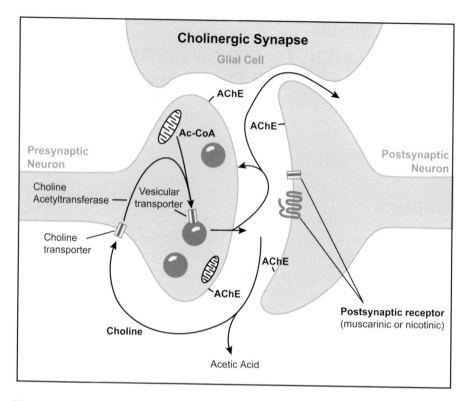

Figure 7.1 Schematic representation of a cholinergic synapse in the central nervous system. The precursor for acetylcholine (ACh) synthesis is choline. ACh is synthesized from choline and acetyl CoA by the enzyme choline acetyltransferase. The ACh is stored in and released from vesicles. Synaptic ACh activates postsynaptic receptors comprised of both muscarinic and nicotinic subtypes. The synaptic action of ACh is terminated by the enzyme acetyl cholinesterase (AChE) through hydrolysis to acetate and choline. The choline is salvaged by a high-affinity transporter for reutilization in the syntheses of ACh.

Figure 7.2). Inhibition of this enzyme prolongs the half-life of acetylcholine in the synapse and therefore enhances cholinergic transmission. Drugs such as tacrine, donepezil (Aricept), and rivastigmine (Exelon) are ACHE inhibitors (ACHEI) that have been used in the treatment of cognitive dysfunction associated with Alzheimer's disease. These drugs produce modest beneficial effects for periods of approximately one year, but do not prevent the progressive deterioration of mental function in Alzheimer's patients. Inhibition of ACHE has, moreover, a high propensity for adverse effects, and a significant fraction of patients withdraw from treatment due to side effects.

Cholinergic receptors that mediate the synaptic actions of acetylcholine are either muscarinic or nicotinic cholinergic receptors. The muscarinic receptors are members of the G protein-coupled receptor family, and five subtypes of muscarinic cholinergic receptors have been cloned and characterized. The alkaloids, atropine and scopolamine, act as nonselective, competitive antagonists of these muscarinic receptors. Both atropine and scopolamine are capable of disrupting working memory in humans and animals through their antimuscarinic actions in the cerebral cortex and hippocam-

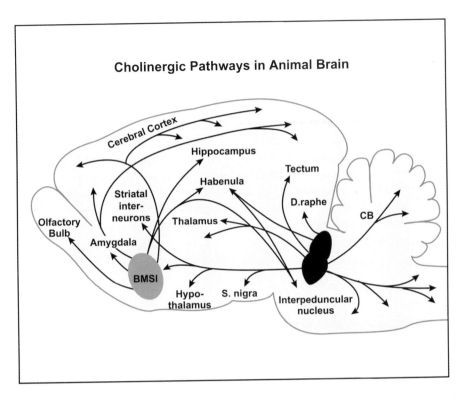

Figure 7.2 Schematic diagram of the cholinergic pathways in the animal brain. Central cholinergic neurons exist as both local circuit interneurons and projection neurons. S. nigra, substantia nigra.

pus. High doses of either drug can produce delirium, hyperactivity, visual hallucinations, and disorientation.

The M_2 muscarinic receptor predominates in hindbrain regions while the M_1 receptor is expressed at high levels in the cerebral cortex and hippocampus, which are brain regions involved with memory and cognition. The M_1 muscarinic receptor has accordingly generated considerable recent interest as a target for drug discovery of agents that might facilitate learning and memory. In animal models M_1 muscarinic receptor agonists restore cognitive impairment associated with damage to cholinergic pathways and may exert additional disease-modifying effects beneficial to Alzheimer's disease (Fisher et al. 2003).

The other class of cholinergic receptors that exist in the central nervous system are nicotinic receptors. These acetylcholine receptors are members of the ligand-gated ion channel super family and are composed of multiple homologous subunits oriented around a central cation channel. Each subtype of nicotinic cholinergic receptor is composed of 5 subunits, of which 2 bind acetylcholine; hence, it takes the binding of two molecules of acetylcholine to open the cation channel and allow Na^+ influx and depolarization of neuronal membranes. A total of 12 neuronal nicotinic receptor subunits have been identified, and the combination of these subunits into a pentameric structure determines its electrophysiological and pharmacological properties. In addition to responding to acetylcholine, these receptors, as their name implies, are also activated by the alkaloid nicotine found in tobacco leaves. Nicotine shares with other drugs of abuse the ability to activate the mesocortical limbic dopaminergic pathways that represent the reward circuitry of mammalian brain. The interaction with nicotinic cholinergic receptors in this pathway underlies the rewarding and dependence-related actions of nicotine. In addition to the adverse addictive properties of nicotine, this naturally occurring product increases mental alertness and improves memory in humans and animals. Chronic transdermal nicotine has indeed been found to improve attentional performance in patients with Alzheimer's disease and in individuals with the precursor age-associated memory impairment syndrome (White and Levin 2004). There is, therefore, a great deal of interest in the pharmaceutical industry directed toward the development of synthetic nicotinic receptor agonists for the treatment of memory deficits and cognitive dysfunction. There are currently several nicotine analogs in various stages of preclinical and clinical development for use in neurodegenerative and Alzheimer's disease.

Norepinephrine

The neurotransmitter norepinephrine is distributed throughout the brain. The relatively low concentration of norepinephrine in brain, however, initially led physiologists to question its functional importance. Application of a fluorescent histochemical technique subsequently permitted visualization of norepinephrine containing neurons and pathways in both the central and peripheral nervous system. Norepinephrine, dopamine, and epinephrine are catecholamines. The microanatomy of catecholamine-containing neurons in the central nervous system is distinct from amino acid and cholinergic fibers in that they possess varicosities along the axons in terminal fields. These varicosities contain all the machinery for neurotransmitter synthesis, storage, and release and are therefore the points of synaptic contact with target neurons. This unique microanatomy therefore allows a single catecholamine neuron with long terminal branches to possess thousands of varicosities. One catecholamine neuron consequently can influence the activity of thousands of target neurons.

The biosynthesis of norepinephrine in central neurons begins with the precursor tyrosine (See Figure 7.3). This tyrosine is converted to dopa by the soluble enzyme tyrosine hydroxylase. Tyrosine hydroxylase is the rate-limiting step in the biosynthesis of norepinephrine, and the activity of this enzyme is closely coupled to neuronal firing rate. The dopa is in turn converted to dopamine by the enzyme dopa decarboxylase. In noradrenergic, but not dopaminergic, neurons the dopamine is converted into norepinephrine by dopamine-β-hydroxylase and stored in vesicles for release. Once the norepinephrine is released into the synaptic cleft, the signaling action of this transmitter is terminated by the selective, high affinity of reuptake of norepinephrine by a distinct transporter expressed on noradrenergic neurons. Amphetamine and related psychostimulants exert their sympathomimetic and central stimulant properties through inhibition of norepinephrine reuptake and facilitation of transmitter release.

Norepinephrine interacts with both α- and β-adrenergic receptors expressed in the brain. There are eight subtypes of adrenergic receptors expressed in brain, including $\alpha_{1A^-, 1B^-, 1D}$-adrenergic receptors; $\alpha_{2A^-, 2B^-, 2C}$-adrenergic receptors; β_1- and β_2-adrenergic receptors. All adrenergic receptors are G protein-coupled receptors. While

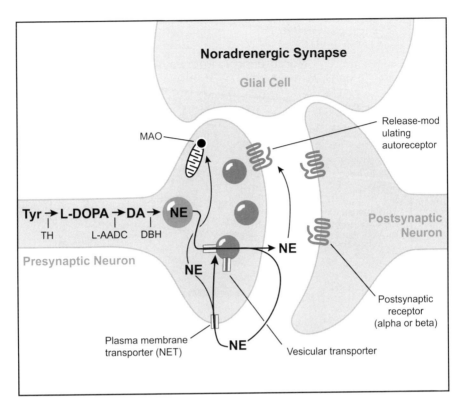

Figure 7.3 Schematic representation of a noradrenergic synapse. The amino acid precursor tyrosine is converted to L-dopa by the enzyme tyrosine hydroxylose (TH) in noradrenergic neurons. The L-dopa is converted to dopamine by L-aromatic amino acid decarboxylase (L-AADC), and the dopamine is in turn converted to norepinephrine (NE) by dopamine-β-hydroxylase (DBH). The NE is stored in and released from vesicles, and synaptic NE activates a complement of pre- and postsynaptic receptors. Synaptic NE action is terminated by the reuptake of the transmitter into the presynaptic terminal. This reuptake is mediated by the plasma membrane NE transporter (NET). Cytoplasmic NE can be degraded by the mitochondrial enzyme monoamine oxidase (MAO). Presynaptic release modulating autoreceptors are the α_2-adrenergic subtype.

the release of all neurotransmitters is regulated by presynaptic autoreceptors that respond to the released transmitter, this was first demonstrated in noradrenergic neurons. The noradrenergic neuron autoreceptors are members of the α_2-adrenergic receptor class. Agonists for α_2-adrenergic receptors, such as clonidine, produce an inhibition of norepinephrine release, while α_2 antagonists such as yohimbine increase the amount of norepinephrine released from presynaptic terminals. Given the existence of three subtypes of α_2-adrenergic receptors, the identity of the subtypes representing presynaptic autoreceptors was addressed using gene knockout strategies in mice. This approach has shown that both α_{2A}- and α_{2C}-adrenergic receptors are involved in the presynaptic control of transmitter release in noradrenergic neurons (Hein et al. 1999).

Noradrenergic neurons in the brain emanate from cell bodies in the pons (see Figure 7.4). The primary nuclear complex from which noradrenergic neurons arise in mammalian brain is the locus ceruleus. Norepinephrine neurons belonging to this nuclear

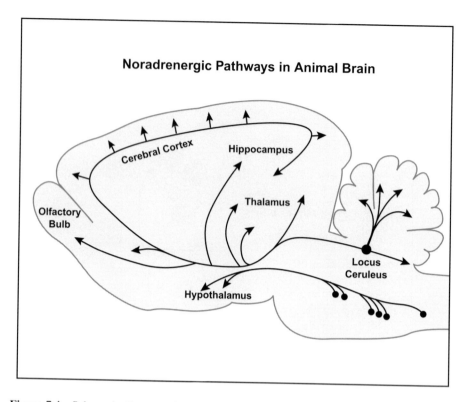

Figure 7.4 Schematic diagram of the noradrenergic pathways in the animal brain. Noradrenergic cell bodies are localized to the caudal pons in the locus ceruleus and also distributed more diffusely in the ventral tegmentum.

complex branch widely in their terminal fields, allowing, for example, a single norepinephrine axon to innervate a large fraction of the cerebral cortex. Locus ceruleus noradrenergic efferents innervate target cells in cerebral cortical, subcortical, and spinomedullary fields. The sole source of norepinephrine input to the cerebral cortex and hippocampus, brain regions critical for cognitive and affective processes, is derived from the locus ceruleus. Collectively, this noradrenergic system places a critical role in the regulation of vigilance, mood, and cardiovascular function. An additional group of noradrenergic neurons lie outside the locus ceruleus where they are sparsely distributed throughout the lateral ventral tegmental area of the pons (Cooper et al. 1996).

Selective α_2 receptor agonists such as clonidine, xylazine, and medetomidine produce sedation, analgesia, and muscle relaxation in animals. The sedative effects of these drugs are mediated by activation of α_2 receptors on locus ceruleus noradrenergic neurons. The sedative actions of medetomidine (Domitor) in dogs is most likely mediated by the α_{2A}-adrenergic receptor subtype inasmuch as this receptor was the only α_2 subtype recently shown to be expressed in the canine brain stem (Schwartz et al. 1999). The actions of medetomidine may be reversed through the administration of atipamezole (Antisedan) due to the α_2-adrenergic receptor competitive antagonist properties of the latter compound. Medetomidine also affects the cardiovascular system of dogs and cats producing marked bradycardia. The medetomidine-induced bradycardia is produced by a central action where activation of α_{2A}-adrenergic receptors in the nucleus tractus solitarius reduces sympathetic outflow (Cullen 1996). These nucleus tractus solitarius α_{2A}-adrenergic receptors are most likely postsynaptic receptors on dendrites of target neurons receiving input from noradrenergic neurons (Glass et al. 2001). The more variable effects of medetomidine on blood pressure of dogs and cats is produced by a combination of stimulation of central α_{2A} sites and peripheral postsynaptic α_{2A} receptors in vascular smooth muscle.

Although throughout the 1990s the emergence of selective serotonin reuptake inhibitors (SSRIs) as the primary treatment of depressive illness focused attention on serotonergic mechanisms, traditional antidepressants such as the tricyclic antidepressants (TCAs) and monoamine oxidase inhibitors (MAOIs) increase synaptic concentrations of both norepinephrine and serotonin. Similarly, newer drugs such as venlafaxine that block the reuptake of both serotonin and norepinephrine (SNRIs) are effective antidepressants (Hardy et al. 2002). When coupled with the recent introduction of the selective norepinephrine reuptake inhibitor (NRI) reboxetine as an antidepressant, there has been a resurgence of interest into the role of noradrenergic mechanisms in depression and affective disorders in general.

The renewed attention on noradrenergic pathways is consistent with the original formulation of the biogenic amine theory of affective disorders that posited that depressive symptoms arose from a deficiency of biogenic amines such as norepinephrine (Schidkraut and Kety 1967). This hypothesis arose from the observations in the 1950s that iproniazid, an MAOI, elevated mood in depressed patients being treated for tuberculosis, and that imipramine, developed as an antipsychotic, elevated mood in patients with depressive illness. Imipramine was subsequently shown to inhibit the reuptake of the biogenic amines norepinephrine and serotonin. The demonstration of the effectiveness of imipramine as an antidepressant led to the development of an array of TCAs that remain in use in human and veterinary medicine. The TCAs that remain in clinical use are the tertiary amines amitriptyline, clomipramine, doxepin, and imipramine and the secondary amines desipramine and nortriptyline. While the tertiary amines were originally proposed to have some selectivity for inhibiting the serotonin transporter *in vitro*, their secondary amine metabolites generated *in vivo* preferentially inhibit the norepinephrine transporter. The differential affinities of TCAs for the norepinephrine (NET) and serotonin transporters (SERT) *in vitro* have been well characterized and indicate that several of these antidepressants are relatively selective inhibitors of norephinephrine reuptake. As indicated in Table 7.1, the TCAs desipramine and nortriptyline have selectivity for the norepinephrine transporter, while amitriptyline and imipramine display little selectivity. In contrast, the SSRIs fluoxetine, sertraline, and paroxetine preferentially inhibit the serotonin transporter.

Although technically a tricyclic compound, the structurally unique drug reboxetine is quite selective as an inhibitor of norepinephrine reuptake. The human literature indicates that there is no significant difference between the antidepressant efficacies of norepinephrine- and serotonin-selective antidepressant drugs (Brunello et al. 2002). These data suggest that both noradrenergic and serotonergic mechanisms are involved in depressive symptomatology, and, as a consequence, chronic inhibition of either NET- or SERT-mediated reuptake leads to improvement in the symptoms of clinical depression. An interesting observation from a preclinical investigation recently indicated that the behavioral effects of the SSRIs fluoxetine, sertraline, and paroxetine were either absent or severely attenuated in transgenic mice incapable of producing

Table 7.1 Interaction of antidepressants with the norepinephrine and serotonin transporters *in vitro*

Drug	K_I (nM) NET	K_I (nM) SERT	NET Selectivity (ratio SERT/NET)
Desipramine	0.77	288	374
Reboxetine	8	1070	130
Nortriptyline	4.34	190	44
Doxepin	40	355	9
Amitriptyline	27	107	4
Imipramine	28	37.2	1.3
Fluoxetine	1235	17.7	0.014
Sertraline	220	3.4	0.015
Paroxetine	161	0.033	0.0002

Note: These antidepressants are listed in decreasing order of NET selectivity. Norepinephrine, NET; serotonin, SERT

Source: Rothman and Bauman 2003; Brunello et al. 2002.

norepinephrine (Cryan et al. 2004). These results indicate that norepinephrine may play an important role in mediating the acute behavioral and neurochemical effects of many antidepressants, including some widely used SSRIs.

An important concept that is germane to our current understanding of the mechanism of action of antidepressants is that the original biogenic amine theory of affective disorders is an over simplification. A critical discrepancy in the view that mental depression is simply due to a deficiency in synaptic levels of biogenic amines is that TCAs, MAOIs, SSRIs, and norephinephrine-serotonin reuptake inhibitors (NSRIs) all act to increase the levels of biogenic amines in the synapse within hours, whereas the therapeutic response does not manifest until two to three weeks of chronic drug administration. Newer theories of the mechanism of therapeutic action of antidepressant drugs have accordingly focused on adaptive changes in receptor sensitivities with temporal patterns that agree with those of the clinical therapeutic response. Thus chronic, but not acute, administration of antidepressants produces changes in both noradrenergic and serotonergic receptor systems. These adaptive changes provoked by chronic antidepressant drug administration include down-regulation of β-adrenergic, α_1-adrenergic, α_2-adrenergic, 5-HT$_2$-serotonergic, and 5-HT$_{1A}$-serotonergic receptors in various brain regions (Brunello et al. 2002). These adaptive changes in receptor sensitivity typically require 14–21 days of chronic antidepressant drug treatment that mimics the time course for the therapeutic response.

Although the TCAs, MAOIs, SSRIs, and NSRIs do not appear to differ significantly with respect to the temporal pattern for onset of therapeutic response or for clinical efficacy, they do differ with respect to side effect profiles. The adverse effects of TCAs are manifold and are a function of the affinities of these compounds for α_1-adrenergic, α_2-adrenergic, H$_1$ histamine, and muscarinic-cholinergic receptors. Newer antidepressants such as the SSRIs and NSRIs have negligible affinities for these neurotransmitter receptors and therefore possess a much more favorable side effect profile (Kent 2000). First generation TCAs commonly produce constipation, urinary retention, dry mouth, sedation, and postural hypotension and are highly toxic on overdose. The latter side effects of sedation and postural hypotension are well correlated with

Table 7.2 Antidepressant affinities for H_1-histaminic, muscarinic cholinergic, α_1 and α_2 adrenergic receptors

Antidepressant	Receptor Affinity (nM)			
	H_1	M	α_1	α_2
Doxepin	0.17	23	23	1,270
Amitriptyline	0.95	9.6	24	690
Nortriptyline	6.3	37	55	2,030
Desipramine	60	66	100	5,500
Fluoxetine	1,000	1,300	5,900	>10,000
Sertraline	>10,000	500	300	5,000
Paroxetine	1,000	89	>10,000	>10,000
Reboxetine	1,400	3,900	>10,000	>10,000

Source: Brunello et al. 2002; Kent 2000.

affinity for α_1-adrenergic receptors, whereas the other autonomic responses are correlated with their respective affinities for muscarinic cholinergic receptors. TCAs also exhibit cardiac toxicities such as enhancing or slowing of cardiac conduction and arrhythmias that are potentially lethal on overdose or in vulnerable populations.

As depicted in Table 7.2, the SSRIs and NSRIs have much lower affinities for muscarinic and α_1-adrenergic receptors and are accordingly nonsedating and do not produce hypotension, dry mouth, constipation, or other side effects typical of TCAs. MAOIs share with TCAs the property that they can be lethal on overdose and, in addition, have the added risk of potentially severe hypertensive crisis due to pressor effects of dietary tyramine or the interaction with several over-the-counter and prescription drugs. The newer SSRI and NSRI antidepressants therefore have a much improved therapeutic index and tolerability as compared with TCAs and MAOIs.

Dopamine

Dopamine is a catecholamine neurotransmitter originally believed to function only as a precursor for norepinephrine and epinephrine biosynthesis. It is now established, however, that dopamine functions as an important neurotransmitter in the brain that accounts for approximately 50% of the catecholaminergic neurons in the central nervous system (CNS). These dopaminergic neurons exist in discrete pathways that are distinct from the distribution of noradrenergic neurons.

Similar to synthesis of norepinephrine in the CNS, dopamine is formed from the precursor tyrosine (see Figure 7.5). The tyrosine is converted into dopa by tyrosine hydroxylase, and the dopa is metabolized to dopamine by the enzyme L-aromatic amino acid decarboxylase. Dopaminergic neurons are, however, distinct from noradrenergic neurons in that they do not express dopamine β hydroxylase and hence do not convert dopamine into norepinephrine.

Two important nuclei containing dopaminergic cell bodies are located in the mesencephalon. (See Figure 7.6.) One of these nuclei is the substantia nigra, with long axon projections to the striatum. This nigrostriatal dopamine pathway contains the

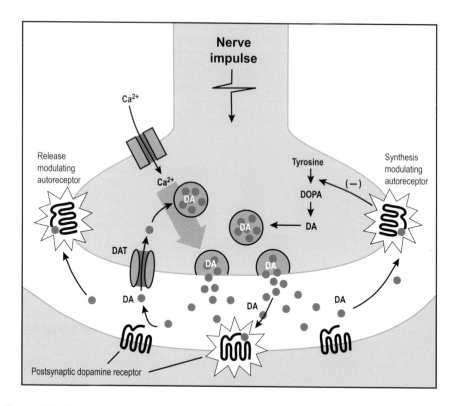

Figure 7.5 Schematic representation of a dopaminergic synapse. As in NE neurons, tyrosine is converted to L-dopa and then to dopamine (DA) in dopaminergic neurons. These neurons lack the enzyme dopamine-β-hydroxylase, and DA therefore functions as the neurotransmitter in these cells. The DA is stored in and released from vesicles, and synaptic DA activates both pre- and postsynaptic receptors. Synaptic DA action is terminated by the reuptake of the transmitter into the presynaptic terminal. This reuptake is mediated by the plasma membrane DA transporter (DAT). Cytoplasmic DA can be degraded by the mitochondrial enzyme monoamine oxidase (MAO). The presynaptic DA autoreceptors are primarily D_2 dopamine receptors.

majority of total brain dopamine and is the pathway that degenerates in Parkinson's disease. Parkinsonian patients with only mild symptoms are thought to have as much as a 70–80% reduction in striatal dopamine content, whereas patients with severe symptoms have greater than 90% loss of nigrostriatal dopaminergic neurons. The other major mesencephalic nucleus containing dopaminergic cell bodies is the ventral tegmental area (VTA); this nucleus lies medial to the substantia nigra in the mesencephalon. The VTA projects to limbic structures such as the nucleus accumbens and to the cerebral cortex (prefrontal cortex). These dopaminergic pathways are therefore termed, respectively, the mesolimbic and mesocortical dopamine systems. Due to the fundamental involvement of the VTA dopaminergic projection to the nucleus accumbens in the regulation of reward-related behavior, this system has been characterized as the neuroanatomical reward center in the brain (Spanagel and Weiss, 1999). Synaptic dopaminergic transmission in the nucleus accumbens is increased in response to natural rewards such as food, water, and sex, and also by drugs of abuse such as amphetamine, cocaine, opioids, and nicotine. Other dopaminergic projections in

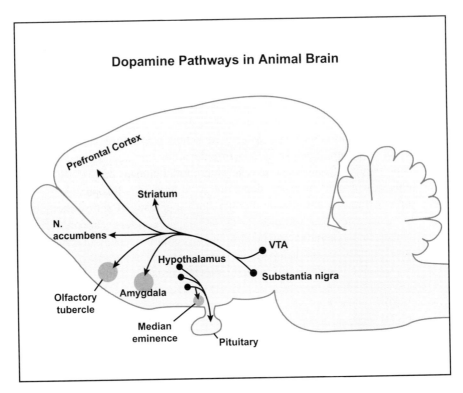

Figure 7.6 Schematic diagram of the dopaminergic pathways in animal brain. Dopaminergic cell bodies are localized to midbrain structures including the ventral tegmental area (VTA) and substantia nigra. Additional DA cell bodies are in the arcuate and periventricular nuclei projecting to the median eminence and intermediate lobe of the pituitary. The mesolimbic DA pathway from the VTA to the nucleus accumbens represents a component of the reward circuitry of the brain. N. accumbens, nucleus accumben.

the brain include those of the arcuate nucleus in the hypothalamus with axons terminating in the intermediate lobe of the pituitary, where dopamine acts as a key inhibitory regulator of prolactin release.

Within dopaminergic presynaptic terminals the mitochondrial enzyme MAO can degrade free dopamine. At these axon terminals dopamine is released by action potential-driven exocytosis from vesicles into the synaptic cleft. The synaptic action of dopamine is terminated by the high-affinity reuptake of dopamine mediated by the dopamine transporter (DAT) expressed on the presynaptic terminal. The use of dopamine transporter knockout mice has indicated that the absence of this transporter produces a 300-fold increase in the amount of time required to clear dopamine from the synapse (Gainetdinov et al. 2001). Inasmuch as the dopamine transporter protein is the molecular target for psychostimulant drugs such as cocaine, methylphenidate, and amphetamine; the actions of these drugs are blunted in mice lacking the transporter. Dopamine in the synapse interacts with a family of dopamine receptors (D_1, D_2, D_3, D_4, and D_5) that are localized to either presynaptic or postsynaptic membranes. Dopamine receptors are all G protein-coupled receptors whose cell-signaling actions are mediated by stimulation or inhibition of adenylyl cyclase or activation of phospholipase C. Dopamine D_2 receptors are expressed as both pre- or postsynaptic receptors. As autoreceptors at the cell body they decrease the firing rate of dopaminergic neurons, and as autoreceptors on axon terminals the D_2 receptors regulate the release of dopamine (Schmitz et al. 2002).

The dopamine hypothesis of schizophrenia was originally formulated in the late 1960s by VanRossum (VanRossum 1967). He suggested that the pathophysiology of schizophrenia may involve an overstimulation of dopamine receptors. Key elements of this hypothesis were that drugs used to treat schizophrenia acted as dopamine receptor antagonists, and indirect acting dopaminergic agonists such as amphetamine could produce features of a psychosis in normal humans or exacerbate certain symptoms in schizophrenics. The dopamine hypothesis of schizophrenia has also derived support from the observation that the clinical potency of antipsychotic drugs is well correlated with their affinities for D_2 dopamine receptors. These antipsychotic drugs include first-generation compounds such as chlorpromazine (Thorazine), trifluoperazine (Stelazine), and haloperidol (Haldol), as well as second-generation drugs such as clozapine (Clozaril) and risperidone (Risperdal). Therapeutic doses of most antipsychotic drugs produces levels of D_2 receptor occupancy in the striatum of 60–80%, while atypical antipsychotics such as clozapine produce lower levels of striatal D_2 receptor occupancy ranging from 10–66% (Seeman and Kapur 2000; Lidow et al. 1998). Recent positron emission tomography studies in human patients with schizophrenia have demonstrated an increased occupancy of striatal D_2 receptors by endogenous dopamine (Abi-Dargham et al. 2000). This observation supports the dopaminergic hyperactivity hypothesis of schizophrenia.

While much attention has been focused on striatal D_2 dopamine receptors in schizophrenia, these receptors are unlikely to be the primary target for the therapeutic action of antipsychotic drugs to mitigate the thought disorder of schizophrenic patients. Striatal D_2 dopamine receptors certainly are the target for the Parkinson-like extrapyramidal side effects of typical antipsychotic drugs. Antipsychotic drugs such as fluphenazine have been reported to cause extrapyramidal symptoms in horses when this drug is used to produce sedation (Kauffman et al. 1989; Langlois et al. 1990). In horses the extrapyramidal symptoms manifest as akathisia and repetitive pawing.

The D_2 receptor representing the target for the therapeutic effects of antipsychotic drugs are likely to be those expressed in the cerebral cortex (Lidlow et al. 1998). The cerebral cortex possesses higher densities of D_1 than D_2 dopamine receptors, and these D_1 receptors are down-regulated after chronic antipsychotic drug treatment (Lidlow et al. 1998). These D_1 dopamine receptors may be linked to some of the negative symptoms of schizophrenia, such as chronic apathy, and cognitive deficits, such as memory impairment. The activation of prefrontal cortical D_1 receptors in a narrow occupancy range has been shown to enhance signaling in prefrontal cortex neurons engaged in working memory in nonhuman primates (Lidlow et al. 1998). This observation points to an essential role of D_1 dopamine receptor function in prefrontal cortex during working memory.

Germane to the function of dopaminergic pathways in the brain is the recent introduction of L-deprenyl (or selegiline) (Anipryl) to control canine cognitive dysfunction syndrome. Deprenyl is a selective irreversible inhibitor of the enzyme MAO-B. Monoamine oxidase exists in two forms termed MAO-A and MAO-B. MAO is a mitochondrial enzyme that is widely expressed in tissues including gastrointestinal tract, liver, platelets, smooth muscle, and brain. In the brain the preferred substrates for MAO-A are norepinephrine and serotonin, whereas the preferred substrate for MAO-B is phenylethylamine. Dopamine and tyramine are metabolized at equivalent rates by the two forms of MAO. MAO enzymes are localized to the outer membranes of mitochondria in both neuronal and non-neuronal cells. In neuronal cells these enzymes are responsible for the oxidative deamination of monoamines.

In the late 1980s deprenyl was shown to delay the onset of disability and hence the need for L-dopa therapy, associated with early, untreated cases of Parkinson's disease (Parkinson Study Group 1989). This observation suggested that deprenyl may exert a neuroprotective action to ameliorate an underlying disease process in Parkinson's disease. Neuroprotection in this context refers to an intervention that protects or rescues vulnerable neurons and slows the progression of the neurodegenerative disease. MAO activity could contribute to neural degeneration by producing hydrogen peroxide, which, although normally detoxified by glutathione, can react with ferrous iron to generate the highly reactive and cytotoxic hydroxyl (OH) radical. Thus, by inhibiting MAO-B, deprenyl may exert a neuroprotectant action through a reduction in the generation of free radicals. Environmental chemicals may also contribute to the development of neurodegenerative disorders such as Parkinson's disease, and chemicals structurally related to the designer drug precursor MPTP (1-methyl-4-phenyl-1,2,3,6-tetrahydropyridine) may require metabolism by MAO to produce active neurotoxins. In this case MAO inhibitors such as deprenyl would be neuroprotective due to inhibition of the formation of neurotoxic metabolites. Postmortem studies have consistently implicated oxidative damage in Parkinson's disease, and the source of reactive oxygen species may also derive from dysfunction of mitochondria caused by either environmental or genetic mechanisms (Greenamyre and Hastings 2004).

The ability of deprenyl to act as a neuroprotectant may therefore be involved in its therapeutic actions in canine cognitive dysfunction. Chronic deprenyl treatment elevates dramatically brain levels of the trace amine β-phenylethylamine and also produces modest increases in striatal dopamine content (Youdim and Weinstock 2004). The elevation of β-phenylethylamine may also contribute to the pharmacological actions of deprenyl inasmuch as this compound promotes the release of dopamine and inhibits dopamine reuptake. The administration of β-deprenyl leads to the appearance of L-methamphetamine as a major metabolite in animals, and this compound may contribute to the clinical benefits of this drug (Engberg et al. 2001). Chronic administration of deprenyl to elderly dogs improves decrements in hearing, activity, attention, and ability to navigate stairs (Ruehl et al. 1995). The combined neuroprotectant and indirect actions to facilitate dopaminergic neurotransmission may account for its effects on behavior and cognitive function in elderly dogs (Milgram et al. 1993).

References

Abi-Dargham A, Rodenhiser J, Printz D, Zea-Ponce Y, Gil R, Kegeles LS, Weiss R, Cooper TB, Mann JJ, Van Heertum RL, Gorman JM, and Laruelle M 2000. Increased baseline occupancy of D$_2$ receptors by dopamine in schizophrenia. *Proceedings of the National Academy of Science* 97(14): 8104–8109.

Brunello N, Mendlewicz J, Kasper S, Leonard B, Montgomery S, Nelson JC, Paykel E, Versiani M, and Racagni G 2002. The role of noradrenaline and selective noradrenalie reuptake inhibition in depression. *European Neuropsychopharmacology* 12: 461–475.

Coffield JA 2003. Botulinum Neurotoxin: The Neuromuscular Junction Revisited. *Critical Reviews in Neurobiology* 15(3&4): 175–195.

Cooper JR, Bloom FE, and Roth RH 1996. *The biochemical basis of neuropharmacology.* Oxford University Press, New York.

Cryan JF, O'Leary OF, Jin S-H, Friedland JC, Ouyang M, Hirsch BR, Page ME, Dalvi A, Thomas SA and Lucki I 2004. Norepinephrine-deficient mice lack responses to antidepressant drugs, including selective serotonin reuptake inhibitors. *Proceedings of the National Academy of Science* 101(21): 8186–8191.

Cullen, LK 1996. Medetomidine Sedation in Dogs and Cats: A Review of its Pharmacology, Antagonism and Dose. *British Veterinary Journal* 152: 519–535.

Engberg G, Elebring T and Nissbrandt H 2001. Deprenyl (selegiline), a selective MAO-B inhibitor with active metabolites; effects on locomotor activity, dopaminergic neurotransmission and firing rate of nigral dopamine neurons. *Journal of Pharmacology and Experimental Therapeutics* 259(2): 841–847.

Fisher A, Pittel Z, Haring R, Bar-Ner N, Kliger-Spatz M, Natan N, Egozi I, Sonego H, Marcovitch I and Brandeis R 2003. M_1 muscarinic agonists can modulate some of the hallmarks in Alzheimer's disease: implications in future therapy. *Journal of Molecular Neuroscience* 20(3): 349–356.

Gainetdinov RR, Mohn AR and Caron MG 2001. Genetic animal models: focus on schizophrenia. *Trends in Neurosciences* 24(9): 527–533.

Glass MJ, Huang J, Aicher SA, Milner TA and Pickel VM 2001. Subcellular localization of alpha-2A-adrenergic receptors in the rat medial nucleus tractus solitarius: regional targeting and relationship with catecholamine neurons. *Journal of Comparative Neurology* 433(2): 193–207.

Greenamyre JT and Hastings TG 2004. Parkinson's—Divergent Causes, Convergent Mechanisms. *Science* 304: 1120–1122.

Hardy J, Argyropouos S and Nutt DJ 2002. Venlafaxine: a new class of antidepressant. *Hospital Medicine* 63(9): 549–552.

Hein L, Altman JD and Kobilka BK 1999. Two functionally distinct α_2-adrenergic receptors regulate sympathetic neurotransmission. *Nature* 402: 181–184.

Kauffman VG, Soma L, Divers TJ and Perkons SZ 1989. Extrapyramidal side effects caused by fluphenazine decanoate in a horse. *Journal of the American Veterinary Medical Association* 195(8): 1128–1130.

Kent JM 2000. SNaRIs, NaSSAs, and NaRIs: new agents for the treatment of depression. *The Lancet* 355: 911–918.

Langlois JF, Brewer BD, Hines MT and Stewart JT 1990. Fluphenazine induced Parkinson-like syndrome in a horse. *Equine Veterinary Journal* 22(2): 136–137.

Lidow MS, Williams GV and Goldman-Rakic PS 1998. The cerebral cortex: a case for a common site of action of antipsychotics. *Trends in Pharmacological Science* 19: 136–140.

Milgram NW, Ivy GO, Head E, Murphy MP, Wu PH, Ruehl WW, Yu PH, Durden DA, Davis BA, Paterson IA and Boulton AA 1993. The effect of L-deprenyl on behavior, cognitive function, and biogenic amines in the dog. *Neurochemical Research* 18(12): 1211–1219.

Parkinson Study Group 1989. Effect of deprenyl on the progression of disability in early Parkinson's disease. *The New England Journal of Medicine* 321: 1364–1371.

Rothman RB and Baumann MH 2003. Monoamine transporters and psychostimulant drugs. *European Journal of Pharmacology* 479: 23–40.

Ruehl WW, Bruyette DS, DePaoli A, Cotman CW, Head E, Milgram NW and Cummings BJ 1995. Canine cognitive dysfunction as a model for human age-related cognitive decline, dementia and Alzheimer's disease: clinical presentation, cognitive testing, pathology and response to L-deprenyl therapy. *Progress in Brain Research* 106: 217–225.

Sarter M and Bruno JP 1999. Abnormal regulation of corticopetal cholinergic neurons and impaired information processing in neuropsychiatric disorders. *Trends in Neurosciences* 22(2): 67–74.

Schildkraut JJ and Kety SJ 1967. Biogenic amines and emotion. *Science* 156: 21–37.

Schmitz Y, Schmauss C and Sulzer D 2002. Altered Dopamine Release and Uptake Kinetics in Mice Lacking D_2 Receptors. *The Journal of Neuroscience* 22(18): 8002–8009.

Schwartz DD, Jones WG, Hedden KP and Clark TP 1999. Molecular and pharmacological characterization of the canine brainstem alpha-2A adrenergic receptor. *Journal of Veterinary Pharmacology and Therapeutics* 22: 380–386.

Seeman P and Kapur S 2000. Schizophrenia: More dopamine, more D_2 receptors. *Proceedings of the National Academy of Science* 97(14): 7673–7675.

Spanagel R and Weiss F 1999. The dopamine hypothesis of reward: past and current status. *Trends in Neurosciences* 22(11): 521–527. Van Rossum J 1967. In *Neuropsychopharmacology, Proceedings Fifth Collegium Internationale Neuropsychopharmacologicum*, pp. 321–329, edited by H Brill, J Cole, P Deniker, H Hippius, and PD Bradley, Excerpta Medica, Amsterdam.

Van Rossum, J. (1967) in *Neuropsychopharmacology, Proceedings Fifth Collegium Internationale Neuropsychopharnacologicum*, eds. Brill, H., Cole, J., Deniker, P., Hippius, H. & Bradley, P.D. (Excerpta Medica, Amsterdam), pp. 321–329.

White HK and Levin ED 2004. Chronic transdermal nicotine patch treatment effects on cognitive performance in age-associated memory impairment. *Psychopharmacology* 171: 465–471.

Youdim MBH and Weinstock M 2004. Therapeutic applications of selective and non-selective inhibitors of monoamine oxidase A and B that do not cause significant tyramine potentiation. *NeuroToxicology* 25: 243–250.

Chapter Eight
Monoamine Oxidase Inhibitors

Action

Monoamine oxidase (MAO) is an enzyme of the outer mitochondrial membrane that occurs in a variety of tissues, including heart, liver, kidneys, spleen, platelets, peripheral nervous system, and central nervous system (CNS) (Obata et al. 1987). In the CNS, MAO, primarily MAO-B, catabolizes the oxidative deamination of catecholamines, including dopamine, norepinephrine, epinephrine, β-phenylethylamine (2-phenylethylamine), and serotonin. In the intestinal tract and liver, MAO, primarily MAO-A, is also important in catabolizing exogenous amines, for example, tyramine, derived from various foods and drugs. The name is not entirely accurate since MAO enzymes can also deaminate long-chain diamines (Gerlach et al. 1993).

MAO inhibitors prevent the action of MAO-A, MAO-B, or both. Drugs in this category, while classified according to their action of inhibiting MAO, also have a variety of other actions, many of which enhance activity of catecholamines. For example, L-deprenyl, in addition to inhibiting MAO activity, inhibits presynaptic catecholamine receptors, inhibits the uptake of catecholamines, induces the release of catecholamines from their intraneuronal stores, and stimulates action potential-transmitter release coupling (Knoll et al. 1996). Thus, they should not be considered to be drugs that just have a simple and specific activity.

They are also likely to exhibit substantially different actions on different species because there are species differences in the ratios of MAO-A to MAO-B, both overall and in given organ systems. For example, in humans and monkeys, dopamine in the brain is a substrate of both MAO-A and MAO-B (Glover et al. 1977; O'Carroll et al. 1983). As a consequence, basal levels of brain dopamine increase with chronic administration of L-deprenyl in these species (Riederer and Youdim 1986; Boulton et al. 1992). MAO-B has little effect on dopamine metabolism in the rat brain, however. Thus, dopamine levels in the brain of the rat are less affected by L-deprenyl treatment than those of humans (Kato et al. 1986; Paterson et al. 1991). The guinea pig appears to be a better model of dopamine metabolism by MAO in humans than either mice or rats (Ross 1987). Human platelet MAO is primarily or entirely of the B form, while dog platelet MAO is of both the A and B form (Collins and Sandler 1971; Donnelly and Murphy 1977; Obata et al. 1987). As a consequence of these species variations in metabolism, initiation of use of a MAO inhibitor in a new species should be done cautiously.

Overview of Indications

MAO-B inhibitors, specifically selegiline, have been shown to increase life span when given to healthy mice, rats, and dogs (Knoll 1988; Knoll et al. 1989; Milgram et al. 1990; Kitani et al. 1992; Ivy et al. 1994; Ruehl et al. 1997). Selegiline also increases the survival of human patients with Parkinson's disease (Birkmayer et al. 1985). Selegiline likewise causes a decreased accumulation of lipofuscin in various parts of the brain of aging rats (Amenta et al. 1994a, 1994b, 1994c; Zeng et al. 1994). It also appears to facilitate activation of astrocytes that are associated with increased secretion of trophic factors, resulting in increased neuronal survival and growth (Biagini et al. 1994). It blocks the pathological changes induced by the neurotoxin 1-methyl,4,phenyl-1,2,3,6-tetrahydropyridine (MPTP) (Battistin et al. 1987).

Medications that significantly inhibit MAO-A exist but are not used in the treatment of behavior problems in animals. Only the MAO-B inhibitor selegiline will be discussed in detail. Therefore, all discussion of contraindications, side effects, adverse drug interactions, and treatment of overdose is presented in coverage of that drug.

Specific Medications

I. Selegiline Hydrochloride

Chemical Compound: (R)-(-)-*N*,2-dimethyl-*N*-2-propynylphenethylamine hydrochloride

DEA Classificaton: Not a controlled substance

Preparations: generally available as 2-, 5-, 10-, 15-, and 30-mg tablets and as 5-mg capsules. FDA approved for use in dogs with canine cognitive dysfunction.

Clinical Pharmacology

Selegiline is an irreversible inhibitor of MAO. It has a substantially greater affinity for MAO-B than for MAO-A and therefore functions as a selective MAO-B inhibitor when given at clinically appropriate doses (Knoll and Magyar 1972; Yang and Neff 1974; Glover et al. 1977; Pfizer Animal Health 2000). It was the first drug to be developed that was specific in its inhibition of MAO-B (Knoll 1983). Inhibition of MAO happens in two steps: an initial reversible reaction followed by a second irreversible reaction (Heinonen et al. 1994). However, selectivity is not absolute, and rare patients may exhibit signs of MAO-A inhibition. In average adult humans, the selectivity of selegiline's MAO inhibition appears to disappear at a dose of about 30–40 mg total dose per day (Somerset Pharmaceuticals, Inc. 2003).

Following administration of 1 mg/kg of selegiline PO, absorption in dogs is rapid, with peak plasma concentration occurring after 20–30 minutes. Measurable concentrations are detectable in the plasma up to three hours later. The absorption half-life is about 41 minutes whereas the elimination half-life is about 78 minutes (Mahmood et al. 1994).

Selegiline also inhibits the reuptake of dopamine, norepinephrine, and serotonin into presynaptic nerves, inhibits dopamine autoreceptors, increases the turnover of dopamine, reduces oxidative stress caused by the degradation of dopamine, increases free radical elimination by enhancing superoxide dismutase and catalase activity, potentiates neural responses to dopamine by the indirect mechanism of elevating phenylethylamine, a neuromodulator of dopaminergic responses, and enhances scavenger function in the CNS. At clinically appropriate doses, it does not have the "cheese effect," that is, does not potentiate the hypertensive effects of tyramine, which is characteristic of MAO-A and mixed MAO inhibitors (Lai et al. 1980; Knoll 1983; Fagervall and Ross 1986; Knoll 1987; Heinonen and Lammintausta 1991; Berry et al. 1994; Fang and Yu 1994; Hsu et al. 1996; Pfizer Animal Health 2000). Nevertheless, it is probably best to avoid regular use of cheese as a treat for dogs on selegiline, since a rare dog may, as happens in humans, exhibit a cheese response despite selegiline generally being very MAO-B specific.

Selegiline has three principal metabolites: l-(-)amphetamine, l-(-)methamphetamine, and *N*-desmethylselegiline (Reynolds et al. 1978a, 1978b; Philips 1981; Yoshida et al. 1986; Dirikolu et al. 2003), and some of its pharmacological actions appear to be the result of the sympathomimetic properties caused by its metabolites (Fozard et al. 1985). See chapter 10, CNS Stimulants, for further discussion of amphetamine. Phenylethylamine, a modulator of catecholamine neurotransmission in the CNS, is a substrate of MAO-B, and levels of this molecule also increase following treatment with selegiline (Philips and Boulton 1979; Philips 1981; Paterson et al. 1990; Durden and Davis 1993).

Uses in Humans

Selegiline is used to treat Parkinson's disease, in which it potentiates the effects of L-dopa, and Alzheimer's disease (see, for example, Tariot et al. 1987; Parkinson Study Group 1989, 1993; Tariot et al. 1993; Olanow et al. 1995; Sano et al. 1997; Heikkila 1981).

Contraindications

Selegiline is contraindicated in patients with a known history of sensitivity to this drug.

Severe CNS toxicity, potentially resulting in death, can ensue from combining selegiline with various other drugs, particularly tricyclic antidepressants (TCAs), for example, amitriptyline, clomipramine, and selective serotonin reuptake inhibitors (SSRIs), for example, fluoxetine and paroxetine. The phenomenon is called serotonin syndrome (see Chapter 15 for further discussion). The detailed mechanism of this serious drug interaction is poorly understood. Therefore, these drugs should never be combined. Because of medication half-life, no TCA or SSRI should be given for at least two weeks following discontinuation of selegiline. Due to fluoxetine's long half-life, selegiline should not be given for at least five weeks following discontinuation of that drug. Even after a five-week washout period, MAO inhibitors should be initiated with caution and the patient closely monitored, because metabolites of fluoxetine may remain in the system for longer periods of time and still induce serotonin syndrome (Coplan and Gorman 1993; Pfizer Animal Health 2000; Somerset Pharmaceuticals 2003).

Selegiline should not be given with potential MAO inhibitors including amitraz, a topical ectoparasiticide (Pfizer Animal Health 2000).

Possible drug interactions have been observed in dogs concurrently on metronidazole, prednisone, and trimethoprim sulfa.

Combining selegiline with meperidine, a synthetic narcotic analgesic, is also contraindicated in humans due to the occurrence of stupor, muscular rigidity, severe agitation, and elevated temperature in some patients receiving this combination. While it is not known if this will occur in veterinary patients, it is recommended that this combination also be avoided in nonhuman animals as well (Somerset Pharmaceuticals, Inc. 2003).

Also in humans concurrent use of MAO inhibitors in conjunction with α-2 agonists sometimes results in extreme fluctuations of blood pressure (Somerset Pharmaceuticals, Inc. 2003). Blood pressure monitoring is therefore recommended in veterinary patients concurrently given selegiline and any α-2 agonist.

Side Effects

In one clinical trial of dogs treated with selegiline, 4% of the study population experienced events sufficiently adverse to result in a reduction of dose or withdrawal from medication. Side effects experienced by these dogs included restlessness, agitation, vomiting, disorientation, diarrhea, and diminished hearing. Also during clinical trials conducted on dogs as a part of safety and efficacy testing, three dogs showed an increase in aggression (Pfizer Animal Health 2000).

Studies to date have not identified any mutagenic or chromosomal damage potential.

No evidence of teratogenic effects were identified in rats given 4, 12, or 36 mg/kg selegiline daily during pregnancy or in rabbits given 5, 25, or 50 mg/kg during pregnancy. However, in the two higher doses given to rats, fetuses exhibited a decreased body weight. At the highest dose given to rabbits, there was an increase in resorption and percentage of postimplantation losses, with a concurrent decrease in the number of live fetuses. In another study in which pregnant rats were given 4, 16, or 64 mg/kg daily there was an increase in the number of stillbirths and a concurrent decrease in pup body weight, the number of pups per dam, and pup survival. At the highest dose (64 mg/kg) no pups survived to postpartum day 4 (Somerset Pharmaceuticals, Inc. 2003).

Overdose

In early overdose induction of emesis or gastric lavage may be helpful, otherwise provide supportive treatment. Convulsions and other signs of CNS overstimulation should be treated with diazepam. Avoid use of phenothiazine derivatives and all CNS stimulants. Treat hypotension and vascular collapse with IV fluids.

Discontinuation

Because selegiline is used to treat an irreversible, degeneration of the CNS, it should not be discontinued in patients that respond to it.

Other Information

The term cognitive dysfunction (CD) as used in veterinary behavior refers to geriatric onset changes in behavior that cannot be attributed to medical conditions such as neoplasia or organ failure. In dogs, a number of categories of behavior may be altered. First, dogs with CD often exhibit various behaviors that suggest disorientation, for example, they may wander around the house in an aimless fashion, appear not to be able to find something, such as their bed, or get stuck behind open doors. Second, there is often altered social interaction. Usually, this is noted as a decrease in social interaction with human family members, other pets in the household, or both. Third, there is a loss of prior training, including house-training and basic obedience commands, such as "sit." Fourth, sleep habits change. Total sleep increases, but nighttime wakefulness may develop. Finally, overall activity, particularly purposeful activity, decreases.

Histologic lesions identified postmortem in the brains of dogs with CD closely resemble lesions in the brains of humans with Alzheimer's disease (Cummings et al. 1996b). Specifically, dogs that exhibited geriatric behavior problems before death have been identified as having meningeal fibrosis, lipofuscinosis, generalized gliosis, and ubiquitin-containing granules in the white matter upon postmortem histological examination (Ferrer et al. 1993). There are also age-related cerebral vascular changes and gliosis, dilation of the ventricles, and thickening of the meninges (Uchida et al. 1992; Shimada et al. 1992). β-Amyloid plaques develop in the brains of old dogs that are similar to those found in the brains of humans with Alzheimer's disease (Cummings et al. 1993). Deficits in discrimination learning, reversal learning, and spatial learning are strongly associated with degree of deposition of β-amyloid in the dog brain (Cummings et al. 1996a).

Dogs with CD have hypothalamic-pituitary-adrenal axis dysregulation that occurs without typical signs of Cushing's syndrome or other medical conditions expected to activate the hypothalamic-pituitary-adrenal axis (Ruehl et al. 1997).

The mechanisms by which selegiline reverses CD are not fully understood. It increases dopamine activity by several mechanisms, inhibition of MAO-B (a dopamine metabolizer), increasing the impulse-mediated release of catecholamines, decreasing presynaptic dopamine reuptake, increasing concentrations of phenylethylamine, which potentiates dopamine action, and increasing synthesis of aromatic L-amino acid decarboxylase, which results in increasing dopamine synthesis (e.g., Heinonen and Lammintausta 1991; Knoll et al. 1996; Jurio et al. 1994). Selegiline also decreases free radical production and increases activity of superoxide dismutase, which scavenges free radicals (Carillo et al. 1994). These actions are beneficial to the aging brain since free radicals contribute to the pathogenesis of neurodegenerative disorders (Gerlach et al. 1993).

Geriatric cognitive decline also occurs in the cat, although it is not as well studied as in the dog. Doses and approximate costs for treating cats and dogs with selegiline are given in Table 8.1.

Effects Documented in Nonhuman Animals
Cats

Although selegiline is not approved for use in cats, signs of Alzheimer's disease pathology have been reported in them (Cummings et al. 1996b). Cats have been treated with up to 10 times the therapeutic dose with no toxicity (Ruehl et al. 1996),

Table 8.1   Doses and cost of selegiline for dogs and cats.

	Dose	One month	Cost for one-month treatment
Cat	0.5–1.0 mg/kg	5 mg daily	$$$
Dog	0.5–1.0 mg/kg	10 mg daily	$$$

Note: Cost example is for a 5-kg cat and a 20-kg dog for one month.

and geriatric cats treated with selegiline for signs of cognitive decline have shown improvement (Landsberg 1999).

Dogs

In dogs, selegiline hydrochloride is used to treat canine cognitive dysfunction (CCD) at a dose of 0.5–1.0 mg/kg given once daily in the morning, and pituitary-dependent hyperadrenocorticism is treated at a dose of 1.0–2.0 mg/kg daily. It has also been shown to have anticataplectic activity in research dogs, though this effect is due to activity of the stimulant metabolites rather than by MAO-B inhibition (Milgram et al. 1993; Nishino et al. 1996; Nishino and Mignot 1997). Activity is specific to certain brain regions. In dogs, three weeks of medication with 0.1, 0.5, or 1.0 mg/kg/day PO caused significant, dose-dependent increases in superoxide dismutase activity in the striatum but not in the hippocampus (Carrillo et al. 1994).

Dogs given 1 mg/kg of selegiline daily PO for one year do not show any sign of hepatic damage or dysfunction. There was no significant difference in bile acid concentrations between treated and placebo groups (Ruehl et al. 1993).

A detailed discussion of its use in the treatment of pituitary-dependent hyperadrenocorticism is beyond the scope of this book. Further discussion can be found in Bruyette et al. (1995), Bruyette et al. (1997a; 1997b), Peterson (1999), Reusch et al. (1999).

Selegiline prolongs life in otherwise healthy elderly dogs (>10 years) when given at a dose of 1 mg/kg daily (Ruehl and Hart 1998).

In clinical trials of the treatment of CDS with selegiline at recommended doses, dogs show improvement in sleeping patterns, house-training, and activity level after four weeks of treatment (Ruehl et al. 1994), with treated dogs showing significant improvement over dogs receiving placebo (Head et al. 1996). Individual response varies substantially and some dogs continue to show additional improvement for up to three months. Geriatric, but not young, dogs given L-deprenyl exhibit improved spatial short-term memory over dogs given placebo. The best effect occurred at 0.5–1.0 mg/kg, with smaller or larger doses being less effective (Head et al. 1996).

Selegiline causes a dose-dependent inhibition of MAO-B activity in the striatum, hippocampus, liver, and kidney of dogs. When selegiline is given at doses of 0.5–1.0 mg/kg over a two-week period it has no detectable effect on MAO-A activity in the same tissues (Milgram et al. 1995). This contrasts with the rat, in which a single dose of selegiline does not cause MAO-A inhibition, but repeated doses do cause MAO-A inhibition (Waldmeier et al. 1981; Zsilla et al. 1986; Terleckyi et al. 1990; Murphy et al. 1993). Likewise, there are no significant changes in levels of dopamine, 3,4-dihydroxyphenylacetic acid, homovanillic acid, 3-methoxy-turamine, 5-hydroxytryptamine, or 5-hydroxyindoleactic acid in the striatum or cortex (Milgram et al. 1995). At least in the rat, sex, as well as dose and route of administration, affect activity of selegiline on MAO-A and MAO-B. Females respond to selegiline at a lower dose than do males, and subcutaneous injection is more efficient than oral dosing (Murphy et al. 1993).

Healthy adult dogs given 0, 0.1, 0.5, or 1 mg/kg of selegiline for two weeks exhibit no changes in locomotor activity, inactivity, sniffing, or urination as assessed in an open field test. At this dose range, the development of repetitive behavior has not been observed (Milgram et al. 1995). However, a single dose of 3 mg/kg produces repetitive locomotion in females, decreased frequency of urination in males, and decreased exploratory sniffing in both genders (Head and Milgram 1992).

In safety studies, beagle dogs have been given selegiline at doses of 0, 1, 2, 3, and 6 mg/kg daily, that is, up to three times the maximum recommended daily doses. Dogs at the 3 and 6 mg/kg dose exhibited increased salivation, decreased pupillary response, and decreased body weight. The latter occurred despite normal to increased feed consumption. Additionally, at the 6 mg/kg dose, the dogs exhibited increased panting, dehydration, and increased stereotypic behaviors, that is, weaving. Interestingly, this latter problem was observed several hours after dosing but was no longer present 24 hours later. There were no changes in blood pressure, ophthalmic assessment, heart rate, or electrocardiogram parameters. The drug was assessed as being safe in the dogs given 2 mg/kg daily or less.

Plasma levels of the L form of amphetamine in dogs given selegiline are detectable within 2 hours of medication and exhibit a significant dose-dependent effect (Salonen 1990; Milgram et al. 1995). Levels continue to increase for the seven days of daily dosing until the end of the first week of medication, after which there is no further increase. Plasma levels of amphetamine after two weeks of administration of selegiline at 1.0 mg/kg daily are about 30 ng/ml. This level of amphetamine is unlikely to have significant behavioral effects (Milgram et al. 1995). Within 24 hours of discontinuation of selegiline, plasma amphetamine levels are substantially decreased and are undetectable five days after discontinuation of selegiline.

When dogs are given 3 mg/kg of selegiline, amphetamine and metamphetamine are detectable in the serum for 48 hours, while desmethylselegiline is detectable for only about 80 minutes. When dogs are given 10 mg/kg, desmethylselegiline is detectable in the serum for up to 4 hours (Salonen 1990).

Plasma levels of phenylethylamine likewise increase in dogs given selegiline, although it is only by the second week of treatment that plasma levels are significantly greater than dogs given placebo. Plasma phenylethylamine levels decrease within 24 hours of administration. Levels of phenylethylamine in the hypothalamus and striatum, but not the cortex, are significantly elevated in dogs given 0.1 mg/kg for two weeks, with levels in the striatum increasing almost 400% and levels in the hypothalamus increasing about 1000% (Milgram et al. 1995).

Selegiline appears to have beneficial effects on learning even in young, healthy dogs. Specifically, in a study conducted on various breeds aged one to seven years, dogs given 0.5 mg/kg daily for three weeks prior to training and testing exhibited greater success when trained with motivationally significant cues, that is, lures, were more likely to walk near novel objects and were less distractible than a placebo group (Mills and Ledger 2001). Selegiline has been shown to improve spatial short-term memory in aged dogs in a dose-dependent fashion (Ivy et al. 1994).

Pageat (1996) reported an 85% success rate when treating cocker spaniels with "rage syndrome" with selegiline.

In a study of 141 dogs of various breeds, ages, and sexes, with a variety of behavior problems considered to be based on dysfunctional emotional status, 80% of the cases were considered improved or cured after treatment with 0.5 mg/kg of selegiline daily for periods of time ranging from 36 days to over a year. Behavior modification specific to the case was also used. Improvement at 30 days after initiation of treatment was a good predictor of the final outcome of treatment. Vomiting or diarrhea was occasionally observed in dogs in this study (Pobel and Caudrillier 1997).

Selegiline, at a dose of 2 mg/kg PO, suppresses cataplexy in dogs (Nishino et al. 1996).

Horses

Selegiline is considered to have high abuse potential in race horses and is classified as a class 2 agent by the Association of Racing Commissioners International (ARCI). Traces of selegiline, amphetamine, and methamphetamine can be recovered in thoroughbred horse urine when a single oral dose of 40 mg is given. Relatively higher urinary concentrations of *N*-desmethylselegiline (2-methyl-*N*-2-propynylphenethylamine) are found in the horse. *N*-desmethylselegiline concentration peaks in horse urine at 480 ng/ml at 2 hours. Amphetamine peaks in the urine at 38 ng/ml 24 hours after oral dosing, while methamphetamine peaks in the urine at 6.1 ng/ml after 4 hours. Horses given 30 mg/kg of selegiline orally or intravenously while confined to box stalls (3.4 × 3.4 m) do not exhibit any significant changes in heart rate or motor activity (Dirikolu et al. 2003).

Clinical Examples

Case 1

Signalment and Chief Complaint

An 11-year-old, 30-kg, neutered female Staffordshire pit bull terrier, Sarah, was presented with a chief complaint of sporadic destructiveness of two years' duration.

History

Sarah had previously been trained in agility, tracking, search and rescue, and had been used as a therapy dog. Until approximately nine years of age she was alert, attentive, learned well, and had no notable behavior problems. Additional problems had begun and gradually worsened over the previous 2 years, including development of aloofness in her relationship with both the owner and other dogs in the household, staring into space, humping her dog bed and the air, wandering aimlessly through the house, decreased response to verbal cues and wandering attention, increased total sleep, decreased purposeful activity, forgetting to urinate when she was outside, and persistent barking. Sometimes Sarah would develop a rhythm of barking and would spend five minutes or longer barking, apparently oblivious to her environment. Within the previous month, Sarah had begun having periods of having a "vacant look."

The destructive behavior occurred almost entirely during the owner's absence. When the owner was leaving, Sarah watched her and appeared anxious. Once the owner had left the house, Sarah would watch her through a window and persistently bark. If the owner realized she had forgotten something and returned to the house within a few minutes, she would often find that something was already damaged by Sarah. The items damaged were usually small, such as pens or pieces of paper, but there had been one incident of damaging furniture. When the owner was home, Sarah followed her from room to room, but at the time of presentation ignored her or turned away when the owner paid attention to her. The owner gave her a toy stuffed with food upon departure.

At the time of presentation, Sarah was on Cosequin DS and occasional buffered aspirin for arthritis, phenylpropanolamine for urinary incontinence, Sentinel, and Advantage. The owner had begun feeding Sarah B/D approximately 6 weeks previously.

Diagnosis

Sarah was diagnosed with CCD with concurrent separation anxiety.

Treatment Plan

It was recommended that the owner continue B/D and begin selegiline at 15 mg (0.5 mg/kg) daily. Because Sarah was also on phenylpropanolamine for urinary incontinence, her blood pressure was measured at initiation of treatment, one week after beginning selegiline, and every few weeks thereafter. Because Sarah had reached a stage where her apparent awareness of her environment was severely compromised, behavior modification was delayed pending assessment of the response to selegiline. In the meantime, the owner was to stay outside with her when she went out to eliminate and was to give her clear cues to attempt to stimulate her to urinate appropriately. For Sarah's anxiety upon the owner's departure, diazepam, 10 mg, was to be given as needed. Clomipramine was not used specifically because it is contraindicated for concurrent use with selegiline. Treatment with selegiline was considered more important because it would be necessary for Sarah to have improved cognitive function before behavior modification could be effectively initiated.

Follow-up

Two months after initiation of treatment, Sarah's cognitive function was clearly improving, and behavior modification for separation anxiety was initiated. Eight months after initiation of treatment, a plateau appeared to have been reached, and the dose was increased to 22.5 mg daily (0.75 mg/kg). This resulted in further improvement. Sarah entirely discontinued episodes of vacant staring. She consistently eliminated outside and had discontinued engaging in episodes of persistent barking. The owner reported that her personality was "coming back," that is, she was returning to her previous behavior of being sociable to both the owner and several canine housemates, responded to cues, and appeared to be aware of and interact appropriately with her environment. Her response to verbal cues began declining while other symptoms were improving, and it was determined that she was experiencing a decline in hearing ability.

At 14 months after initiation of treatment, a further increase in selegiline dose to 30 mg daily (1.0 mg/kg) was attempted when a second plateau in improvement occurred. Within three weeks of increasing the dose, Sarah developed excessive licking behavior directed at both herself and another dog in the household. Although further improvement in cognition appeared to be occurring, it was decided that the excessive licking was sufficiently detrimental that the higher dose should not be continued. The dose was reduced to 22.5 mg daily. Twenty months after beginning treatment, Sarah is now 13.5 years old and continues to maintain good cognitive function. Sarah is physically active and interacts with her environment in a fairly normal fashion. Sarah's blood pressure has remained normal throughout treatment.

References

Amenta F, Bograni S, Cadel S, Ferrante F, Valsecchi B and Vega JA 1994a. Microanatomical changes in the frontal cortex of aged rats: Effect of L-deprenyl treatment. *Brain Research Bulletin* 34(2): 125–131.

Amenta F, Bongrani S, Cadel S, Ferrante F, Valsecchi B and Zeng Y-C 1994b. Influence of treatment with L-deprenyl on the structure of the cerebellar cortex of aged rats. *Mechanisms of Ageing and Development* 75: 157–167.

Amenta F, Bongrani S, Cadel S, Ricci A, Valsecchi B and Zeng Y-C 1994c. Neuroanatomy of aging brain: Influence of treatment with L-deprenyl. *Annals of the New York Academy of Sciences* 717: 33–44.

Battistin L, Rigo A, Bracco F, Dam M and Pizzolato G 1987. Metabolic aspects of aging brain and related disorders. *Gerontology* 33: 253–258.

Berry MD, Scarr E, Zhu MY, Paterson IA and Jourio AV 1994. The effects of administration of monoamine oxidase-B inhibitors on rat striatal neurone responses to dopamine. *British Journal of Pharmacology* 113(4): 1159–1166.

Biagini G, Frasoldati A, Fuxe K and Agnati LF 1994. The concept of astrocyte-kinetic drug in the treatment of neurodegenerative diseases: Evidence for L-deprenyl-induced activation of reactive astrocytes. *Neurochemistry International* 25(1): 17–22.

Birkmayer W, Knoll J, Riederer P, Youdim MBH, Hars V and Marton J 1985. Increased life expectancy resulting from addition of L-deprenyl to Madopar® treatment in Parkinson's disease: A long term study. *Journal of Neural Transmission* 64: 113–127.

Boulton AA, Ivy G, Davis B, Durden D, Juorio AV and Yu P 1992. Inhibition of MAO-B alters dopamine metabolism in primate caudate. *Transactions of the American Society for Neurochemistry* 23: 225. Houston, TX, March 16–20.

Bruyette DS, Ruehl WW, Entriken TL, Darling LA and Griffin DW 1997a. Treating canine pituitary-dependent hyperadrenocorticism with L-deprenyl. *Veterinary Medicine* 92(8): 711–727.

Bruyette DA, Ruehl WW, Entriken T, Griffin D and Darling L 1997b. Management of canine pituitary-dependent hyperadrenocorticism with l-deprenyl (Anipryl). In *Veterinary clinicals of North America: small animal practice; Adrenal Disorders* 27(2), pp. 273–285, edited by PK Kintzer, Philadelphia, WB Saunders.

Bruyette DS, Ruehl WW and Smidberg TL 1995. Canine pituitary-dependent hyperadrenocorticism: a spontaneous animal model for neurodegenerative disorders and their treatment with l-deprenyl. In *Progress in Brain Research* 106, edited by PM Yu, KF Tipton and AA Boulton: pp. 207–215, Elsevier Science.

Carillo MC, Ivy GO, Milgram NW, Head E, Wu P and Kitani K 1994. (-)deprenyl increases activities of superoxide dismutase (SOD) in striatum of dog brain. *Life Sciences* 54(20): 1483–1489.

Collins GGS and Sandler M 1971. Human blood platelet monoamine oxidase. *Biochemical Pharmacology* 20: 289–296.

Coplan JD and Gorman JM 1993. Detectable levels of fluoxetine metabolites after discontinuation: An unexpected serotonin syndrome. The *American Journal of Psychiatry* 150 (5): 837.

Cummings BJ, Su JH, Cotman CW, White R and Russell MJ 1993. β-Amyloid accumulation in aged canine brain: A model of early plaque formation in Alzheimer's disease. *Neurobiology of Aging* 14: 547–560.

Cummings BJ, Head E, Afagh AJ, Milgram NW and Cotman CW 1996a. β-Amyloid accumulation correlates with cognitive dysfunction in the aged canine. *Neurobiology of Learning and Memory* 66: 11–23.

Cummings BJ, Head E, Ruehl W, Milgram NW and Cotman CW 1996b. The canine as an animal model of human aging and dementia. *Neurobiology of Aging.* 17: 259–268.

Cummings BJ, Satou T, Head E, Milgram NW, Cole GM, Savage MJ, Podlisny MB, Selkoe DJ, Siman R, Greenberg BD and Cotman CW. 1996. Diffuse plaques contain C-terminal Aβ_{42} and not AB$_{40}$: Evidence from cats and dogs. *Neurobiology of Aging* 17(4): 653–659.

Dirikolu L, Lehner AF, Karpiesiuk W, Hughes C, Woods WE, Boyles J, Harkins JD, Troppmann A and Tobin T 2003. Detection, quantification, metabolism, and behavioral effects of selegiline in horses. *Veterinary Therapeutics.* 4(3): 257–268.

Donnelly CH and Murphy DL 1977. Substrate and inhibitor-related characteristics of human platelet monoamine oxidase. *Biochemical Pharmacology* 26: 853–858.

Durden DA and Davis BA 1993. Determination of regional distributions of phenylethylamine and meta-and para-tyramine in rat brain regions and presence in human and dog plasma by an ultra-sensitive negative chemical ion gas chromatography-mass spectrometric (NCI-GC-MS) method. *Neurochemical Research* 18(9): 995–1002.

Fagervall I and Ross SB 1986. Inhibition of monoamine oxidase in monoaminergic neurons in the rat brain by irreversible inhibitors. *Biochemical Pharmacology* 35 (8): 1381–1387.

Fang J and Yu PH 1994. Effect of L-deprenyl, its structural analogues and some monoamine oxidase inhibitors on dopamine uptake. *Neuropharmacology* 33(6): 763–768.

Ferrer I, Pumarola M, Rivera R, Zújar MJ, Cruz-Sánchez F and Vidal A 1993. Primary central white matter degeneration in old dogs. *Acta Neuropathologica* 86: 172–175.

Fozard JR, Zreika M, Robin M and Palfreyman MG 1985. The functional consequences of inhibition of onoamine oxidase type B: comparison of the pharmacological properties of L-deprenyl and MDL 72145. *Naunyn-Schmiedeberg's Archives of Pharmacology* 331(2–3): 186–193.

Gerlach M, Riederer P and Youdim MBH. 1993. The mode of action of MAO-B inhibitors. In *Inhibitors of monoamine oxidase B: pharmacology and clinical use in neurodegenerative disorders*, pp. 183–200, edited by I. Szelenyi. Birkhauser Verlag, Basel; Boston.

Glover V, Sandler M, Owen F and Riley GJ 1977. Dopamine is a monoamine oxidase B substrate in man. *Nature* 265: 80–81.

Head E and Milgram NW. 1992. Changes in spontaneous behavior in the dog following oral administration of L-deprenyl. *Pharmacology Biochemistry and Behavior* 43: 749–757.

Head E, Hartley J, Kameka AM, Mehta R, Ivy GO, Ruehl WW and Milgram NW. 1996. The effects of L-deprenyl on spatial, short term memory in young and aged dogs. *Progress in Neuro-Psychopharmacology and Biological Psychiatry* 20: 515–530.

Heikkila RE, Cabbat FS, Manzino L and Duvoisin RC. 1981. Potentiation by deprenil of L-dopa induced circling in nigral-lesioned rats. *Pharmacology Biochemistry and Behavior* 15(1): 75–79.

Heinonen EH, Anttila MI and Lammintausta RAS 1994. Pharmacokinetic aspects of L-deprenyl (selegiline) and its metabolites. *Clinical Pharmacology and Therapeutics* 56(6): 742–749.

Heinonen EH and Lammintausta R 1991. A review of the pharmacology of selegiline. *Acta Neurologica Scandinavia*. 84 (suppl. 136): 44–59.

Hsu K-S, Huang C-C, Su M-T and Tsai J-J 1996. L-deprenyl (selegiline) decreases excitatory synaptic transmission in the rat hippocampus via a dopaminergic mechanism. *Journal of Pharmacology and Experimental Therapeutics* 279(2): 740–747.

Ivy GO, Rick JT, Murphy MP, Head E, Reid C and Milgram NW 1994. Effects of L-deprenyl on manifestations of aging in the rat and dog. *Annals of the New York Academy of Sciences* 717: 45–59.

Jurio AV, Li XM, Paterson A and Boulton AA 1994. Effects of monoamine oxidase B inhibitors on dopaminergic function: role of 2-phenylethylamine and aromatic l-amino acid decarboxylase. In *Monoamine oxidase inhibitors in neurologic diseases*, pp. 181–200, edited by A Lieberman, CW Olanow, MBH Youdim and K Tipton, Marcel Dekker, New York.

Kato T, Dong B, Ishii K and Kinemuchi H 1986. Brain dialysis: In vivo metabolism of dopamine and serotonin by monoamine oxidase A but not B in the striatum of unrestrained rats. *Journal of Neurochemistry* 46 (4): 1277–1282.

Kitani K, Kanai S, Sato Y, Ohta M, Ivy GO and Carillo M-C 1992. Chronic treatment of (-) deprenyl prolongs the life span of male Fischer 344 rats. Further evidence. *Life Sciences* 52: 281–288.

Knoll J 1983. Deprenyl (selegiline): The history of its development and pharmacological action. *Acta Neuroligica Scandinavica*. (Suppl.) 95: 57–80.

Knoll J 1987. R-L-deprenyl (Selegiline, Movergan®) facilitates the activity of the nigrostriatal dopaminergic neuron. *Journal of Neural Transmission* [suppl.] 25: 45–66.

Knoll J 1988. The striatal dopamine dependency of life span in male rats. Longevity study with (-) deprenyl. *Mechanisms of Ageing and Development* 46 (1–3): 237–262.

Knoll J, Dallo J and Yen TT 1989. Striatal dopamine, sexual-activity and life span-longevity of rats treated with (-) deprenyl. *Life Sciences* 45: 525–531.

Knoll J and Magyar K 1972. Some puzzling pharmacological effects of monoamine oxidase inhibitors. *Advances in Biochemical Psychopharmacology* 5: 393–408.

Knoll J, Miklya I, Knoll B, Marko R and Kelemen K 1996. (-) Deprenyl and (-) 1-phenyl-2-propylaminopentane, [(-) PPAP], act primarily as potent stimulants of action potential-transmitter release coupling in the catecholaminergic neurons. *Life Sciences* 58 (10): 817–827.

Lai JCK, Leung TKC, Guest JF, Lim L and Davison AN 1980. The monoamine oxidase inhibitors clorgyline and L-deprenyl also affect the uptake of dopamine, noradrenaline and serotonin by rat brain synaptosomal preparations. *Biochemical Phmarmacology* 29: 2763–2767.

Landsberg G 1999. Feline house soiling: Marking and inappropriate elimination. *Proceedings of the Atlantic Coast Veterinary Conference*, Atlantic City, New Jersey, pp. 315–320.

Mahmood I, Peters DK and Mason WD 1994. The pharmacokinetics and absolute bioavailability of selegiline in the dog. *Biopharmaceutics & Drug Disposition* 15: 653–664.

Milgram NW, Racine RJ, Nellis P, Mendonca A and Ivy GO 1990. Maintenance on L-deprenyl prolongs life in aged male rats. *Life Sciences* 47: 415–420.

Milgram NW, Ivy GO, Head E, Murphy MP, Wu PH, Ruehl WW, Yu PH, Durden DA, Davis BA, Paterson IA and Boulton AA 1993. The effect of L-deprenyl on behavior, cognitive function, and biogenic amines in the dog. *Neurochemical Research* 18(12): 1211–1219.

Milgram NW, Ivy GO, Murphy MP, Head E, Wu PW, Ruehl WW, Yu PH, Durden DA, Davis BA and Boulton AA 1995. Effects of chronic oral administration of L-deprenyl in the dog. *Pharmacology Biochemistry and Behavior* 51 (2/3): 421–428.

Mills D and Ledger R 2001. The effects of oral selegiline hydrochloride on learning and training in the dog: A psychobiological interpretation. *Progress in Neuro-psychopharmacology & Biological Psychiatry* 25: 1597–1613.

Murphy DL and Donelly CH 1974. Monoamine oxidase in man: enzyme characteristics in human platelets, plasma and other tissues. *Advances in Biochemical Psychopharmacology* 12: 71–86.

Murphy P, Wu PH, Milgram NW and Ivy GO 1993. Monoamine oxidase inhibition by L-deprenyl depends on both sex and route of administration in the rat. *Neurochemical Research* 18(12): 1299–1304.

Nishino S, Arrigoni J, Kanbayashi T, Dement WC and Mignot E 1996. Comparative effects of MAO-A and MAO-B selective inhibitors on canine cataplexy. *Sleep Research* 25: 315.

Nishino S and Mignot E 1997. Pharmacological aspects of human and canine narcolepsy. *Progress in Neurobiology*. 52: 27–78.

Obata T, Egashira T and Yamanaka Y 1987. Evidence for existence of A and B form monoamine oxidase in mitochondria from dog platelets. *Japanese Journal of Pharmacology* 44: 105–111.

O'Carroll AM, Fowler CJ, Phillips JP, Tobbia I and Tipton KF 1983. The deamination of dopamine by human brain monoamine oxidase: Specificity for the two enzyme forms in seven brain regions. *Naunyn-Schmiedebergs Archives of Pharmacology* 322: 198–202.

Olanow CW, Hauser RA, Gauger L, Malapira T, Koller W, Hubble J, Bushenbark K, Lilienfeld D and Esterlitz J 1995. The effect of deprenyl and levodopa on the progression of Parkinson's disease. *Annals of Neurology*. 38(5): 771–777.

Pageat P 1996. Rage syndrome in cocker spaniel dog. In *Proceedings and Abstracts of the XXIst Congress of the World Small Animal Veterinary Association*, pp. 138–139. Jerusalem, Israel, Oct. 20–23.

Parkinson Study Group 1989. Effect of deprenyl on the progression of disability in early Parkinson's disease. *New England Journal of Medicine* 321(20): 1364–1371.

Parkinson Study Group 1993. Effects of tocopherol and deprenyl on the progression of disability in early Parkinson's disease. *New England Journal of Medicine* 328: 176–183.

Paterson IA, Juorio AV, Berry MD and Zhu MY 1991. Inhibition of monoamine oxidase-B by (-)-deprenyl potentiates neuronal responses to dopamine agonists but does not inhibit dopamine catabolism in the rat striatum. *The Journal of Pharmacology and Experimental Therapeutics* 258: 1019–1026.

Paterson IA, Juorio AV and Boulton AA 1990. 2-Phenylethylamine: A modulator of catecholamine transmission in the mammalian central nervous system? *Journal of Neurochemistry* 55: 1827–1837.

Peterson ME 1999. Medical treatment of pituitary-dependent hyperadrenocorticism in dogs: Should L-deprenyl (Anipryl) ever be used? *Journal of Veterinary Internal Medicine* 13: 289–290.

Philips SR 1981. Amphetamine, *p*-hydroxyamphetamine and B-phenethylamine in mouse brain and urine after (-) and (+) deprenyl administration. *The Journal of Pharmacy and Pharmacology* 33: 739–741.

Philips SR and Boulton AA 1979. The effect of monoamine oxidase inhibitors on some arylalkylamines in rat striatum. *Journal of Neurochemistry* 33: 159–167.

Pfizer Animal Health and Product Information 2000. Anipryl®.

Pobel T and Caudrillier M 1997. Evaluation of the efficacy of selegiline hydrochloride in treating behavioural disorders of emotional origin in dogs. *Proceedings of the First International Conference on Veterinary Behavioural Medicine*, edited by DS Mills, SE Heath and LJ Harrington, pp. 42–50. Birmingham, UK.

Reusch CD, Steffen T and Hoerauf A 1999. The efficacy of L-deprenyl in dogs with pituitary-dependent hyperadrenocorticism. *Journal of Veterinary Internal Medicine* 13: 291–301.

Reynolds GP, Elsworth JD, Blau K, Sandler M, Lees AJ and Stern GM 1978a. Deprenyl is metabolized to methamphetamine and amphetamine in man. *British Journal of Clinical Pharmacology* 6(6): 542–544.

Reynolds GP, Riederer P, Sandler M, Jellinger K and Seemann D 1978b. Amphetamine and 2-phenylethylamine in post-mortem Parkinsonian brain after (-) deprenyl administration. *Journal of Neural Transmission* 43: 271–277.

Riederer P and Youdim MBH 1986. Monoamine oxidase activity and monoamine metabolism in brains of Parkinsonian patients treated with L-deprenyl. *Journal of Neurochemsitry* 46: 1359–1365.

Ross SB 1987. Distribution of the two forms of monoamine oxidase within monoaminergic neurons of the guinea pig brain. *Journal of Neurochemistry* 48(2): 609–614.

Ruehl WW, Bruyette DS, Entriken TL and Hart BL 1997. Adrenal axis dysregulation in geriatric dogs with cognitive dysfunction. *Journal of Veterinary Internal Medicine* (Abstract)11: 119.

Ruehl W, Bruyette D and Muggenburg B 1993. Effects of age and administration of the monoamine oxidase inhibitor L-deprenyl on total fasting bile acid concentration in laboratory beagles. *Veterinary Pathology* 30: 432.

Ruehl WW, DePaoli AC and Bruyette DS 1994. L-deprenyl for treatment of behavioural and cognitive problems in dogs: preliminary report of an open label trial. *Applied Animal Behaviour Science* 39(2): 191.

Ruehl WW, Entriken TL, Muggenburg BA, Bruyette DS, Griffith WC, and Hahn FF 1997. Treatment with L-deprenyl prolongs life in elderly dogs. *Life Sciences* 61(11): 1037–1044.

Ruehl WW, Griffin D, Bouchard G and Kitchen D 1996. Effects of L-deprenyl in cats in a one month dose escalation study. *Veterinary Pathology* 33(5): 621.

Ruehl WW and Hart BL 1998. Canine cognitive dysfunction. In *Psychopharmacology of animal behavior disorders*, edited by Nicholas H. Dodman and Louis Shuster, pp. 283–303, Blackwell Science, Inc., Malden, MA.

Salonen JS 1990. Determination of the amine metabolites of selegiline in biological fluids by capillary gas chromatography. *Journal of Chromatography* 527: 163–168.

Sano M, Ernesto C, Thomas RG, Klauber MR, Schafer K, Grundman M, Woodbury P, Growdon J, Cotman CW, Pfeiffer E, Schneider LS and Thal LJ 1997. A controlled trial of selegiline, alpha-tocopherol, or both as treatment for Alzheimer's disease. *The New England Journal of Medicine* 336(17): 1216–1222.

Shimada A, Kuwamura M, Awakura T, Umemura T, Takada K, Ohama E and Itakura C 1992. Topographic relationship between senile plaques and cerebrovascular amyloidosis in the brain of aged dogs. *Journal of Veterinary Medical Science* 54: 137–144.

Somerset Pharmaceuticals, Inc 2003. Eldepryl® product information. In *2003 Physicians desk reference*, pp. 3171–3171, Montvale, New Jersey.

Tariot PN, Cohen RM, Sunderland T, Newhouse PA, Yount D, Mellow AM, Weingartner H, Mueller EA and Murphy DL 1987. L-Deprenyl in Alzheimer's disease: Preliminary evidence for behavioral change with monoamine oxidase B inhibition. *Archives of General Psychiatry* 44: 427–433.

Tariot PN, Schneider LS, Patel SV and Goldstein B 1993. Alzheimer's disease and L-deprenyl: rationales and findings. In *Inhibitors of monoamine oxidase B*, pp. 301–317, edited by I. Szelenyi, Birkhauser Verlag, Basel; Boston.

Terleckyi IA, Sieber BA and Heikkila RE 1990. Loss of selective MAO-B inhibition with long-term administration of L-deprenyl in rodents: Crossover to MAO-A inhibition and clinical considerations. *Society for Neuroscience Abstracts*. 66: 1109.

Uchida K, Nakayama H, Tateyama S and Goto N 1992. Immunohistochemical analysis of constituents of senile plaques and cerebrovascular amyloid in aged dogs. *Journal of Veterinary Medical Science* 54: 1023–1029.

Waldmeier PC, Felner AE and Maitre L 1981. Long-term effects of selective MAO inhibitors on MAO activity and amine metabolism. In *Monoamine oxidase inhibitors—the state of the art,* pp. 87–102, edited by MBH Youdim and ES Paykel, John Wiley and Sons Ltd., New York.

Yang HYT and Neff NH 1974. The monoamine oxidases of brain: selective inhibition with drugs and the consequences for the metabolism of the biogenic amines. *Journal of Pharmacology and Experimental Therapeutics* 189(3): 733–740.

Yoshida T, Yamada Y, Yamamoto T, and Kuroiwa Y 1986. Metabolism of deprenyl, a selective monoamine oxidase (MAO) B inhibitor in rat: Relationship of metabolism to MAO-B inhibitory potency. *Xenobiotica* 16: 129–136.

Zeng YC, Bongrani S, Bronzetti E, Cadel S, Ricci A, Valsecchi B and Amenta F 1994. Influence of long-term treatment with L-deprenyl on the age-dependent changes in rat brain microanatomy. *Mechanisms of Ageing and Development* 73(2): 113–126.

Zsilla G, Földi P, Held G, Székely AM and Knoll J 1986. The effect of repeated doses of (-) deprenyl on the dynamics of monoaminergic transmission. Comparison with clorgyline. *Polish Journal of Pharmacology and Pharmacy* 38: 57–67.

Chapter Nine
Antipsychotics

Antipsychotics are used to treat most forms of psychosis, including schizophrenia, in humans. They do not have the same significance in animal behavior therapy and are usually most appropriately used on a short-term, intermittent basis. The first antipsychotic, chlorpromazine, was developed in 1950. Individual antipsychotic drugs show a wide range of physiological effects, resulting in tremendous variation in side effects. The most consistent pharmacological effect is an affinity for dopamine receptors. In humans, antipsychotics produce a state of relative indifference to stressful situations. In animals, antipsychotics reduce responsiveness to a variety of stimuli, exploratory behavior, and feeding behavior. Conditioned avoidance responses are lost in animals that are given antipsychotics.

Antipsychotic agents are divided into two groups based on side effect profiles (low-potency and high-potency drugs) or by structural classes (Table 9.1). Low-potency antipsychotics have a lower affinity at D2 receptor sites, higher incidence of anticholinergic effects (sedation), stronger α-adrenergic blockade (cardiovascular side effects), and require larger doses (1–3 mg/kg), but have a lower incidence of extrapyramidal side effects. High-potency antipsychotics show a greater affinity for D2 receptor sites, fewer autonomic effects, less cardiac toxicity, a higher incidence of extrapyramidal signs, and are effective in smaller doses (0.5–1 mg/kg) (Simpson and Simpson 1996). The phenothiazine neuroleptics are antipsychotics that are commonly used in veterinary medicine for sedation and restraint.

Action

Antipsychotic agents block the action of dopamine, a catecholamine neurotransmitter that is synthesized from dietary tyrosine. Dopamine regulates motor activities and appetitive behaviors. Dopamine depletion is associated with behavioral quieting, depression, and extrapyramidal signs. Excess dopamine is associated with psychotic symptoms and the development of stereotypies. A large proportion of the brain's dopamine is located in the corpus striatum and mediates the part of the extrapyramidal system concerned with coordinated motor activities. Dopaminergic neurons project to the basal ganglia and extrapyramidal neuronal system. Side effects associated with blockade of this system are called extrapyramidal responses. Dopamine is also high in some regions of the limbic system (Marder and Van Putten 1995).

The nigrostriatal pathway consists of cell bodies originating in the substantia nigra and mediates motor activities. The mesolimbic pathway consists of neuronal cell bodies that originate in the ventral tegmental area, project to ventral striatum and limbic structures, and mediate appetitive behaviors. Dopamine is broken down by mono-

Table 9.1 Classes of antipsychotic drugs

Phenothiazine tranquilizers
    High potency
        Fluphenazine (Prolixin)
    Low potency
        Acepromazine (Promace)
        Chlorpromazine (Thorazine)
        Promazine (Sparine)
        Thioridizine (Melleril)
Butyrophenones
    Haloperidol (Haldol)
    Droperidol (Innovar)
    Azaperone (Stresnil, Suicalm)
Diphenylbutylpiperidines
    Pimozide (Orap)
Dibenzoxazepines
    Clozapine (Clozaril)
Atypical antipsychotics
    Sulpiride (Sulpital)

amine oxidase inside the presynaptic neuron or by catechol-*O*-methyltransferase outside the presynaptic neuron. There are five dopamine receptor subtypes. Traditional antipsychotics are D2 receptor antagonists and block 70–90% of D2 receptors at therapeutic doses.

Antipsychotics have a wide spectrum of physiological actions. Traditional antipsychotics have antihistaminic activity, dopamine receptor antagonism, α-adrenergic blockade, and muscarinic cholinergic blockade. Blockade of dopamine receptors in the basal ganglia and limbic system produces behavioral quieting, as well as depression of the reticular-activating system and brain regions that control thermoregulation, basal metabolic rate, emesis, vasomotor tone, and hormonal balance. Antipsychotics produce ataraxia: a state of decreased emotional arousal and relative indifference to stressful situations. They suppress spontaneous movements without affecting spinal and pain reflexes.

Overview of Indications

Antipsychotic agents are most often used in veterinary practice when chemical restraint is necessary. Antipsychotic agents are used for restraint or the temporary decrease of motor activity in cases of intense fear or stereotypic behavior. A complete behavioral and medical history is necessary to determine which pharmacological agents will be the most beneficial for any given case. A comprehensive treatment plan that includes behavior modification exercises and environmental modifications, along with drug therapy, has the best chance for success (Overall 1997a).

Antipsychotic agents have poor anxiolytic properties and should not be the sole treatment for any anxiety-related disorder. Therefore, while they can be useful in preventing self-injury or damage to the environment by an animal exhibiting a high-intensity fear response, they are not appropriate for long-term therapy and treatment of phobias.

Antipsychotic agents are indicated for the treatment of intense fear responses requiring heavy sedation to prevent self-injury or property damage. Sedation to the point of ataxia may be necessary to control frantic responses in storm-phobic dogs, but owners often report that their dogs still appear to be frightened.

Antipsychotic agents have also been used in game capture operations and to allow physical examination in intractable animals. Antipsychotics can also be used as antiemetics and for the treatment and prevention of motion sickness. When used as preanesthetic agents, antipsychotics may induce a state of indifference to a stressful situation.

Antipsychotic agents produce inconsistent results for the treatment of aggressive behavior, and in some cases have induced aggressive behavior in animals with no history of aggressiveness (Overall 1997a).

General Pharmacokinetics

Antipsychotic agents have a high hepatic extraction ratio. Metabolites are generally inactive compounds and excreted in the urine. Maximal effect occurs about 1 hour after administration. Duration of action ranges from 4 to 24 hours. Half-lives range from 10 to 30 hours in humans. These agents are highly lipid soluble and highly protein bound.

Contraindications, Side Effects, and Adverse Events

Significant side effects can occur with acute antipsychotic use because of decreased dopaminergic activity in the substantia nigra. Side effects may include motor deficits or Parkinsonian-like symptoms, such as difficulty initiating movements (akinesis), muscle spasms (dystonia), motor restlessness (akathisia), and increased muscle tone resulting in tremors or stiffness.

Behavior effects include indifference (ataraxia), decreased emotional reactivity, and decreased conditioned avoidance responses. Antipsychotic agents may also cause a suppression of spontaneous movements, a decrease in apomorphine-induced stereotypies, a decrease in social and exploratory behaviors, a decrease in operant responding, and a decrease in responses to non-nociceptive stimuli.

Tardive dyskinesia occurs as a result of upregulation of dopamine receptors with chronic antipsychotic use. An increase in postsynaptic receptor density due to dopamine blockade can result in the inability to control movements or torticollis, and hyperkinesis. The dopaminergic system is unique in that intermittent use of antipsychotic medications can result in up-regulation of postsynaptic receptors. Chronic side effects may occur after three months of treatment. At least 10–20% of human patients treated with antipsychotics for more than one year develop tardive dyskinesia, and the symptoms are potentially irreversible even after the medication is discontinued.

Bradycardia and transient hypotension due to α-adrenergic blocking effects can occur. Syncope has been reported, particularly in brachycephalic breeds. Hypertension is possible with chronic use.

Endocrine effects include an increase in serum prolactin, luteinizing hormone, follicle-stimulating hormone suppression, gynecomastia, gallactorhea, infertility, and weight gain. Parasympatholytic autonomic reactions are possible. Other side effects include lowered seizure threshold, hematological disorders (thrombocytopenia), hyperglycemia, and electrocardiographic changes. Priapism has been reported in stallions.

Antipsychotic agents should be used with caution, if at all, in patients with seizure disorders, hepatic dysfunction, renal impairment, or cardiac disease, and in young or debilitated animals, geriatric patients, pregnant females, giant breeds, greyhounds, and boxers.

Overdose

Neuroleptic malignant syndrome is a rare, but potentially fatal, complex of symptoms associated with antipsychotic use. It results in muscular rigidity, autonomic instability, hyperthermia, tachycardia, cardiac dysrhythmias, altered consciousness, coma, increased liver enzymes, creatine phosphokinase, and leukocytosis. Mortality reaches 20–30% in affected humans. Treatment includes discontinuation of the antipsychotic medication, symptomatic treatment, and medical monitoring.

Clinical Guidelines

Antipsychotic agents will typically have an immediate effect on behavior and so do not require chronic dosing, but can be used as needed for their behavioral quieting effects. When used intermittently, antipsychotic agents do not need to be gradually withdrawn. An owner consent form is helpful to outline potential adverse events and ensure that the owner is aware of these.

Specific Medications

I. Acepromazine Maleate

Chemical Compound: 2-Acetyl-10-(3-dimethylaminopropyl) phenothiazine hydrogen maleate
DEA Classification: Not a controlled substance
Preparations: Generally available in 5-, 10-, 25-mg tablets and 10 mg/ml injectable forms

Clinical Pharmacology
Acepromazine is a low-potency phenothiazine neuroleptic agent that blocks postsynaptic dopamine receptors and increases the turnover rate of dopamine. Acepromazine has a depressant effect on the central nervous system (CNS) resulting in sedation, muscle relaxation, and a reduction in spontaneous activity. In addition, there are anticholinergic, antihistaminic, and α-adrenergic blocking effects.

Acepromazine, like other phenothiazine derivatives, is metabolized in the liver. Both conjugated and unconjugated metabolites are excreted in urine. Metabolites can be found in the urine of horses up to 96 hours after dosing. Horses should not be ridden within 36 hours of treatment.

Indications

Acepromazine is indicated as a preanesthetic agent, for control of intractable animals, as an antiemetic agent to control vomiting due to motion sickness in dogs and cats, and as a tranquilizer in horses.

Contraindications

Acepromazine can produce prolonged depression when given in excessive amounts or when given to animals that are sensitive to the drug. The effects of acepromazine may be additive when used in combination with other tranquilizers and will potentiate general anesthesia. Tranquilizers should be administered in smaller doses during general anesthesia and to animals that are debilitated, animals with cardiac disease, or animals with sympathetic blockage, hypovolemia, or shock. Phenothiazines should be used with caution during epidural anesthetic procedures because they may potentiate the hypotensive effects of local anesthetics. Phenothiazines should not be used prior to myelography.

Acepromazine should not be used in patients with a history of seizures and should be used with caution in young or debilitated animals, geriatric patients, pregnant females, giant breeds, greyhounds, and boxers. Studies in rodents have demonstrated the potential for embryotoxicity. Phenothiazines should not be used in patients with bone marrow depression.

Side Effects

Phenothiazines depress the reticular activating system and brain regions that control vasomotor tone, basal metabolic rate, and hormonal balance. They also affect extrapyramidal motor pathways and can produce muscle tremors and akathisia (restlessness, pacing, and agitation).

Cardiovascular side effects include hypotension, bradycardia, cardiovascular collapse, and reflex tachycardia. Hypertension is possible with chronic use. Syncope, collapse, apnea, and unconsciousness have been reported. Other side effects include hypothermia, ataxia, hyperglycemia, excessive sedation, and aggression. Paradoxical excitability has been reported in horses, cats, and dogs.

Hematological disorders have been reported in human patients taking phenothiazines, including agranulocytosis, eosinophilia, leukopenia, hemolytic anemia, thrombocytopenia, and pancytopenia.

There is anecdotal evidence that chronic use may result in exacerbation of noise-related phobias. Startle reactions to noise can increase with acepromazine use. Acepromazine is contraindicated in aggressive dogs, because it has been reported to facilitate acute aggressiveness in rare cases.

Priapism, or penile prolapse, may occur in male large animals. Acepromazine should be used with caution in stallions, as permanent paralysis of the retractor muscle is possible.

In a safety study, no adverse reactions to acepromazine occurred when it was administered to dogs at three times the upper limit of the recommended daily dosage (1.5 mg/lb). This dose caused mild depression that resolved within 24 hours after termination of dosing. The LD_{50} (the dose that kills half of the animals [mice] tested) is 61 mg/kg for intravenous administration and 257 mg/kg for oral administration.

Adverse Drug Interactions

Additive depressant effects can occur if acepromazine is used in combination with anesthetics, barbiturates, and narcotic agents. Concurrent use of propranolol can increase blood levels of both drugs. Concurrent use of thiazide diuretics may potentiate hypotension.

Overdose

Gradually increasing doses of up to 220 mg/kg PO were not fatal in dogs, but resulted in pulmonary edema. Hypotension can occur after rapid intravenous injection causing cardiovascular collapse. Epinephrine is contraindicated for the treatment of acute hypotension produced by phenothiazine tranquilizers because further depression of blood pressure can occur.

Overdosage of phenothiazine antipsychotics in human patients is characterized by severe CNS depression, coma, hypotension, extrapyramidal symptoms, agitation, convulsions, fever, dry mouth, ileus, and cardiac arrhythmias. Treatment is supportive and symptomatic, and it may include gastric lavage, airway support, and cardiovascular support.

Doses in Nonhuman Animals

Dosages should be individualized depending upon the degree of tranquilization required. Generally, as the weight of the animals increases, the dosage requirement in terms of milligram of medication per kilogram weight of the animal decreases. Doses that are 10 times lower than the manufacturer's recommended dose may be effective.

Arousal is most likely in the first 30 minutes after dosing. Maximal effects are generally reached in 15–60 minutes, and the duration of effect is approximately 3–7 hours. There may be large individual variation in response (Tables 9.2 and 9.3).

Table 9.2 Doses for antipsychotics for dogs and cats

Drug	Canine	Feline
Acepromazine	0.5–2.0 mg/kg PO q8h or prn	1.0–2.0 mg/kg PO prn
Chlorpromazine	0.8–3.3 mg/kg PO q6h	3.0–6.0 mg/kg PO
Promazine	2.0–6.0 mg/kg IM or IV q4–6h prn	2.0–4.5 mg/kg IM
Thioridizine	1.0–3.0 mg/kg PO q12–24h	
Haloperidol	0.05–2.0 mg/kg PO q12h	0.1–1.0 mg/kg PO
Pimozide	0.03–0.3 mg/kg PO	
Clozapine	1.0–7.0 mg/kg PO	
Sulpiride	5.0–10.0 mg/kg PO	

prn, according to need.

Table 9.3 Doses of antipsychotics for horses

Drug	Dose
Acepromazine	0.02–0.1 mg/kg IM
Promazine	0.4–1.0 mg/kg IV or 1.0–2.0 mg/kg PO q4–6h
Haloperidol decanoate	0.004 mg/kg IM

Effects Documented in Nonhuman Animals

Several incidences of idiosyncratic aggression in dogs and cats treated with acepromazine have been reported (Meyer 1997; Waechter 1982). In an incident report received by the United States Pharmacopeia Veterinary Practitioners' Reporting Program, a German shepherd dog being treated with acepromazine following orthopedic surgery attacked and killed the other dog in the household, with no prior history of aggression. There were two incidences of aggression following acepromazine administration identified by the FDA Adverse Drug Experience Summary between 1987 and 1994. There are reports of aggressive behavior following oral and parenteral administration of acepromazine. While this is a rare side effect, the potential for serious injury should prompt practitioners to educate owners about this possibility and suggest appropriate precautions.

In horses, acepromazine can be detected in the urine for at least 25 hours after injection of 0.1 mg/kg (Smith and Chapman 1987).

II. Azaperone

Chemical Compound: 4′-Fluoro-4-[4-(2-pyridyl)-1-piperazinyl]butyrophenone
DEA Classification: Not a controlled substance
Preparations: Generally available as a 40 mg/ml injectable form

Clinical Pharmacology

Azaperone is a butyrophenone antipsychotic agent that blocks dopamine receptors. The peak sedative effect occurs approximately 30 minutes after intramuscular injection, and the effects last 2–4 hours. Azaperone is metabolized by the liver, with 13% excreted in feces.

Indications

Azaperone is labeled for control of aggression when mixing or regrouping weanling or feeder pigs and as a general tranquilizer for swine. It is not approved for use in other species and should not be used in horses.

Doses in Nonhuman Animals

Azaperone is administered at a dose of 1.0 mg/kg IM for sedation, 2.2 mg/kg IM for mixing feeder pigs, 2.0–4.0 mg/kg IM as a preanesthetic, and 5.0–10.0 mg/kg for immobilization.

III. Chlorpromazine

Chemical Compound: 10-(3-Dimethylaminopropyl)-2-chlorphenothiazine
DEA Classification: Not a controlled substance
Preparations: Generally available as 10-, 25-, 50-, 100-, 200-, and 300-mg tablets; 30-, 75-, 150-, 200-, and 300-mg capsules; 2 mg/ml, 30 mg/ml, and 100 mg/ml oral orange-flavored syrup; 25 mg and 100 mg suppositories; and a 25 mg/ml injectable dose

Clinical Pharmacology

Chlorpromazine is a phenothiazine antipsychotic agent with properties similar to acepromazine. It has anticholinergic, antiadrenergic, antihistaminic, and antiserotonin activity. It is less potent than acepromazine and has a longer duration of action. It is highly protein bound and metabolized extensively in the liver, with greater than 100 potential metabolites, some that are active.

Uses in Humans

Chlorpromazine is indicated in humans for the treatment of psychotic disorders, nausea and vomiting, mania, intractable hiccups, and as an adjunct in the treatment of tetanus.

Indications in Veterinary Medicine

Chlorpromazine is used primarily as an antiemetic, but also as a preanesthetic agent in dogs and cats. It is not recommended for use in horses.

Contraindications

Contraindications and precautions are similar to acepromazine. Horses given chlorpromazine may develop ataxia and excitability with potentially violent consequences. In human patients being administered lithium in combination with chlorpromazine, an encephalopathic syndrome has been reported, which resulted in irreversible brain damage in a few cases.

Side Effects

Side effects are similar to acepromazine. Chlorpromazine may cause significant extrapyramidal side effects in cats if given in high doses, including tremors, rigidity, lethargy, and loss of sphincter tone. Electrocardiographic changes include prolongation of Q-T and P-R intervals, S-T depression, and T wave blunting. There is evidence that chlorpromazine is excreted in breast milk of nursing mothers.

Effects Documented in Nonhuman Animals

The effects of chlorpromazine, compared with diazepam, were evaluated in dogs in a placebo-controlled trial (Hart 1985). Friendliness, excitability, and fearfulness were measured in response to human handling. Chlorpromazine significantly reduced excitability, but did not affect fear responses or friendliness.

IV. Clozapine

Chemical Compound: 8-Chloro-11-(4-methyl-1-piperazinyl)-5H-dibenzo[b,e][1,4] diazepine
DEA Classification: Not a controlled substance
Preparations: Generally available as 25- and 100-mg tablets

Clinical Pharmacology

Clozapine is an atypical antipsychotic agent, a tricyclic dibenzodiazepine derivative. Clozapine blocks dopaminergic activity at D1, D2, D3, and D5 receptors and has high affinity for D4 receptor subtypes. It is more active at limbic system sites than at nigrostriatal receptors, resulting in fewer extrapyramidal symptoms. In addition to dopaminergic receptors, clozapine has blocking activity at serotonergic receptors. It is an adrenergic, cholinergic, and histaminergic antagonist. Traditional neuroleptic agents block 70–90% of D2 receptors at therapeutic doses. Clozapine blocks 30–60% of D2 receptors and 85–90% of 5-HT2 receptors (Tarsy et al. 2002).

Clozapine is highly protein bound and almost completely metabolized by the liver prior to excretion. The major metabolites have been measured in dogs following single dose administration of clozapine (Mosier et al. 2003).

Uses in Humans

Clozapine is indicated for the treatment of severe psychotic disorders in human patients who have failed to respond to traditional therapy.

Contraindications

Clozapine is contraindicated in patients with myeloproliferative disease or seizure disorder.

Side Effects

Clozapine can cause life-threatening bone marrow suppression or agranulocytosis. In human patients, 32% of agranulocytosis cases were fatal. White blood cell counts must be monitored during treatment. Cardiac side effects are also possible. Anticholinergic effects may include increased intraocular pressure, urinary retention, constipation, and ileus.

Doses in Nonhuman Animals

Reliable dose-response data have not been established for veterinary patients (Table 9.2).

Effects Documented in Nonhuman Animals

According to Dodman (1998), preliminary results of treatment of aggressive dogs with clozapine were disappointing. Antiaggressive properties of clozapine have been reported in other species (Chen et al 2001; Garmendia and Sanchez 1992).

In a review of animal models of acute neuroleptic-induced akathisia, Sachdev and Brune (2000) compared the effects of haloperidol and clozapine in dogs. Haloperidol (0.3 mg/kg) induced more hyperkinesia and stereotypic movements than clozapine (7 mg/kg), measured 4 hours after administration. Persistent scratching, licking, rotating, self-grooming, and continuous walking were considered evidence of extrapyramidal symptoms.

The effects of orally administered neuroleptic agents on conditioned avoidance tasks in dogs were evaluated for chlorpromazine, thioridazine, haloperidol, and clozapine (Cohen 1981). All drugs blocked conditioned avoidance responses, inhibited escape behavior, and caused ataxia. Clozepine produced excessive salivation. Sedation was most common with chlorpromazine and thioridazine, and haloperidol and thioridazaine produced tremors.

V. Fluphenazine

Chemical Compound: 10-[3-[4-(2-Hydroxyethyl)-piperazin-1-yl] propyl]-2-(trifluoromethyl)-phenothiazine; 4-[3-2-(trifluoromethyl) phenothiazin-2-yl] propyl-1-piperazine ethanol

DEA Classificaton: Not a controlled substance

Preparations: Generally available as 1-, 2.5-, 5-, and 10-mg tablets; 2.5 mg/ml, 5 mg/ml, and 25 mg/ml solution; a 2.5 mg/5 ml elixir; a 2.5 mg/ml short-acting injectable; and 25 mg/ml and 100 mg/ml long-acting injectables (fluphenazine decanoate or enanthate)

Clinical Pharmacology

Fluphenazine is a high-potency phenothiazine agent, showing a greater affinity for D2 receptor sites, fewer autonomic effects, less cardiac toxicity, but a higher incidence of extrapyramidal signs.

Contraindications and Side Effects

Contraindications and side effects are similar to those noted for other phenothiazines.

Effects Documented in Nonhuman Animals

Fluphenazine was used as a sedative in an equine patient (thoroughbred filly) at a dose of 0.1 mg/kg IM (Brewer et al. 1990). The onset of extrapyramidal symptoms occurred at 15 hours after injection when the horse began sweating, pawing at the air, circling, head swinging, and licking her forelimbs. Rhythmic neck flexion, facial grimacing, and muscle fasciculations were observed. Periods of hyperexcitability were interspersed with periods of immobility. Serum fluphenazine levels were 20.3 ng/ml at admission and <1 ng/ml 24 hours after admission. Symptoms persisted 45 hours after the initial intramuscular dose. The horse was treated with 250 mg intravenous diphenhydramine (centrally acting anticholinergic agent), was behaving normally within three minutes, and remained normal for 18 hours. She was retreated with 300 mg diphenhydramine and then required no further treatment.

Fluphenazine has been used successfully in individual cases to treat flank biting in horses (Dodman 1994).

VI. Haloperidol

Chemical Compound: 4-[4-(*p*-Chlorophenyl)-4-hydroxypiperidino]-4'-fluorobutyrophenone

DEA Classificaton: Not a controlled substance

Preparations: Generally available as 0.5-, 1-, 2-, 5-, 10-, and 20-mg tablets; a 2 mg/ml solution (haloperidol lactate); 50 mg/ml and 100 mg/ml long-acting injectables (haloperidol decanoate); and a 5 mg/ml short-acting injectable

Clinical Pharmacology

Haloperidol is a butyrophenone antipsychotic that has dopamine-blocking activity. There is one major metabolite with low activity. Haloperidol decanoate may require three months in human patients to reach steady state. Substantial plasma concentrations can be detected months after treatment has been discontinued. Because it is administered once per month, patients require significantly less medication per month and potentially lower their risk of developing extrapyramidal side effects.

Uses in Humans

Haloperidol is indicated for use in the management of psychotic disorders and to control tics associated with Tourette's disorder.

Contraindications

Neurotoxicity is possible in patients with thyrotoxicosis that are also receiving haloperidol.

Side Effects

The most common side effects experienced by human patients in clinical trials were extrapyramidal reactions, including involuntary facial, arm, leg, and body movements. Tardive dyskinesia is also possible, as well as cardiovascular side effects, hematological disorders, and endocrine abnormalities. Additional side effects reported in human patients include jaundice, anorexia, constipation, diarrhea, hypersalivation, nausea, vomiting, dry mouth, urinary retention, priapism, laryngospasm, bronchospasm, visual disturbances, and sudden death (*Physicians' Desk Reference* 2002).

Reported side effects in psittacine birds include sedation, incoordination, vomiting, agitation, severe depression, and anorexia. Haloperidol may lower the seizure threshold.

The LD_{50} (dog) is 90 mg/kg when given orally, and 18 mg/kg for intravenous injection. A dose of 12 mg/kg/day for 12 months resulted in liver toxicity, tremors, and convulsions in dogs. The therapeutic index for dogs is 900 (50% of the lethal dose/the median effective dose or LD_{50}/ED_{50}).

Fatal cases of bronchopneumonia have been reported in human patients, resulting from lethargy, decreased sensation of thirst leading to dehydration, hemoconcentration, and reduced pulmonary ventilation.

Overdose

Overdose in human patients is characterized by severe extrapyramidal signs, hypotension, sedation, respiratory depression, electrocardiographic changes, and shock. There is no specific antidote, so treatment primarily involves supportive care.

Doses in Nonhuman Animals

Reliable dose-response data have not been established for veterinary patients (Tables 9.2, 9.3, and 9.4).

Effects Documented in Nonhuman Animals

Dodman (1998) has reported minimal success using haloperidol to treat aggression in dogs. Luescher (1998) also reported lack of success and undesirable side effects when using haloperidol in dogs to treat stereotypic behaviors.

Yen et al. (1970) evaluated the effects of antipsychotic agents, chlorpromazine and haloperidol, on conflict-induced behaviors in laboratory cats. In this experimental situation, cats were taught to press a pedal for a food reward and then were later pun-

Table 9.4 Doses of antipsychotics for parrots

Drug	Dose
Haloperidol	0.2 mg/kg–0.4 mg/kg q12h; begin at lowest dose and increase in 0.02 increments q2d to effect
Haloperidol decanoate	1–2 mg/kg IM q14–21d; lower dose for cockatoos, African grey parrots, and Quaker parakeets

ished for opening the reward box with a compressed air blast. Cats displayed a variety of conflict-induced behaviors after four to five weeks, including restlessness, depression, immobility, pupil dilation, altered feeding behavior, and avoidance of the pedal. Chlorpromazine administration resulted in mild improvement of conflict-induced behaviors. Haloperidol administration caused a complete normalization of operant responding, and even increased reward-seeking activity in despite the air blasts. Treatment with amphetamine facilitated the development of conflict-induced behaviors, and pretreatment with neuroleptics blocked the effects of amphetamine-induced behaviors.

There are case reports of haloperidol use for the treatment of self-mutilation in psittacine birds (Lennox and VanDerHeyden 1993; Iglauer and Rasim 1993), but no controlled studies or dose-titration trials are available. Lennox and VanDerHeyden reported that haloperidol was more effective for birds that mutilate soft tissue, when compared with birds that limit self-trauma to feathers. They report agitation, depression, decreased appetite, and excitability in patients treated with haloperidol. Response to treatment occurred within two to three days. Iglauer and Rasim (1993) report great variability in response to haloperidol and length of treatment required. They medicated patients by placing haloperidol in the drinking water, so dosing may have been less reliable. Cockatoo species and Quaker parakeets may require lower doses than other species (Cooper and Harrison 1994).

Haloperidol has been used successfully in game capture operations to increase tractability of wild hoof stock (Hofmeyer 1981). It may be most effective for antelope species. Doses ranging from 0.1 to 0.4 mg/kg IV facilitated handling for 7 to 12 hours, resulting in a decrease in injuries and mortality during transportation. The presence of extrapyramidal signs was species specific and was believed to be exacerbated by hyperthermia, noise, and excitability.

VII. Pimozide

Chemical Compound: 1-[1-[4,4-Bis(4-fluorophenyl)butyl]-4-piperidinyl]-1, 3-dihydro-2H-benzimidazole-2-one
DEA Classification: Not a controlled substance
Preparations: Generally available as 1- and 2-mg tablets

Clinical Pharmacology

Pimozide is a diphenylbutylpiperidine antipsychotic agent with dopamine-blocking activity. It undergoes extensive first-pass metabolism. Two major metabolites are produced by dealkylation in the liver. Pimozide has a long half-life in humans (55 hours).

Uses in Humans

Pimozide is indicated for the treatment of Tourette's syndrome in human patients when other standard treatments have failed.

Contraindications

Pimozide is contraindicated with cardiac disease and in patients taking macrolide antibiotics, antifungal agents, or other drugs metabolized by cytochrome P450 3A enzyme system.

Side Effects

Side effects are similar to those of other antipsychotic agents. Pimozide can cause prolongation of the Q-T interval, predisposing patients to ventricular arrhythmias. Sudden death has been reported. Electrocardiographic monitoring is recommended. Pimozide produces anticholinergic side effects and may lower the seizure threshold.

According to Luescher (1998), the presence of side effects in dogs given relatively low doses of pimozide limits its usefulness. The LD_{50} in dogs is 40 mg/kg. Oral doses as low as 0.16 mg/kg can cause catalepsy and sedation. Chronic dosing at 3 mg/kg resulted in weight loss, muscle tremors, and mammary and gingival dysplasia.

Doses in Nonhuman Animals

Reliable dose response data have not been established for veterinary patients (Table 9.2).

Effects Documented in Nonhuman Animals

The effects of pimozide on human avoidance in the Arkansas line of nervous pointer dogs were evaluated in a placebo-controlled crossover design (Angel et al. 1982). The human interaction test was used to assess behaviors. Positive responses included approaching, wagging tail, sniffing hands, jumping up, and nuzzling the human subject. Negative responses included retreating, circling, trembling, urinating, or defecating. Dogs were given 0.3 mg/kg daily for seven days. Pimozide treatment attenuated avoidance responses. Maximum effect occurred at four days, and the effects persisted nine days past treatment. Pimozide was more effective than a benzodiazepine in attenuating avoidance responses.

Pimozide was not effective in the treatment of a Doberman pinscher with acral lick dermatitis (Dodman 1994). The dog developed head bobbing at a dose of 4 mg per day.

VIII. Promazine

Chemical Compound: 10-[3-(Dimethylamino)propyl]-phenothiazine
DEA Classification: Not a controlled substance
Preparations: Generally available as 25-, 50-, and 100-mg tablets, a 2 mg/ml oral syrup, 2 mg/ml and 5 mg/ml injectables, and granules approved for use in horses

Clinical Pharmacology

Promazine is a phenothiazine agent with properties similar to acepromazine. It is metabolized by the liver to glucuronide conjugates, which are excreted by the kidneys.

Indications

Promazine has been used as a preanesthetic agent, tranquilizer, and antiemetic in dogs and as a tranquilizer in cats, horses, cattle, and swine.

Contraindications

There are reports of violent reactions in horses and increased sensitivity to noise.

Side Effects

Side effects are similar to acepromazine.

IX. Sulpiride

Chemical Compound: *N*-[(1-Ethyl-2-pyrrolidinyl)-methyl]-5-sulfamayl-*o*-anisa-mide

DEA Classification: Not a controlled substance

Preparations: Generally available as 50-mg capsule, 200- and 400-mg tablets, 25 mg/5 ml and 200 mg/5 ml oral solution

Clinical Pharmacology

Sulpiride is a substituted benzamide derivative with selective dopamine D2 antagonist properties. Other benzamide derivatives include metoclopramide, tiapride, and sulto-pride. In contrast to other neuroleptics, sulpiride appears to lack effects on norepi-nephrine, acetylcholine, serotonin, and histamine. Specificity may explain the rela-tively low incidence of extrapyramidal and other adverse effects observed with sulpiride use. Sulpiride also stimulates secretion of prolactin. Sulpiride has also been shown to improve blood flow and mucus secretion in the gastroduodenal mucosa and has been investigated for the treatment of ulcers.

Sulpiride does not appear to be extensively metabolized by the liver and thus is pri-marily excreted renally. No metabolites have been identified. The half-life in humans is six to eight hours and is prolonged with renal insufficiency.

Uses in Humans

Sulpiride is indicated for the treatment of depression, duodenal ulcer, Huntington's disease, inadequate lactation, neuroses, schizophrenia, and Tourette's syndrome, and to suppress the symptoms associated with tardive dyskinesia in human patients.

Contraindications

Sulpiride is contraindicated with pheochromocytoma and Parkinson's disease. Caution is advised in patients with cardiovascular disease, mania, renal insufficiency (dose reductions appropriate for the individual patient and extent of renal insuffi-ciency), patients with epilepsy, hyperthyroidism, pulmonary disease, or urinary reten-tion, and elderly patients.

Side Effects

Side effects are similar to those of other neuroleptic agents.

Doses in Nonhuman Animals

Reliable dose-response data have not been established for veterinary patients (Table 9.2).

Effects Documented in Nonhuman Animals

The effects of neuroleptic drugs in cats were evaluated following intracerebroventric-ular injection (Beleslin et al. 1985). Chlorpromazine, haloperidol, and droperidol in-jection induced profound motor impairment (ataxia). Emotional reactions, including restlessness and aggression, and autonomic changes were inconsistent with chlorpro-mazine, haloperidol, and droperidol administration. Sulpiride injection did not pro-duce any behavioral, autonomic, or motor activity changes.

Bruhwyler and Chleide (1990) evaluated the behavioral, motor, and physiological effects of neuroleptic agents in dogs. Subjects were trained in an operant task and then given chlorpromazine, haloperidol, thioridazine, pimozide, clozapine, sulpiride, and several other anxiolytic agents in a random order prior to each trial. There was a decrease in operant responding and an increase in incomplete responses with neuroleptic administration. The drugs causing the most neurovegetative effects (palpebral ptosis and urination) were clozapine, thioridazine, pimozide, and sulpiride. Low doses of thioridazine and clozapine caused excitation. Loss of motivation was significant for haloperidol, pimozide, clozapine, and sulpiride. Pimozide cause significant hyperkinesia. Ataxia occurred with all drugs except pimozide and sulpiride. Catalepsy was not produced by haloperidol or clozapine. Sulpiride did not produce akinesia.

X. Thioridazine

Chemical Compound: 10-[2-(1-Methyl-2-piperidinyl)ethyl]-2-(methylthio)-phenothiazine
DEA Classification: Not a controlled substance
Preparations: Generally available as 10-, 15-, 25-, 50-, 100-, 150-, and 200-mg tablets; 30 mg/ml and 100 mg/ml solution; and 5 mg/ml and 20 mg/ml suspension

Clinical Pharmacology

Thioridazine has pharmacological activity similar to other phenothiazine agents, but may produce less extrapyramidal symptoms. Thioridazine has minimal antiemetic properties. Some metabolites may be more active than the parent compound.

Uses in Humans

Thioridazine is used to treat psychotic disorders in human patients, and for the short-term treatment of depression, agitation, anxiety, tension, and sleep disturbances.

Contraindications

Contraindications are similar to those noted for acepromazine.

Side Effects

Side effects are similar to acepromazine. Extrapyramidal responses are generally minimal. Electrocardiography abnormalities (marked T-wave effects), arrhythmias, and sudden death are reported.

Doses in Nonhuman Animals

Reliable dose response data have not been established for veterinary patients (Table 9.2).

Effects Documented in Nonhuman Animals

Thioridazine was used in the treatment of a dog with motor disturbances (Jones 1987). A male Pekingese dog that presented with fly biting, barking, restlessness, nocturnal activity, muscular tremor, self-trauma, and unprovoked aggression was treated with 1.1–2.2 mg/kg of thioridazine. The dog's physical examination was unremarkable, skin scrapings were negative, and fluorescent antibody for distemper was negative. The patient had failed to respond to phenobarbital. The patient responded within two days of starting the higher dose of thioridazine. Symptoms recurred with two missed doses. Side effects observed were mild tachycardia and dry feces, but no extrapyramidal signs.

Important Information for Owners of Pets Being Placed on an Antipsychotic

The following should be considered when placing an animal on an antipsychotic.

1. Antipsychotic agents have minimal anxiolytic properties and are not appropriate as the sole treatment for anxiety or phobias.
2. A wide range of side effects is possible, and some may occur acutely with a single dose.
3. Idiosyncratic aggressive responses may occur with some of the drugs in this class and precautions should be taken to prevent injury to humans and other animals.
4. Chronic treatment with antipsychotic agents has been associated with tardive dyskinesia in human patients, which in some cases is irreversible.
5. The effects of antipsychotics in animals vary greatly in the degree of sedation and the duration of effect.

Clinical Examples

Case 1

Signalment

Conan was a 3-year-old neutered male collie mix.

Presenting Complaint

Conan presented with destructive behavior and self-injury during fireworks and thunderstorms.

History

During a New Year's Eve celebration involving fireworks, Conan was alone in the home. The owners returned to find the wood of the front door damaged because of chewing, an 8-foot area of wall in which drywall and trim had been removed, and Conan bleeding from his footpads. In addition, there was evidence of hypersalivation and pacing. Conan vomited foreign material for four days following the incident. In the absence of loud noises, Conan is able to stay at home alone without causing damage to property or himself.

Diagnosis

Conan was diagnosed with noise phobia.

Treatment Plan

Behavior modification was instituted to desensitize Conan to eliciting noise stimuli using commercially available fireworks and thunderstorm CDs. The volume of the audio was gradually increased as Conan relaxed on command for rewards. Thunderstorms were rare in this region, and fireworks were not likely to occur for another six months, so no maintenance anxiolytic medications were prescribed. Due to the severity of the response, the cost of the property damage, and the risk of self-injury, neuroleptic tranquilizers were considered for use during the next incident, in case behavior modification was not yet completed. Acepromazine was prescribed, and the owner was instructed to give a test dose of 0.1 mg/kg and monitor the effects.

Follow-up

Conan progressed with noise desensitization exercises such that even occasional thunder elicited only a mild startle reaction. Conan became very nervous while construction was being done in the neighborhood, and the owner gave a single dose of acepromazine, which allowed Conan to sleep and remain calm throughout the day. After the initial reaction, the construction continued, but the owner was able to redirect Conan with relaxation exercises and did not use any additional medication. Conan received acepromazine during the July 4 holiday and no property damage occurred.

References

Angel C, Luca DC, Newton JEO and Reese WG 1982. Assessment of pointer dog behavior: Drug effects and neurochemical correlates. *Pavlovian Journal of Biological Science* 17(2): 84–88.

Beleslin DB, Jovanovic-Micic D, Japundzic N, Terzic AM and Samardzic R 1985. Behavioral, autonomic and motor effects of neuroleptic drugs in cats: Motor impairment and aggression. *Brain Research Bulletin* 15: 353–356.

Brewer BD, Hines MT and Stewart JT 1990. Fluphenazine induced Parkinsonian-like syndrome in a horse. *Equine Veterinary Journal* 22: 136–137.

Bruhwyler J, and Chleide E 1990. Comparative study of the behavioral, neurophysiological, and motor effects of psychotropic drugs in the dog. *Biological Psychiatry* 27: 1264–1278.

Chen NC, Bedair HS, McKay B, Bowers MB and Mazure C 2001. Clozapine in the treatment of aggression in an adolescent with autistic disorder. *Journal of Clinical Psychiatry* 62(6): 479–480.

Cohen BM 1981. Effects of orally administered psychotropic drugs on dogs' conditioned avoidance responses. *Archives Internationales de Pharmacodynamie et de Therapie* 253: 11–21.

Cooper JE and Harrison GJ 1994. Dermatology. In *Avian medicine: principles and application,* edited by BW Ritchie, GJ Harrison and LR Harrison, pp. 608–639, Wingers, Lake Worth, Florida.

Dodman NH 1998. Pharmacologic treatment of aggression in veterinary patients. In *Psychopharmacology of animal behavior disorders,* edited by NH Dodman and L Shuster, pp. 17–30, Blackwell Sciences, Malden, Massachusetts.

Dodman NH 1994. Equine self-mutilation syndrome: A series of 57 cases. *Journal of the American Veterinary Medical Association* 204(8): 1219–1223.

Dodman NH and Shuster L 1994. Pharmacological approaches to managing behavior problems in small animals. *Veterinary Medicine* 89(10): 960–969.

Garmendia L, Sanchez JR, Azpiroz A, Brain PF and Simon VM 1992. Clozapine: Strong anti-agressive effects with minimal motor impairment. *Physiol Behav* 51(1): 51–54.

Hart BL 1985. Behavioral indications for phenothiazine and benzodiazepine tranquilizers in dogs. *Journal of the American Veterinary Medical Association* 186: 1192–1194.

Hofmeyer JM 1981. The use of haloperidol as a long-acting neuroleptic in game capture operations. *Journal of the South African Veterinary Association* 52(4): 273–282.

Iglauer F and Rasim R 1993. Treatment of psychogenic feather picking in psittacine birds with a dopamine antagonist. *Journal of Small Animal Practice* 34: 564–566.

Jones RD 1987. Use of thioridazine in the treatment of aberrant motor behavior in a dog. *Journal of the American Veterinary Medical Association* 191: 89–90.

Lennox AM and VanDerHeyden N 1993. Haloperidol for use in treatment of psittacine self-mutilation and feather plucking. In *Proceedings of the Association of Avian Veterinarians,* pp. 119–120.

Luescher UA 1998. Pharmacologic treatment of compulsive disorder. In *Psychopharmacology of animal behavior disorders,* edited by NH Dodman and L Shuster, pp. 203–221, Blackwell Sciences, Malden, Massachusetts.

Marder SR and Van Putten T 1995. Antipsychotic medications. In *Textbook of psychopharmacology,* edited by AF Schatzberg and CB Nemeroff, pp 247–262, American Psychiatric Press, Washington, DC.

Meyer KE 1997. Rare, idiosyncratic reaction to acepromazine in dogs. *Journal of the American Veterinary Medical Association* 210(8): 1114–1115.

Mosier KE, Song J, McKay G, Hubbard JW, and Fang J 2003. Determination of clozapine, and its metabolites, N-desmethylclozapine and clozapine N-oxide in dog plasma using high-performance liquid chromatography. *Journal of Chromatography B* 783: 377–382.

Overall KL 1997a. *Clinical behavioral medicine for small animals,* pp. 293–322, Mosby, St. Louis, Missouri.

Overall KL. 1997b. Pharmacologic treatment for behavior problems. In *Veterinary Clinics of North America: Small Animal Practice: Progress in Companion Animal Behavior* 27(3): 637–665.

Physicians' desk reference 2002. Medical Economics Data Production Co., Montvale, New Jersey.

Plumb DC 1998. *Veterinary drug handbook*, 3rd ed. Iowa State University Press, Ames, Iowa.

Sachdev PS and Brune M 2000. Animal models of acute drug-induced akathisia—a review. *Neuroscience and Biobehavioral Reviews* 24(3): 269–277.

Simpson BS and Simpson DM 1996. Behavioral pharmacotherapy. Part I. Antipsychotics and antidepressants. *Compendium on Continuing Education for the Practicing Veterinarian* 18(10): 1067–1081.

Smith ML and Chapman CB 1987. Development of an enzyme-linked immunosorbent assay for the detection of phenothiazine tranquilizers in horses. *Research in Veterinary Science* 42: 415–417.

Tarsy D, Baldessarini RJ, and Tarazi FI 2002. Atypical antipsychotic agents: effects on extrapyramidal function. *CNS Drugs* 16(1): 23–45.

Waechter RA 1982. Unusual reaction to acepromazine maleate in the dog. *Journal of the American Veterinary Medical Association* 180: 73–74.

Yen HCY, Krop S, Mendez HC, and Katz MH 1970. Effects of some psychoactive drugs on experimental "neurotic" (conflict induced) behavior in cats. *Pharmacology* 3(1): 32–40.

Chapter Ten
CNS Stimulants

Action

Central nervous system (CNS) stimulants increase synaptic dopamine and norepinephrine.

Overview of Indications

CNS stimulants are used to treat attention deficit disorder (ADD), also called attention deficit hyperactivity disorder (ADHD), or hyperkinesis in dogs (Corson et al. 1976).

Contraindications, Side Effects, and Adverse Events

While CNS stimulants may decrease overall activity in animals with true hyperkinesis, the effects that give the medications their names will occur in animals that do not have true hyperkinesis. Therefore, during a testing situation, preparations should be made for this possibility. A variety of other side effects can occur in animals with and without hyperkinesis. These include pain and difficulty with urination due to contraction of the urethral sphincter, gastrointestinal disturbance, decreased appetite, anorexia, dry mouth, convulsions, hyperthermia, increased blood pressure, tachycardia, and cardiac arrhythmias. CNS stimulants are contraindicated in animals with cardiovascular disease or glaucoma.

CNS stimulants should not be given to patients with significant anxiety, because these symptoms may be exacerbated.

Adverse Drug Interactions

Do not give CNS stimulants with monoamine oxidase inhibitors (MAOIs) or within 14 days of discontinuing MAOIs.

Overdose

In case of overdose remove stomach contents by gastric lavage. Give activated charcoal and cathartics. A short-acting barbiturate may be given before attempting gastric lavage. Minimize external stimuli that will exacerbate the existing drug-induced hyperexcitement. Provide supportive therapy, including procedures to prevent hyperpyrexia.

Clinical Guidelines

True hyperkinesis, or ADD, appears to be rare in animals, but it has been identified in dogs. In a group of telomian dogs that had hyperkinetic syndrome and were therefore used as research models for the study of ADD in humans, dogs that responded to treatment with amphetamines were identified as being biochemically different from dogs that did not respond. Specifically, they had low levels of norepinephrine, dopamine, and homovanillic acid (HVA) in the brain and low levels of HVA in the cerebrospinal fluid (Bareggi et al. 1979a).

However, if the chief complaint is hyperactivity, care should be taken to ensure that other, more common, possibilities are ruled out before a trial with a CNS stimulant is conducted. Young, healthy animals are normally very active. One possible cause of a complaint of hyperactivity is that the owner is simply not exercising their pet enough. Owners may have unrealistic expectations of how quiet and calm their pet will be or be keeping the pet in an unsuitable environment. For example, an elderly, sedentary couple living in a small apartment may get a Great Dane, supposedly for protection, and then find that they have a "hyperactive," out of control pet on their hands because they are unable to meet the dog's need for basic exercise.

Sometimes owners unintentionally reinforce intensely active behaviors, especially in dogs and parrots. These and other pets may learn that they do not get attention when they are quiet, but they do get attention when they are noisy and rambunctious, specifically engaging in such behaviors as barking, screaming, spinning, running, or jumping. If the pet is primarily motivated by the need for social contact, even reprimands and screaming at the pet may simply make the problem worse.

Owners of pet dogs may focus more on issues of training and consider the dog to be inattentive because it is not learning well in obedience school. In this case, again, environmental factors rather than a true pathology in the pet are likely to be the cause of the problem. Inappropriate training techniques include issues of failure to use appropriate reinforcers, use of inappropriate or excessive punishment, and inappropriate timing on the part of the trainer and/or owner can all result in failure of obedience training. In particular, the use of inappropriate and excessive punishment is quite common in dog training in the United States. This can lead to problems of chronic anxiety that interfere with the dog's ability to learn because of emotional arousal.

If a dog persists in hyperactive and/or inattentive behavior despite adequate exercise, reinforcement of quiet, calm behavior, ignoring of rambunctious behaviors, and appropriate obedience training techniques, it may have true hyperkinesis and respond to medication with CNS stimulants. Specifically look for (1) a short attention span, (2) constant movement, and (3) failure to learn obedience, even with strong rewards. The truly hyperkinetic dog is likely to be unable to learn to sit on command, not because it does not want a delicious treat held over its head, but because it is unable to maintain the sitting position even for the brief moment required to reinforce a sit. Behavioral signs must have been present for an extended period of time and the pa-

Table 10.1 Doses of CNS stimulants for dogs with true hyperkinesis or canine ADD

CNS stimulant	Dose	Cost	Cost based on
Dextroamphetamine	0.2–1.3 mg/kg	$$	10 mg b.i.d.
Levoamphetamine	1–4 mg/kg	Not commercially available	
Methylphenidate	2.0–4.0 mg/kg	$$$	20 mg b.i.d.

Note: Medication should only be given as needed, but can be repeated several times a day. Cost given is for twice a day dosing for a 20-kg dog. b.i.d., two times a day.
Source: Dodman and Shuster 1994; Overall 1994.

tient must have been unresponsive to appropriate attempts to facilitate calmer behavior. Not all humans with ADD respond to medication, and this is likely to be the case with dogs.

If a dog with an appropriate history becomes calmer and more attentive when given a CNS stimulant, the diagnosis of hyperkinesis is confirmed. It is important when working with families that have a hyperkinetic dog to discuss the fact that identifying a useful medication is just the beginning. Historically, the dog is likely to have not learned any basic obedience due to its inability to be attentive. Additionally, its previous hyperactivity may have led to the development of various bad habits that the owners have given up on. Once responsiveness to medication has been identified it is important that appropriate training techniques, using positive reinforcement, be initiated immediately to teach the dog what is acceptable and desirable behavior. Table 10.1 gives the doses and approximate cost of CNS stimulants used for ADD in dogs.

Specific Medications

I. Amphetamine

Chemical Compound: (+)-α-methylphenethylamine; (-)-β-methylphenethylamine and D,L-amphetamine aspartate monohydrate; dextro isomer of the D,L-amphetamine sulfate

DEA Classification: D-Amphetamine is a DEA class II, non-narcotic medication. While there are recognized medical uses, it has a high potential for abuse. D-Amphetamine is more potent than L-amphetamine (e.g., Taylor and Snyder 1970; Angrist and Gershon 1971; Wallach et al. 1971; Balster and Schuster 1973).

Preparations: Generally available in 5-, 7.5-, 10-, 12.5-, 15-, 20-, and 30-mg tablets; Adderall XR available in 5-, 10-, 15-, 20-, and 30-mg extended-release capsules; Dexedrine is available in 5-mg tablets and in 5-, 10-, and 15-mg sustained-release capsules; Spansule available as sustained-release capsules

Extended- and sustained-release capsules are designed for the human digestive system and may not function in an equivalent fashion in dogs and other veterinary patients.

Clinical Pharmacology

Amphetamines are believed to block reuptake of norepinephrine and dopamine into the presynaptic neuron and to increase the release of norepinephrine and dopamine into the extraneuronal space. They are noncatecholamine, sympathomimetic amines that stimulate the CNS. Peripherally, they stimulate both systolic and diastolic blood pressure, stimulate respiration, and dilate the bronchi (Shire US, Inc. 2003).

Gastrointestinal acidifying agents will lower the absorption of any amphetamine, while urinary acidifying agents increase excretion. Thus, either type of medication will decrease the efficacy of amphetamine. In contrast, gastrointestinal alkalinizing agents increase the absorption of amphetamine, while urinary alkalinizing agents decrease the excretion of amphetamines. Either of these types of medications will therefore increase blood levels of amphetamines (GlaxoSmithKline 2003).

In the dog, plasma levels of amphetamine peak at about 1.5 hours after oral administration, while cerebral spinal fluid (CSF) levels peak at about 2.5 hours (Bareggi et al. 1978). However, differences between breeds have been identified. Telomian-beagle hybrids form less of the active metabolite of amphetamine, *p*-hydroxyamphetamine, than do purebred beagles and exhibit less stereotypic behavior and hyperthermia when given the same dose of amphetamine (Bareggi et al. 1979b).

Uses in Humans
Amphetamines are used to treat ADD and narcolepsy.

Contraindications
Do not use amphetamines in patients that have known hypersensitivity to sympathomimetic amines, cardiovascular disease, hyperthyroidism, or glaucoma. Do not give amphetamines with an MAOI or within 14 days of discontinuing medication with an MAOI. Amphetamines can increase the activity of tricyclic antidepressants and any sympathomimetic agents. Avoid using these medications together.

MAOIs and a metabolite of furazolidone decrease the rate of metabolism of amphetamines, thus increasing their effects and side effects. The CNS stimulant effects of amphetamines are blocked by a variety of drugs, including chlorpromazine, haloperidol, and lithium (GlaxoSmithKline 2003).

Side Effects
Patients that do not have hyperkinesis will exhibit increased arousal and activity. Stereotypic behavior may also occur, as well as cardiac effects, including tachycardia, gastrointestinal disturbances, dry mouth, urticaria, and decreased libido. In dogs, D-amphetamine is 1.4 times more potent than levo-amphetamine in inducing stereotypic behavior. Doses of 1–2 mg/kg given as a single intravenous injection induce various stereotyped behavior, including bobbing, head turning, circling, pacing, and sniffing (Wallach et al. 1971).

Amphetamines have been shown to have embryotoxic and teratogenic effects in mice, but not in rabbits. Human infants born to women addicted to amphetamines have increased risk of low birth weight and premature birth. They may also exhibit signs of withdrawal, including both agitation and lassitude. Amphetamines are excreted in milk (GlaxoSmithKline 2003).

Overdose
In case of overdose, conduct gastric lavage and give activated charcoal, cathartics, and sedatives. Acidifying the urine increases renal excretion, but increases the probability

of acute renal myoglobinuria occurring. Chlorpromazine blocks the stimulant effects of amphetamines and can be used in the treatment of overdose. In rats, the LD_{50} (the dose that kills half of the animals tested) is 96.8 mg/kg (GlaxoSmithKline 2003).

Discontinuation

Chronic use can result in both tolerance and dependence. If a patient has been on amphetamines for an extended period, gradual withdrawal is recommended.

Other Information

Do not give amphetamines in the evening, because they may cause nighttime restlessness.

Amphetamines may cause increases in plasma corticosteroid levels and interfere with measurements of urinary steroids (GlaxoSmithKline 2003).

Effects Documented in Nonhuman Animals

Dogs

Healthy, fasted laboratory beagles given 2.5 mg/kg or 0.6 mg/kg amphetamine orally exhibited increased amounts of stereotypic behavior that peaked 2.5 hours after administration, as did CSF levels of amphetamine. Stereotypic behaviors were elevated between 2.5 and 6.5 hours after administration and then began to decrease. The relationship between stereotypic behavior and levels of amphetamine was exponential, suggesting that the amphetamine metabolite *p*-hydroxyamphetamine contributes to stereotypic behavior when this drug is given. Increasing body temperature, on the other hand, has a linear relationship with the amount of amphetamine in the plasma, peaking at about 1.5 hours after administration, suggesting that this phenomenon is related to the presence of amphetamine in the plasma (Bareggi et al. 1978).

In a telomian-beagle hybrid used as a model for research on ADD in children, dogs exhibited hyperactivity, impulsiveness and impaired learning ability. When these dogs are given D-amphetamine, 1.2–2.0 mg/kg by mouth (PO), some dogs show significant improvement. Dogs that improved had higher peak blood levels of amphetamine than those that did not improve, and improvements paralleled blood levels of amphetamine (Bareggi et al. 1979b).

Five of six pet dogs of various breeds diagnosed with canine hyperkinesis responded positively to treatment with D-amphetamine at doses ranging from 0.21 mg/kg twice a day (b.i.d.) to 0.83 mg/kg b.i.d., although the duration of response varied. For some patients, the improvement was only transient, while for others the positive response was both substantial and permanent (Luescher 1993).

Brown et al. (1987), during evaluation of a bull terrier with severe compulsive tail chasing, gave it a test dose of 1.0 mg/kg of D-amphetamine orally. By subjective assessment, clinical signs worsened between two and four hours after administration of the D-amphetamine.

D-Amphetamine has been successfully used to treat narcolepsy in a long-haired dachshund. However, treatment was discontinued because the dog also exhibited undesirable side effects, including hyperactivity, anorexia, excessive sniffing of the ground, and substantially increased activity of climbing into inaccessible spaces (Van Heerden and Eckersley 1989).

Cats

Cats given 13 mg/kg amphetamine IP exhibited stereotyped head movements starting 20 minutes to two hours after injection. Stereotypic behavior subsequently lasted more than four hours. Two of eight cats (25%) vomited and died about two hours after amphetamine administration. One cat, that was otherwise friendly, hissed and spat during the head movements (Randrup and Munkvad 1967).

To date, a behavior problem analogous to human ADD has not been reported in cats, nor has the author had any feline cases in this category.

Other Species

Stereotypic behaviors have been observed in rats given 5 mg/kg subcutaneously (SC), mice given 7.5–10 mg/kg SC, guinea pigs given 5–20 mg/kg SC, and squirrel monkeys given 1.7 mg/kg intramuscularly (Randrup and Munkvad 1967).

II. Atomoxetine HCl

Chemical Composition: R(-) isomer of (-)-*N*-methyl-3-phenyl-3-(o-tolyloxy)-propylamine hydrochloride

DEA Classification: Not a controlled substance. Atomoxetine does not cause dependence or have stimulant or euphoriant properties. While it is not a CNS stimulant, it is included in this section because it is used to treat the same behavioral problem for which stimulants are used.

Preparations: Generally available in capsules containing 10-, 18-, 25-, 40-, or 60-mg of atomoxetine

Clinical Pharmacology

Atomoxetine is a selective inhibitor of the presynaptic norepinephrine transporter. In humans, atomoxetine is rapidly absorbed after oral administration and can be given with or without food. It is metabolized by the P450 enzyme CYP2D6 with subsequent glucuronidation, but does not inhibit the CYP2D6 pathway. In humans it has a mean half-life of 21.6 hours. When doses were standardized to a milligram per kilogram basis, atomoxetine had similar pharmacokinetics in children, adolescents, and adults. There are also no gender effects. Maximum plasma concentrations occur in one to two hours.

The major oxidative metabolite of atomoxetine is 4-hydroxyatomoxetine, which is primarily formed by CYP2D6, but also by other cytochrome P450 enzymes. 4-Hydroxyatomoxetine inhibits transport of norepinephrine as much as the parent compound. CYP2C19 and some other cytochrome P450 enzymes form *N*-Desmethylatomoxetine, which has less pharmacological activity than atomoxetine.

Atomoxetine is excreted primarily in the urine as 4-hydroxyatomoxetine-*O*-glucuronide. Less than 17% is excreted in the feces. There is extensive biotransformation, so that <3% of atomoxetine is excreted in an unchanged form (Eli Lilly 2003).

Uses in Humans

Atomoxetine is used to treat ADHD.

Contraindications

Atomoxetine should not be given to patients with a history of hypersensitivity to the drug. It should not be given concurrently with an MAOI or within 14 days of discontinuing an MAOI. There is an increased risk of mydriasis; therefore, atomoxetine should not be given to patients that have narrow-angle glaucoma. It should be used with caution in patients with cardiovascular disease, because it can cause increased blood pressure and heart rate, and with patients with a history of urinary retention, because it can cause urinary retention.

Paroxetine and fluoxetine can significantly inhibit the CYP2D6 liver enzyme pathway, thus decreasing the rate of metabolism of atomoxetine. Giving these drugs in combination should be avoided or carried out at lower doses.

Atomoxetine doses need to be decreased in patients with hepatic insufficiency, but not in patients with renal disease (Eli Lilly 2003).

Side Effects

Atomoxetine can cause increased blood pressure and heart rate. Occasionally, its use results in orthostatic hypotension or urinary retention. Some patients may have impaired sexual function.

Rats given up to 47 mg/kg/day and mice given up to 458 mg/kg/day for a period of two years exhibit an increased rate of cancer. A variety of tests have not identified atomoxetine as being mutagenic. Rats given doses of 57 mg/kg/day did not exhibit impaired fertility.

Pregnant rabbits given up to 100 mg/kg/day through the period of organogenesis exhibited a decrease in live fetuses and an increase in early resorptions. There was also a small increase in incidents of atypical arterial origin. There were no harmful effects at doses of 30 mg/kg/day.

In studies of rats, females were treated with doses of up to 50 mg/kg/day from 2 weeks prior to mating through all of pregnancy and lactation, while males were treated with comparable doses from 10 weeks prior to mating. This resulted in decreases in pup weight and survival at the highest dose. There was decreased pup survival only at 25 mg/kg and no decrease in survival or weight at 13 mg/kg. In a similar study in which the rats were given 20 mg/kg/day or 40 mg/kg/day only through the period of organogenesis, there was a decrease in the weight of female fetuses and an increase in the occurrence of incomplete ossification of the vertebral arch at the higher dose. However, no adverse effects occurred if pregnant female rats were given up to 150 mg/kg/day only during the period of organogenesis. Atomoxetine is excreted in milk (Eli Lilly 2003).

Overdose

Gastric lavage and repeated administration of activated charcoal, with or without cathartics, may prevent or minimize systemic absorption. Provide supportive therapy (Eli Lilly 2003).

Discontinuation

Atomoxetine does not require dose tapering for discontinuation (Eli Lilly 2003).

Other Information

In humans, atomoxetine does not affect the binding of warfarin, acetylsalicylic acid, phyenytoin, or diazepam to albumin. Drugs that change gastric pH have no effect on atomoxetine bioavailability (Eli Lilly 2003).

Effects Documented in Nonhuman Animals

There are no publications on the use of atomoxetine for the use of clinical behavior disorders in nonhuman animals. In the future, however, it may prove to be useful for the treatment of hyperkinesis in dogs, as it is in the treatment of ADD in humans, without the concomitant problem of using a Class II medication.

III. Methylphenidate Hydrochloride

Chemical Compound: Methyl α-phenyl-2-piperidineacetate hydrochloride

DEA Classification: DEA class II, non-narcotic medication; while there are recognized medical uses, it has a high potential for abuse.

Preparation: Generally available in 5-, 10-, and 20-mg tablets; Ritalin-SR in 20-mg slow-release tablets; Ritalin-LA in 20-, 30-, or 40-mg capsule with an extended-release formulation; Concerta in 18-, 27-, 36-, and 54-mg tablets designed to have 12 hours of effect due to delayed absorption in the human digestive tract. The delay of the SR and LA forms of Ritalin and of Concerta may or may not occur in an equivalent fashion in canine and other veterinary patients.

Clinical Pharmacology

Methylphenidate is a mild CNS stimulant. It is believed to activate the brain stem and cortical arousal system, but the mechanism by which it has its behavioral and mental effects is not truly understood (Novartis Pharmaceuticals Corp. 2003).

Therapeutic activity is mainly due to the parent compound. Methylphenidate is rapidly biotransformed, resulting in rapid de-esterification to α-phenyl-2-piperidine acetic acid (ritalinic acid). Methylphenidate has a low rate of binding to plasma protein, with a range of 10–52%. In human children the average half-life of methylphenidate is 2.5 hours, whereas in adults it is 3.5 hours. The half-life of ritalinic acid is 3–4 hours. After a single, oral dose of immediate-release methylphenidate, almost all is excreted in the urine within 48–96 hours, most as ritalinic acid, although some is excreted as other, minor metabolites. Very little, <1%, is excreted as the parent compound (Novartis Pharmaceuticals Corp. 2003).

Methylphenidate can be given with or without food. The effects of renal impairment and hepatic insufficiency on metabolism of methylphenidate have not been adequately studied. However, renal and hepatic impairment should have little effect on metabolism and excretion of methylphenidate. Metabolism occurs primarily due to activity of nonmicrosomal hydrolytic esterases, which are distributed widely throughout the body.

No gender differences have been identified in the metabolism of methylphenidate (Novartis Pharmaceutals Corp. 2003).

Concerta tablets are designed to use osmotic pressure for delivery of methylphenidate at a controlled rate over an extended period of time. There is an immediate-release outer layer within which lies an osmotically active core with a precision laser-drilled orifice. When the tablet enters the gastrointestinal tract, the outer layer dissolves, providing immediate release. Subsequently, as water enters the interior of the tablet, the osmotically active portion expands, pushing methylphenidate out of the orifice. The inert shell is eliminated in the stool. Obviously, this tablet cannot be split, because doing so would destroy the mechanism for gradual release. In adult humans this medication minimizes the peaks and troughs that result from repeated dosing of the regular, short-acting form of methylphenidate (ALZA Corporation 2003).

Uses in Humans

Methylphenidate is used to treat ADD and narcolepsy. ADD is characterized by impulsivity, emotional lability, moderate to severe distractibility, a short attention span, and, in some cases, hyperactivity (Novartis Pharmaceuticals Corp. 2003).

Contraindications

Do not give to patients that exhibit significant symptoms of anxiety, because these symptoms may be exacerbated. Do not give to patients with any history of intolerance to CNS stimulants, cardiac disease or glaucoma. Do not give with MAOIs or within 14 days of administering MAOIs.

Methylphenidate may decrease metabolism of coumarin anticoagulants, anticonvulsants, tricyclic antidepressants, and phenylbutazone. If these drugs are given concurrently with methylphenidate, the dose should be decreased.

Side Effects

Side effects have not been reported in veterinary patients given clinically relevant doses of methylphenidate, except that patients given test doses may exhibit increased arousal and activity. This finding is interpreted as indicating that the drug will not likely be useful in that particular patient, and no further medication is conducted with this drug. Decreased appetite, tachycardia, and sleeplessness are all side effects that may be expected in the pet population.

In humans, there is some evidence of growth suppression in some cases of long-term use of stimulants. A causal relationship has not been established, and the mechanism of this effect is unknown (Novartis Pharmaceuticals Corp. 2003). The effect identified in humans is not substantial and not likely to be of concern in veterinary patients. While it might theoretically be of concern in animals destined to be show and breeding stock, it is probably not appropriate to show an animal with true hyperkinesis, given the unverified possibility of some degree of genetic effect.

Methylphenidate may lower the seizure threshold in patients with a history of seizures, with abnormal electroencephalograms (EEGs) but no seizures, and, very rarely, patients with no history of seizures and no abnormalities of the EEG. The safety of concurrent use of methylphenidate and anticonvulsants has not been determined; therefore, treatment with methylphenidate should not be initiated in patients with seizures and should be discontinued in patients that develop seizures while on it.

Some humans have reported difficulties of accommodation and blurring of vision when taking methylphenidate. The possibility of worsening of vision should be considered in assessing a nonhuman animal's response to medication.

Methylphenidate is teratogenic in rabbits when given at doses of 200 mg/kg/day, but not when given at 60 mg/kg/day during the period of organogenesis. In rats, the teratogenic effect is not evident at doses of 75 mg/kg/day. Pups of rats given up to 45 mg/kg/day during both pregnancy and lactation exhibited decreased weight gain. Weight gain was normal if the mothers were given 15 mg/kg/day throughout pregnancy and lactation. Methylphenidate has not been found to be mutagenic (ALZA Corp. 2003; Novartis Pharmaceuticals Corp. 2003).

In a study of the effect of methylphenidate on development, rat pups were given doses of up to 100 mg/kg/day, starting at day 7 of life and continuing through week 10. Tests administered at weeks 13 to 14 demonstrated decreased spontaneous loco-motor activity at doses of 50 mg/kg/day and higher. There was a deficit in the acquisition of specific learning tasks in females that had been given the highest dose of 100 mg/kg/day. There were no long-term effects in rats that had been given 5 mg/kg/day (Novartis Pharmaceuticals Corp. 2003).

The fertility of male and female rats given up to 160 mg/day was not impaired (ALZA Corp. 2003).

Carcinogenicity studies carried out on mice resulted in increased frequencies of he-patocellular adenomas in both genders and, in males, an increase in hepatoblastomas when the mice were dosed at 60 mg/kg/day. The total number of malignant hepatic tu-mors did not increase, however. Carcinogenicity studies conducted on rats at doses up to 45 mg/kg/day did not result in any increase in tumor development. A study con-ducted on a transgenic mouse strain that was sensitive to genotoxic carcinogens and using doses of up to 74 mg/kg/day did not reveal any increase in cancers (ALZA Corp. 2003; Novartis Pharmaceuticals Corp. 2003).

Overdose

Various sequelae may be produced by overstimulation of the CNS and excessive sym-pathomimetic arousal. Evacuate the stomach contents with gastric lavage. If neces-sary, give a short-acting barbiturate to allow for this procedure. Also give activated charcoal and cathartics. Place the animal in a dim, quiet location to avoid further stimulation induced by the environment. Monitor vital signs, and provide supportive therapy.

Doses in Nonhuman Animals

When it is effective for a given dog, methylphenidate can be given on an as-needed basis, which is useful given the need to compromise between making the dog a func-tional family pet and minimizing the amount of medication it receives. For example, if the dog is only with the family during the evenings and some weekends, and is kept in a large pen of suitable size and with toys present for it to exercise and play with during the day and weekends when the family is away from home, medication can be given that fits the times that the dog needs to be calm and attentive. When the first adult arrives home in the late afternoon or gets up on a weekend morning, they can medicate the dog, then leave it alone for a minimum of 30 minutes while the methylphenidate has time to take effect. After this time, the dog can be gotten out of its pen to interact with the family.

The slow-release and long-acting forms of methylphenidate (Ritalin-SR, Ritalin-LA, and Concerta) have tremendously benefited humans with ADD because of the drugs' extended activity, such that only one or perhaps two doses need be taken during the day. These forms, however, tend to be substantially more expensive than the regular release form and are not desirable for working families that interact significantly with their dog only in the evenings. Additionally, the various slow-release forms have been designed for the human digestive tract and may act differently in the digestive tracts of veteri-nary patients. In the author's experience, when regular release methylphenidate is used in dogs, they appear to metabolize it very rapidly, with clinical efficacy existing for only two or three hours. Thus, owners need to be aware of the necessity of remedicating regularly so long as the dog is remaining with the family.

For canine cataplexy, methylphenidate is given once daily, in the morning (Shell 1995).

Discontinuation

Chronic administration of methylphenidate can result in dependence. Therefore, discontinuation after administration for several weeks or longer should be done gradually.

Other Information

Periodic complete blood counts, differential and platelet counts are recommended if methylphenidate is prescribed long term.

Effects Documented in Nonhuman Animals

Dogs

A Yorkshire terrier diagnosed with canine hyperkinesis that did not respond to D-amphetamine subsequently responded to treatment with methylphenidate at a dose of 1.25 mg/kg t.i.d.

Methylphenidate, given at a dose of 0.25 mg/kg PO daily has some anticataplectic effects in dogs (Baker et al. 1983; Chrisman 1991; Braund 1994; Shell 1995).

Important Information for Owners of Pets Being Placed on CNS Stimulants

Do not medicate your pet in the evening, because this may result in nighttime restlessness.

Clinical Examples

Case 1

Signalment

Brownie was a tan and white, one-year-old, spayed female cocker spaniel weighing 11.7 kg.

Presenting Complaint

Brownie presented with hyperactivity.

History

The owners had gotten Brownie from a pet store as a 10-week-old puppy. They reported that since they first had her she had been extremely active, climbed onto countertops, chewed clothes and shoes whether the owners were home or absent, did poorly in obedience class, rested very little, and did not seem to be able to focus her attention. The owners reported that, at home, Brownie would only lie down for any significant period of time when she was locked in her crate at night. During the interview, she was almost constantly active, though friendly, investigating and walking around the room. She lay down for about 10 seconds three times, but was panting and looking around alertly while she did so.

Obedience training and paroxetine had been attempted to treat her behavior. The physical exam was unremarkable.

Diagnosis

Brownie was diagnosed with ADHD.

Treatment Plan

The owners were instructed to give Brownie a test dose of 5 mg of methylphenidate and observe her for any changes from her typical behavior. Behavior management of dogs with hyperactivity was discussed. The owners had already raised a child with ADHD and understood that finding a medication that helped was only the beginning and that they would have to put a lot of effort into training Brownie in new ways of behaving.

Follow-up

The owners reported that about 30–45 minutes after being medicated Brownie became calmer and lay down. She subsequently lay still for about 30 minutes. The owners were instructed to increase the methylphenidate to a test dose of 10 mg the next day. Brownie's response to 10 mg was better than to 5 mg, that is, she was even calmer and appeared to be able to focus her attention when one owner attempted a training session using positive reinforcement.

Brownie's behavior continued to improve with the combination of methylphenidate and training using positive reinforcement.

References

ALZA Corporation 2003. *Physicians desk reference,* pp. 1894–1897, Montvale, New Jersey.

Angrist B and Gershon S 1971. A pilot study of pathogenic mechanisms in amphetamine psychosis utilizing differential effect of d- and l-amphetamine. *Pharmacopsychiatry and Neuro-Psychopharmacology* 4: 64–75.

Baker TL, Mitler MM, Foutz AS and Dement WC 1983. Diagnosis and treatment of narcolepsy in animals, in *Current veterinary therapy VIII. Small animal practice,* pp. 755–759, edited by RW Kirk, W.B. Saunders Co., Philadelphia, Pennsylvania.

Balster RL and Schuster CR 1973. A comparison of d-amphetamine, l-amphetamine, and methamphetamine self-administration in Rhesus monkeys. *Pharmacology Biochemistry and Behavior* 1: 67–71.

Bareggi SR, Becker RE, Ginsburg B and Genovese E 1979a. Neurochemical investigation of an endogenous model of the "hyperkinetic syndrome" in a hybrid dog. *Life Sciences* 24: 481–488.

Bareggi SR, Becker RE, Ginsburg B and Genovese E 1979b. Paradoxical effect of amphetamine in an endogenous model of the hyperkinetic syndrome in a hybrid dog: Correlation with amphetamine and p-hydroxyamphetamine blood levels. *Psychopharmacology* 62(3): 217–224.

Bareggi SR, Gomeni R and Becker RE 1978 Stereotyped behavior and hyperthermia in dogs: Correlation with the levels of amphetamine and p-hydroxyamphetamine in plasma and CSF. *Psychpharmacology* 58: 89–94.

Braund KG 1994. *Clinical Syndromes in Veterinary Neurology,* 2nd ed., pp. 196–198, Mosby, St. Louis, Missouri.

Brown SA, Crowell-Davis S, Malcolm T and Edwards P 1987. Naloxone-responsive compulsive tail chasing in a dog. *Journal of the American Veterinary Medical Association* 190(7): 884–886.

Burghardt W 1994. Diagnosis and treatment of hyperactivity in the dog. *Proceedings of the American Veterinary Medical Association Annual Meeting*, San Francisco, California.

Campbell WE 1973. Behavioral modification of hyperkinetic dogs. *Modern Veterinary Practise* 54: 49–52.

Chrisman CL. 1991. *Problems in small animal neurology*, 2nd ed., pp. 223–225, Lea & Febiger, Philadelphia, Pennsylvania.

Corson SA, Corson EO, Arnold LA and Knopp W 1976. Animal models of violence and hyperkinesis: Interaction of psychopharmacologic and psychosocial therapy in behavior modification. In *Animal models in human psychobiology*, edited by G Serban and A Kling, pp. 111–139, Plenum Press, New York.

Eli Lilly 2003. Strattera™. Package insert. Indianapolis, IN. Shire US Inc. 2004. *Physicians Desk Reference*. pp. 3143–3146 Montvale, NJ.

Ginsburg BE, Becker RE, Trattner A and Bareggi SR 1984. A genetic taxonomy of hyperkinesis in the dog. *International Journal of Developmental Neuroscience* 2: 313–322.

GlaxoSmithKline 2003. Adderall product information. *2003 Physicians desk reference,* pp. 1500–1501, Montvale, New Jersey.

Luescher UA 1993. Hyperkinesis in dogs: Six case reports. *Canadian Veterinary Journal* 34: 368–370.

Novartis Pharmaceuticals Corporation. Ritalin product information. 2003 *Physicians desk reference,* pp. 2305–2310, Montvale, New Jersey.

Overall K 1994. State of the art: advances in pharmacological therapy for behavioral disorders. *Proceedings of the North American Veterinary Conference* 8: 43–51.

Poling A, Gadow KD, and Cleary J. Stimulants 1991. In *Drug therapy for behavior disorders: An introduction*, pp. 90–107, edited by AP Goldstein, L Krasner and SL Garfield, Pergamon, New York.

Randrup A and Munkvad I 1967. Stereotypied activities produced by amphetamine in several animal species and man. *Psychopharmacologia* 11(4): 300–310.

Shell L 1995. Sleep disorders, in *Textbook of veterinary internal medicine,* pp. 157–158, edited by SJ Ettinger and EC Feldman, W.B. Saunders, Philadelphia, Pennsylvania.

Shire US 2003. *Physicians Desk Reference,* pp. 3138–3142, Montvale, New Jersey.

Taylor KM and Snyder SH 1970. Amphetamine: Differentiation by d and l isomers of behavior involving brain norepinephrine or dopamine. *Science* 168: 1487–1489.

Van Heerden J and Eckersley GN 1989. Narcolepsy in a long-haired dachshund. *Journal of the South African Veterinary Association* 60: 151–153.

Wallach MB, Angrist BM and Gershon S 1971. The comparison of the stereotyped behavior-inducing effects of d- and l-amphetamine in dogs. *Communications in Behavioral Biology. Part A* 6(2): 93–96.

Wilens TE, Biederman J, Spencer TJ and Prince J 1995. Pharmacotherapy of adult attention deficit/hyperactivity disorder. *Journal of Clinical Psychpharmacology* 15: 270–279.

Chapter Eleven
Tricyclic Antidepressants

Action

The tricyclic antidepressants (TCAs) act as inhibitors of both serotonin and norepinephrine. They also have antihistaminic and anticholergic effects and are α-1 adrenergic antagonists. The extent of these various effects varies widely between the various TCAs (see Table 11.1). Some have strong serotonin reuptake inhibition and weak norepinephrine reuptake inhibition. Others have strong norepinephrine reuptake inhibition and weak serotonin reuptake inhibition. Other molecular activities vary widely as well. For example, amitriptyline has much stronger antihistaminic effects than clomipramine.

Chronic administration of TCAs results in decreased numbers of β-adrenoceptors and serotonin receptors and altered function of various serotonin receptors in the forebrain (Vetulani and Sulser 1975; Sulser et al. 1978; Heninger and Charney 1987; Potter et al. 1995). These long-term changes in receptor number and function are believed to contribute to the significant changes in behavior that evolve over time when a pet is maintained on these medications.

All of the TCAs are readily absorbed from the gastrointestinal tract. Peak plasma levels occur over a wide range of time, 2–6 hours being the mean peak time for various drugs. Half-lives vary widely as well, but are long, somewhere in the range of 24 hours. In the liver, they undergo demethylation, aromatic hydroxylation, and glucuronide conjugation of the hydroxy metabolite (Potter et al. 1995).

Tricyclic antidepressants are so named because of their central three-ring structure. The tertiary amines have two methyl groups at the end of their side chain, while the secondary amines have only one. The type of side chain is substantially related to the molecular action. Tertiary amines have a proportionately greater effect on blocking serotonin transport, while the secondary amines have a proportionately greater effect on blocking norepinephrine transport (Bolden-Watson and Richelson 1993; Tatsumi et al. 1997; Nelson 2004). Only the six TCAs that have been most commonly used in veterinary behavior will be discussed in this chapter; the tertiary amines amitriptyline, clomipramine, doxepin, and imipramine, and the secondary amines desipramine and nortriptyline.

Overview of Indications

Like the selective serotonin reuptake inhibitors (SSRIs), the TCAs have anxiolytic, anticompulsive, and antiaggressive effects, in addition to antidepressant effects. In veterinary behavior practice, they are used primarily for the first three effects. As with the SSRIs, the onset of effect takes several days to several weeks, and clients whose

Table 11.1 Acute *in vitro* biochemical activity of selected tricyclic antidepressants

TCA	NE	5-HT	α-1	α-2	H$_1$	Musc
Amitriptyline	±	++	+++	±	++++	++++
Clomipramine	+	+++	++	0	+	++
Desipramine	+++	0	+	0	0	+
Doxepin	++	+	++	0	+++	++
Imipramine	+	+	++	0	+	++
Nortriptyline	++	±	+	0	+	++

Source: Potter 1984; Potter et al. 1991; Richelson and Nelson 1984a; Richelson and Pfenning 1984b; Potter et al. 1995.

pets are placed on a TCA need to be cautioned of that so that they do not have unrealistic expectations. While occasional pets have a rapid response to a single dose, as a general rule they should not be prescribed on an as-needed basis.

One of the TCAs, clomipramine, is the only psychoactive medication with anxiolytic properties to be FDA approved for an anxiety disorder. Specifically, Clomicalm is approved for the treatment of separation anxiety in dogs, when used in combination with behavior modification. Clomipramine is the most serotonin-selective of the commercially available TCAs.

Common uses in domestic animals include anxiety, affective aggression, compulsive disorder, and urine marking.

Contraindications, Side Effects, and Adverse Events

Side effects vary widely, as there is a substantial range of effect on serotonin and norepinephrine between the various TCAs, as well as substantial variation between the TCAs in molecular effects other than those on serotonin and norepinephrine. In general, side effects may include sedation, constipation, diarrhea, urinary retention, appetite changes, ataxia, decreased tear production, mydriasis, cardiac arrhythmias, tachycardia, and changes in blood pressure.

There is some evidence from the human literature that antidepressant drugs that have a sedative action and an antimuscarinic effect can interfere with memory. Amitriptyline is an example of one such medication that has both a high occurrence of antimuscarinic and sedative effects. Clomipramine, on the other hand, has some antimuscarinic and sedative effects, but not as much as amitriptyline, and has no measurable effect on learning and memory (Liljequist et al. 1974; Thompson 1991). However, mice injected with 10 mg/kg of either amitriptyline or clomipramine did not show any deficits in learning or memory when tested in a maze test (Nurten et al. 1996).

Adverse Drug Interactions

TCAs should never be given in combination with MAOIs. This includes such various compounds as selegiline, which is used for the treatment of canine cognitive dysfunction, and amitraz, which is used for the treatment of demodicosis and is also a common compound in collars designed to prevent infestation with ticks.

Overdose

There is no antidote for overdose of any of the TCAs, although physostigmine given intravenously, has been shown to be useful in alleviating cardiac and central nervous system (CNS) toxic effects in humans (Falletta et al. 1970; Slovis et al. 1971). Treatment must consist of decontamination and supportive therapy; however, emesis is contraindicated.

Discontinuation

While discontinuation of a TCA does not generally produce significant withdrawal symptoms per se, it is generally recommended that a patient that has been medicated with a TCA for several months be weaned off gradually. It may be that, while a behavior problem has resolved at a given dose, it recurs when the patient is off medication or even on a lower dose. Therefore, tapering of the dose while monitoring can allow for identification of dose levels at which the problem returns, and initiation of appropriate management and behavior modification protocols.

Clinical Guidelines

As with the SSRIs, the TCAs should not be given on an as-needed basis, because they act by producing a gradual shift in levels of serotonin and/or norepinephrine and by down-regulation of the postsynaptic neurons. While some patients may begin to exhibit a response after just a few days of daily administration, others that ultimately have a good response may not respond for several weeks.

Specific Medications

Doses of selected TCAs in cats, dogs, horses, and parrots, and the approximate costs for cats and dogs, are given in Tables 11.2, 11.3, and 11.4.

I. Amitriptyline

Chemical Compound: 3-(10,11-Dihydro-5*H*-dibenzo [a,*d*]cycloheptene-5-ylidene)-*N*, *N*-dimethyl-1-propanamine hydrochloride
DEA Classification: Not a controlled substance
Preparations: Generally available in 10-, 25-, 50-, 75-, 100-, and 150-mg tablets and as a sterile solution for intramuscular injection

Clinical Pharmacology

Amitriptyline inhibits the reuptake of norepinephrine and serotonin. It is rapidly absorbed and metabolized. Plasma concentrations correlate with total intake of amitriptyline (Rudorfer and Robins 1982). It undergoes *N*-demethylation and bridge hydroxylation in humans, rabbits, and rats (Merck 1998). It is metabolized into nortriptyline and a variety of other metabolites (Diamond 1965).

Table 11.2   Doses of selected tricyclic antidepressants in dogs and cats

TCA	Cat	Dog
Amitriptyline	0.5–2.0 mg/kg q12–24h	1–6 mg/kg q12h
Clomipramine	0.25–1.3 mg/kg q24h	1.0–3.0 mg/kg q12h
Desipramine		1.5–3.5 mg/kg q24h
Doxepin	0.5–1.0 mg/kg q12h	3.0–5.0 mg/kg q8–12h
Imipramine	0.5–1.0 mg/kg q12–24h	0.5–2.0 mg/kg q8–12h
Nortriptyline	0.5–2.0 mg/kg q12–24h	1.0–2.0 mg/kg q12h

Note: Always start with a low dose and titrate up as necessary if the patient does not exhibit side effects. All doses are given orally.

Table 11.3   Doses of selected tricyclic antidepressants in horses and parrots

Animal	Dose
Parrots	
Clomipramine	2.0–4.0 mg/kg q12h
Doxepin	0.5–5.0 mg/kg q12h
Horses	
Imipramine	0.75–2.0 mg/kg

Note: Always start with a low dose and titrate up as necessary if the patient does not exhibit side effects. All doses are given orally.

Table 11.4   Cost of selected tricyclic antidepressants, based on one-month treatment for a 5-kg cat or a 20-kg dog

	Dog	Cat
Amitriptyline	$	$
Clomipramine	$$	$
Desipramine	$$	
Doxepin	$$	
Imipramine	$	
Nortriptyline	$$	$

The half-life in humans is 5–45 hours (Nelson 2004), and the half-life in dogs is 6–8 hours (Shanley and Overall 1992).

Amitriptyline is excreted in the milk. In rabbits given carbon-14-labeled amitriptyline, the concentration of radioactivity in the milk is equivalent to concentrations in the serum. Concentrations of radioactivity in neonates consuming the milk are substantially lower than concentrations in the equivalent organs in the mother (Aaes-Jørgensen and Jørgensen 1977).

Uses in Humans

Amitriptyline is approved for the treatment of depression.

Contraindications

Amitriptyline is contraindicated in patients with a history of sensitivity to this or other TCAs. It should not be given concurrently with MAOIs, because serious side effects, including convulsions and death, may result. If a patient is to be changed from an MAOI to amitriptyline, discontinue the MAOI for at least two weeks before beginning amitriptyline. Avoid or use it cautiously in patients with a history of seizures, urinary retention, or glaucoma. In humans, amitriptyline has been shown to cause cardiac arrhythmias, tachycardia, and prolonged conduction time. While dogs do not appear to be as susceptible to cardiotoxic side effects as humans (e.g., Reich et al. 2000), it should be avoided or used cautiously in veterinary patients with existing cardiac disease. Sufficiently large doses can induce cardiotoxicity. In a study in which anesthetized dogs were given a continuous intravenous infusion of amitriptyline until cardiotoxicity occurred, toxic effects were observed at an average of 25 mg/kg (range 15–80 mg/kg) in one study and an average 36 mg/kg in another study (Lheureux et al. 1992a, 1992b). Rabbits given amitriptyline by intravenous injection exhibit decreased blood pressure and increased heart rate (Elonen et al. 1974). Amitriptyline may enhance the effects of barbiturates and other CNS depressants (Merck 1998).

Amitriptyline is metabolized in the liver and excreted through the kidneys. It should therefore be used cautiously and at lowered doses in patients with mild to moderate liver disease and avoided entirely in patients with severe liver disease.

Levels of amitriptyline may be elevated in patients concomitantly given drugs that are metabolized by cytochrome P450 2D6 (Merck 1998).

Systemic absorption of amitriptyline is poor when administered transdermally as opposed to orally. Therefore, transdermal administration of amitriptyline is not recommended at this time (Mealey et al. 2004).

Side Effects

The most common side effects in cats and dogs are sedation, miosis, and urinary retention. Weight gain, decreased grooming, and transient cystic calculi may also occur (Chew et al. 1998). A variety of cardiovascular, CNS, anticholinergic, hematologic, gastrointestinal, and endocrine side effects are reported in humans.

Amitriptyline has teratogenic effects in mice and hamsters when pregnant females are given doses of 28–100 mg/kg/day. In the rat, medicating pregnant females with 25 mg/kg/day results in delayed ossification in the fetal vertebrae. In rabbits, if pregnant females are medicated with 60 mg/kg/day, ossification of the cranial bones is delayed. Amitriptyline crosses the placenta, and there have been some reports of adverse events in human babies when the mother was medicated with amitriptyline during pregnancy. However, there is insufficient documentation to determine if the amitriptyline was the cause of the adverse events.

Amitriptyline is also excreted into breast milk. Because of the potential for adverse effects on fetuses or young, pregnant or lactating females should not be medicated with amitriptyline.

The intravenous LD_{50} (the dose that kills 50% of the animals tested) is 18–22 mg/kg in mice and 6–11 mg/kg in rabbits. The oral LD_{50} is 286–359 mg/kg in rats and 100–216 mg/kg in mice (Ribbentrop and Schauman 1965). Toxic signs include respiratory depression, ataxia, tremors, convulsions, and prostration.

Overdose

There is no specific antidote for overdose of amitriptyline. Decontaminate and provide supportive therapy. Emesis is contraindicated.

Discontinuation

Patients that have been on amitriptyline daily for several weeks should be withdrawn gradually.

Other Information

Amitriptyline has historically been commonly used in general practice for the treatment of anxiety disorders in dogs and cats, apparently initially for economic reasons and, later, because of familiarity with the medication. However, compared with other drugs such as fluoxetine and clomipramine, which have become much more economically feasible for the pet owner in recent years, amitriptyline has a relatively low clinical efficacy and high incidence of side effects.

Effects Documented in Nonhuman Animals
Cats

In a retrospective study, two of three cats with psychogenic alopecia that were treated with amitriptyline at doses of 2.5 mg q12h or 5.0 mg q24h (total dose) responded (Sawyer et al. 1999).

Amitriptyline has been used successfully to treat hypervocalization in a cat (Houpt 1994).

Amitriptyline (2 mg/kg orally [PO], daily) may decrease clinical signs of severe recurrent idiopathic cystitis in cats, possibly in part because of analgesic effects such as those that occur in human patients (Hanno et al. 1989; Chew et al. 1998).

High doses of amitriptyline, 7–10 mg/kg intravenously (IV) result in loss of electroencephalogram changes in cats that are subjected to loud tones or pinching. Lower doses result in attenuation of the response (Vernier 1961).

Dogs

Dogs given amitriptyline at a dose range of 0.74–2.5 mg/kg q12h for $\geq$ 45 days do not exhibit any electrocardiogram (EKG) changes. P-wave duration has a significant negative correlation with serum concentration of amitriptyline at clinically usual doses, but remains within normal parameters (Reich et al. 2000).

In a retrospective study of 103 dogs with various presentations of compulsive disorder, amitriptyline was found to be significantly less effective than clomipramine (Overall and Dunham 2002).

In a prospective, randomized, double-blind, placebo-controlled trial of treatment of canine aggression with amitriptyline plus behavior modification versus clomipramine plus behavior modification, amitriptyline was no more effective than placebo (Virga et al. 2001). One dog diagnosed with a combination of dominance aggression and food-defense aggression responded positively to a combination of amitriptyline and behavior modification (Reich 1999).

In an open trial, 15 of 27 dogs (56%) with separation anxiety that were treated with amitriptyline in addition to behavior modification improved (Takeuchi et al. 2000).

Horses

Amitriptyline is rapidly metabolized in the horse. A single dose of 750 mg followed by collection of urine through a catheter during the zero- to three-week period after administration revealed that almost all of the medication being excreted during this period was nortriptyline (Fenwick 1982).

II. Clomipramine Hydrochloride

Chemical Compound: 3-Chloro-5-[3-(dimethyl-amino)propyl]-10,11-dihydro-5H-dibenz[b,f]azepine monohydrochloride

DEA Classification: Not a controlled substance

Preparations: Generally available as 25-, 50-, and 75-mg capsules (Anafranil and generic), and as 20-, 40-, and 80-mg chewable tablets (Clomicalm)

Clinical Pharmacology

Clomipramine affects both the serotonergic and noradrenergic neural transmission in the CNS. The primary mechanism of action is probably prevention of reuptake of serotonin in the CNS, and it is the most serotonin specific of the commercially available TCAs (Table 11.1). It is highly lipophilic and therefore passes easily through lipophilic membranes. The major route of biotransformation is demethylation, resulting in desmethylclomipramine. Subsequently, further metabolic processes produce various water-soluble substances that are eliminated through the bile or the urine (Faigle and Dieterle 1973). In humans, the half-life is 15–60 hours (Nelson 2004).

In the dog, it is almost totally absorbed when given orally. In the dog and the rat, the main mode of excretion is through the bile, with the dog eliminating about 80% of an oral or intravenous dose of 5 mg/kg of clomipramine via the bile within four days, most of the remainder being excreted via the kidneys in the same amount of time. In humans, more clomipramine is excreted via the kidneys than the bile (Faigle and Dieterle 1973).

Following intravenous injection, clomipramine is rapidly distributed throughout the body, penetrating various tissues and organs, as demonstrated by whole-body autoradiography performed on mice given 10 mg/kg. High concentrations initially occur in the lung, adrenal gland, thyroid, kidney, pancreas, heart, and brain, which would be predicted based on clomipramine's lipophilic nature. The affinity of clomipramine for tissues containing fat results in rapid decreases in blood levels (Faigle and Dieterle 1973).

In humans, there is no relation between dose and plasma level of clomipramine, but plasma concentrations of desmethylclomipramine, the primary active metabolite, are correlated with dose (Jones and Luscombe 1977).

After both single-dose and multiple-dose oral treatment of dogs with clomipramine, peak concentrations of clomipramine occur in the plasma within 3 hours, while peak concentrations of the primary active metabolite, desmethylclomipramine, usually occur within 4–6 hours. Subsequently, plasma levels decline rapidly, with a plasma half-life for clomipramine of about 4 hours. However, there is a substantial range in elimination half-life, and it can be as great as 16 hours. The measured plasma half-life for desmethylclomipramine is likewise about 4 hours, but since this is a combination of the interaction between generation of new desmethylclomipramine as clomipramine is metabolized, and elimination of desmethylclomipramine, the actual half-life of desmethylclomipramine is shorter. With intravenous administration in dogs, the mean elimination half-life is 5 hours (Hewson et al. 1998a; King et al. 2000a, 2000b). The half-life in humans is longer, with a mean of about 20 hours when given orally (Nagy and Johansson 1977; Evans et al. 1980).

In dogs, plasma concentrations of clomipramine are higher than concentrations of desmethylclomipramine (about 3:1), which is the opposite of humans, in which plasma concentrations of clomipramine are lower than those of desmethyl-clomipramine (about 1:2.5) (Broadhurst et al. 1977; Jones and Luscombe 1977; Kuss and Jungkunz 1986; Hewson et al. 1998a; King et al. 2000a; King et al. 2000b). This may be one of the reasons that adverse events appear to be less frequent in dogs than in humans, since clomipramine is the molecule that acts predominantly on serotonin whereas desmethylclomipramine has stronger anticholinergic activity (Benfield et al. 1980). When dogs are dosed daily with clomipramine, steady-state plasma levels are achieved within four days (King 2000a).

Normal dogs treated with 3 mg/kg clomipramine daily, PO, have a lower ratio of 5-hydroxyindoleacetic acid (HIAA) to 3-methyl 4-hydroxyphenylglucol (MHPG) in the cerebrospinal fluid than do dogs treated with placebo (Hewson et al. 1995).

Desmethylclomipramine has anticholinergic effects on gastrointestinal smooth muscle, inhibiting motility and antagonizing muscarinic receptors, but does not do so as much as clomipramine. It is a more potent inhibitor of norepinephrine and dopamine reuptake than clomipramine. It has antidepressant activities that are probably due to its monoamine uptake inhibition (Benfield et al. 1980).

There is a faster rate and higher levels of absorption in dogs that are fed than in dogs that are fasted. Overall bioavailability is about 25% greater in dogs that are fed as opposed to fasted. Plasma half-life is 2 to 9 hours in fed dogs, but 3 to 21 hours in fasted dogs, presumably due to delayed absorption (Novartis 2000; King et al. 2000b).

When dogs are repeatedly dosed, the half-lives of clomipramine and desmethyl-clomipramine increase with increased dosage. At doses of 1, 2, and 4 mg/kg twice a day (b.i.d.), the accumulation ratios for clomipramine are 1.4, 1.6, and 3.8, respectively, while for desmethylclomipramine they are 2.1, 3.7, and 7.6. There are two main possibilities for this observation. First, the main route of elimination of both clomipramine and desmethylclomipramine may be saturable. Second, the increasing numbers of molecules may themselves directly inhibit the elimination process (King et al. 2000a).

Uses in Humans

Clomipramine is used to treat obsessive-compulsive disorder in humans.

Contraindications

Clomipramine should not be given to patients with a history of sensitivity to clomipramine or other TCAs. It should not be given in conjunction with an MAOI or within two weeks of discontinuation of administration of an MAOI. Avoid or use cautiously in patients with a history of epilepsy, cardiac arrhythmias, glaucoma, or urine or stool retention.

While clomipramine is not as cardiotoxic in dogs as it is in humans, sufficiently large doses can induce cardiotoxicity. In a study in which anesthetized dogs were given a continuous intravenous infusion of clomipramine until cardiotoxicity occurred, toxic effects were observed at an average of 65 mg/kg (range 53–72). This is much higher than the dose at which cardiotoxicity occurred in dogs infused with amitriptyline (Lheureux et al. 1992a).

Clomipramine should not be given to male breeding dogs, as testicular hypoplasia may occur (Novartis 2000).

In humans, concurrent administration of phenobarbital with clomipramine results in increased plasma levels of clomipramine.

Side Effects

Side effects include sedation, mydriasis, regurgitation, appetite changes, and urinary retention (Pfeiffer et al. 1999; Litster 2000). Clomipramine may also potentiate the side effects of various CNS depressants, including benzodiazepines, barbiturates, and general anesthetics. In humans, on which there is much more data than in the veterinary population, a broad spectrum of side effects has been reported, including cardiovascular effects, mania, hepatic changes, hematologic changes, CNS disorders, sexual dysfunction, and weight changes (Novartis 1998).

Rats given approximately 5 times the maximum daily human dose exhibited no impairment of fertility, while rats given up to 20 times the maximum daily human dose exhibited no clear evidence of carcinogenicity of clomipramine. A rare tumor, hemangioendothelioma, did occur in a small number of the rats. When pregnant rats and mice were given up to 20 times the maximum daily human dose, there were no teratogenic effects, although there was some evidence of fetotoxic effects. Clomipramine does enter the milk (Novartis 1998). Use in pregnant and nursing females should be avoided if possible.

Overdose

There is no specific antidote for overdose with clomipramine. Decontaminate and provide supportive therapy. Emesis is contraindicated.

Discontinuation

Animals that have been given clomipramine daily for several weeks should be withdrawn gradually.

Effects Documented in Nonhuman Animals

Cats

Cats given up to five times the clinical dose for 28 days exhibited mild sedation, occasional pupillary dilatation, and a slight decrease in food consumption (Landsberg 2001).

In an open trial of cats with various anxiety-related and compulsive disorders, six cases of urine spraying, three cases of over-grooming, and one case of excessive vocalization resolved or were substantially improved when treated with clomipramine at a dose of 0.2–0.55 mg/kg daily, combined with behavior modification. Some cats became sedated at the higher dose range, but were successfully treated when the dose was lowered (Seksel and Lindeman 1998, 1999).

In a single-blind trial Dehasse (1997) reported a 75% decrease in the number of urine-spraying incidents in 80% of cats given 5 mg/day of clomipramine as opposed to when they were on placebo. A few of the cats were mildly sedated while on medication. Landsberg (2001) has likewise had improvement in over 80% of patients given 0.5 mg/kg for one month.

Clomipramine has also been used to successfully treat cats with psychogenic alopecia. In a retrospective study, five of five cats treated with clomipramine at doses of 1.25–2.5 mg (total dose) q24h responded (Sawyer et al. 1999). In a prospective, double-blind, placebo-controlled, randomized trial, clomipramine, at a dose of 0.5 mg/kg q12h PO was more effective than placebo in the treatment of feline psychogenic alopecia (Mertens and Torres 2003).

Of 14 cats treated with clomipramine for a variety of anxiety-related behavior problems, including spraying (12 cats), tail-chasing (1 cat), nocturnal vocalization (1 cat), and aggression to the owner (1 of the cats that sprayed), the problem resolved in 6 cats and was improved in the remaining 8 cats. The total daily dose ranged from 0.4 to 1.32 mg/kg (Litster 2000).

The most definitive results on the efficacy of clomipramine in the treatment of urine spraying in cats were obtained in a randomized, double-blind, placebo-controlled, multicenter clinical trial. Sixty-seven neutered cats were treated with placebo, 0.125–0.25 mg/kg daily (low dose), 0.25–0.5 mg/kg daily (moderate dose), or 0.5–1.0 mg/kg daily (high dose) for three months. Various other treatments had been tried previously and been unsuccessful, including pheromones (17 cats), amitriptyline (7), buspirone (2), diazepam (4), megestrol acetate (12), progestogens (4), and corticosteroids (1).

At all doses, clomipramine was more effective than placebo. The moderate and high doses were more effective than the low dose. There was no effect of age, sex, whether or not previous attempts had been made to treat the urine spraying and whether or not the cat lived in a single-cat household versus a multicat household. Aggression toward familiar cats, unfamiliar cats, and animals other than cats was significantly decreased in the high-dosage group. During the third month of treatment, the amount of time spent in stereotypic behaviors other than licking or grooming was also significantly decreased in both the moderate and high-dosage groups as compared with the low-dosage group. Sedation was the most common side effect and always occurred during the first month of treatment. The frequency and severity of sedation was dose related. However, the overall behavior patterns were not changed, and it is possible that some of what the owners were reporting as sedation was simply the consequence of the cat being less confrontational and more relaxed with its housemates. This possibility requires further study (King et al. 2004a).

Dogs

In humans, only moderate overdoses of clomipramine are cardiotoxic, with such sequelae as increased heart rate, decreased blood pressure, and slow intracardiac conduction. Research conducted on dogs has demonstrated that this drug is more benign in this species. Dogs given 20 mg/kg daily for 7 days, which is five times the maximum recommended label dose, exhibited a significant reduction in heart rate, with the peak effect occurring about 12 hours after medication. Doses of 4 or 12 mg/kg of clomipramine did not induce any changes in heart rate. There were no significant changes in the EKG (Pouchelon et al. 2000). In another study, canine patients given clomipramine at doses of 1.5–2.49 mg/kg q12h for ≥45 days did not exhibit EKG changes. Duration of the P-wave significantly positively correlates with serum concentration of clomipramine, but in studies to date has remained within the clinically normal range for dogs given clinically appropriate doses (Reich et al. 2000).

In healthy dogs given 3 mg/kg of clomipramine q12h for 112 days, there are significant decreases in total thyroxin (T_4), free thyroxin (fT_4), and $3,3',5'$–triiodothyronine (reverse T_3, rT_3). T_4 decreased 35% while fT_4 decreased 38%. However, clinical hypothyroidism was not reported at this dose. There was no change in basal or post-thyrotropin-releasing hormone stimulation serum thyroid-stimulating hormone concentrations (Gulikers and Panciera 2003).

Testicular hypoplasia has occurred in male dogs given 12.5 times the maximum daily dose for one year (Novartis 2000). It is not known whether usual clinical doses induce some degree of compromise of testicular function.

Clomicalm, a chewable tablet form of clomipramine, is FDA approved for the treatment of separation anxiety in dogs, but only in conjunction with behavior modification. In a prospective, randomized, double-blind, placebo-controlled, parallel-group, international, multicenter clinical trial, clomipramine, given at a dose of 1–<2 mg/kg PO q12h plus behavior modification was shown to be more effective than behavior modification alone. Only dogs that exhibited both anxiety when their owner was absent and hyperattachment when their owner was present were included in this study. A low-dose group, given 0.5 to <1 mg/kg PO q12h did not have a better response than dogs given placebo. Mild and transient vomiting due to gastritis and mild and transient sleepiness, attributable to clomipramine, occurred in some dogs. One greyhound collapsed with hyperthermia, which may or may not have been an idiosyncratic response to the clomipramine. Beagle dogs given doses of up to 50 mg/kg PO q24h have never exhibited this response (Simpson 1997; King et al. 2000c).

Long-term follow-up of the dogs in the trial described above did not identify any undesirable effects in the dogs given the highest dose (1–2 mg/kg q12h). Acute worsening of separation anxiety occurred in three dogs that had been given the low-dose clomipramine (King et al. 2004b).

Another study compared four different dose ranges for the treatment of separation anxiety with clomipramine. A total daily dose of 2.1–4.0 mg/kg was found to be more effective than 1.1–2 mg/kg, 0.51–1 mg/kg, or 0.25–0.5 mg/kg (Petit et al. 1999).

One trial comparing placebo with clomipramine at 0.5–1.0 mg/kg q12h or clomipramine at 1.0–2.0 mg/kg q12h failed to find a significant effect of clomipramine (Podberscek et al. 1999). Problems in this trial include that the total sample size was small and the authors only evaluated very specific behaviors, which only a small sample of the already small trial exhibited. The authors did not evaluate whether or not the dogs had improved in some fashion that was relevant to the particular case based on baseline symptoms, that is, there was no global assessment.

Clomipramine is also used in the treatment of various forms of compulsive disorder, including acral lick dermatitis (ALD), a condition in which the dog persistently licks itself, producing a dermatitis. In an 11-week-long crossover trial, clomipramine has been shown to be more effective than desipramine in the treatment of ALD, when both drugs were titrated up to 3 mg/kg daily (Rapoport et al. 1992). Similarly, in a 15-week A-B-A design study, clomipramine was more effective than desipramine in the treatment of canine acral lick dermatitis (Goldberger and Rapoport 1991). Subsequently, in a retrospective open trial, clomipramine given at 2 mg/kg q24h resulted in decreased self-licking and the healing of ALD lesions in 8 of 10 cases (Mertens and Dodman 1996).

Clomipramine given at 3 mg/kg PO q12h for four weeks has been shown to be more effective than placebo in the treatment of compulsive disorder. However, treatment for such a short period of time was not curative (Hewson et al. 1998b).

In a prospective study of tail-chasing terriers (bull terrier, miniature bull terrier, American Staffordshire terrier and Jack Russell terrier), 18 dogs were started on treatment with clomipramine at 1 mg/kg q24h, which was subsequently titrated upward depending on side effects and clinical response. Four dogs were withdrawn from the study between four and eight weeks. Of the remaining 14 dogs, 9 had a 75% or greater improvement in tail chasing when given doses of clomipramine ranging between 1–5 mg/kg total daily dose (Moon-Fanelli and Dodman 1998). In a separate case report, a Cairn terrier exhibiting stereotypic tail chasing was successfully treated with clomipramine titrated up to 3 mg/kg q24h (Thornton 1995).

Three dogs with compulsive disorder manifested as stereotypic motor behavior were successfully treated with clomipramine titrated up to a maximum dose of approximately 3 mg/kg PO q12h. One dog had previously been unsuccessfully treated with phenobarbital, while the other two had previously been unsuccessfully treated with amitriptyline. Treatment was conducted over a period of months (Overall 1994).

A dog that exhibited stereotypic motor behavior whenever the owner departed or was out of the dog's sight, that had not responded to previous treatment with amitriptyline or buspirone, did respond well to treatment with clomipramine combined with behavior modification. In this case, an increasing dosage schedule of 1 mg/kg PO q12h for two weeks, then 2 mg/kg PO q12h for two weeks, then 3 mg/kg PO q12h, was used (Overall 1998).

A randomized, double-blind, placebo-controlled, clinical trial of the use of clomipramine (1.5 mg/kg q12h) to treat human-directed dominance-motivated aggression in dogs failed to demonstrate a significant difference between medicated and placebo-treated dogs. In this trial, medication was the only treatment; there was no behavior modification at all (White et al. 1999). Therefore, this trial only addressed the question of whether or not clomipramine is better than nothing, not whether it facilitates improvement if given in conjunction with behavior modification. Clomipramine's licensure for the treatment of separation anxiety is specifically *with* behavior modification, precisely because of the expectation that clomipramine will allow and facilitate learning taking place that ultimately results in changed behavior. Again, as discussed in chapter 1, all medications for the treatment of behavior problems in nonhuman animals should be used only in conjunction with appropriate environmental management and behavior modification.

In a retrospective study of 103 dogs with various presentations of compulsive disorder, clomipramine was found to be significantly more effective than amitriptyline (Overall and Dunham 2002).

Clomipramine has also been used, at a dose of 2 mg/kg b.i.d., in combination with the benzodiazepine alprazolam to successfully treat storm phobia in dogs. Over 90% of dogs treated with this combination improved. Improvement over baseline continued for at least eight months after discontinuation of treatment, which was as long as the dogs were followed. Storm phobia, while problematic when dogs exhibit intense fear of even light rain, is not a behavior that can be expected to be totally resolved, because some degree of fear of intense storms is normal behavior (Crowell-Davis et al. 2003; see also case 1).

Horses

Clomipramine (2.2 mg/kg IV) combined with xylazine (0.5 mg/kg IV) has been used to successfully obtain semen from a stallion that was disabled due to a fracture of the radius (Turner et al. 1995b).

Parrots

In an open trial of the treatment of feather-picking disorder in various parrot species (five Moluccan cockatoos, one umbrella cockatoo, one sulfur-crested cockatoo, two cockatiels, one yellow-headed Amazon, and one scarlet macaw), birds were titrated over several weeks up to 1.0 mg/kg daily. The sulfur-crested cockatoo, the yellow-headed Amazon, and the scarlet macaw all exhibited dramatic decreases in feather-picking and/or self-mutilation within the first month of treatment. The two cockatiels and the Moluccan cockatoo had positive personality changes, but the feather-picking did not improve. The other five birds exhibited no response. Three birds exhibited post-treatment regurgitation. Drowsiness was observed in three birds, and one Moluccan cockatoo exhibited ataxia for one day (Ramsay and Grindlinger 1992). Some birds on clomipramine gain weight (Grindlinger and Ramsay 1991). Later research (see below) suggests that the poor response rate may have been due to the dose being too low.

Seibert et al. (2004) conducted a double-blind, placebo-controlled trial of the treatment of feather-picking disorder in cockatoos. A dose of 3 mg/kg q12h, suspended in raspberry syrup with 2% carboxymethyl cellulose as a suspending agent, was more effective than placebo, based on the evaluations of both the owner and an avian veterinarian who was blinded to treatment. Species used in this study included Goffin's, umbrella, Moluccan, sulphur-crested, and citron-crested cockatoos. No adverse events were reported.

A Congo African grey parrot with feather-picking and self-injurious behavior responded well to treatment with 9.47 mg/kg of clomipramine combined with 0.5 mg/kg buspirone q12h. The initial dose of clomipramine was 4 mg/kg PO q12h, and the dose was subsequently titrated to effect. At a dose of 18.8 mg/kg q12h PO the bird became paradoxically fearful and appeared to be hallucinating. It was at this time that buspirone was added to the treatment regimen, with the dose of clomipramine being concurrently titrated downward. Seventeen months after initiation of treatment, the bird was fully feathered except for its wing tips (Juarbe-Diaz 2000).

III. Desipramine

Chemical Compound: 5*H*-Dibenz[*bf*]azepine-5-propanamine, 10,11-dihydro-*N*-methyl-monohydrochloride
DEA Classification: Not a controlled substance
Preparations: Generally available in 10-, 25-, 50-, 75-, 100-, and 150-mg tablets

Clinical Pharmacology

Desipramine inhibits reuptake of norepinephrine and serotonin. Desipramine is the opposite of clomipramine in that it has substantially more effect on norepinephrine than on serotonin, and is the most norepinephrine selective of the TCAs. The primary metabolite is 2-hydroxydesipramine. In humans, the half-life is 10–30 hours (Nelson 2004).

Desipramine is rapidly absorbed from the gastrointestinal tract, metabolized in the liver, and, primarily, excreted through the kidneys. In humans, 70% is excreted through the kidneys (Merrell Pharmaceuticals 2000), and the half-life is about 18 hours (Potter et al. 1995).

Desipramine is metabolized by the P450 2D6 cytochrome. Therefore, levels may be elevated in patients concurrently being given drugs that also use this pathway (Merrell Pharmaceuticals 2000).

Uses in Humans

Desipramine is used in humans to treat depression.

Contraindications

Desipramine should not be given to patients with a history of sensitivity to TCAs, to patients currently taking MAOIs or within two weeks of taking a MAOI. It should be avoided or used cautiously in patients with cardiovascular disease, a history of urinary retention or glaucoma, thyroid disease, or a seizure disorder (Merrell Pharmaceuticals 2000).

Side Effects

A variety of side effects have been reported in humans, including adverse cardiovascular effects, neurologic effects, anticholinergic effects, gastrointestinal effects, endocrine effects, and hematologic effects (Merrell Pharmaceuticals 2000).

The oral LD_{50} in male mice is 290 mg/kg, while in female rats it is 320 mg/kg (Merrell Pharmaceuticals 2000).

Overdose

There is no specific antidote. Decontaminate and provide supportive therapy. Emesis is contraindicated.

Effects Documented in Nonhuman Animals
Dogs

One small trial has been conducted comparing desipramine to clomipramine and placebo for the treatment of compulsive licking behavior in dogs. Desipramine was not as effective as clomipramine and was no more effective than placebo (Rapoport et al. 1992).

Desipramine has also been shown to be effective in the treatment of cataplexy in dogs. However, it is not as effective as nortriptyline for this disorder (Mignot et al. 1993).

IV. Doxepin

Chemical Compound: 1-Propanamine, 3-dibenz [*b,e*]oxepin-11(6H)ylidene-*N*, *N*-dimethyl-, hydrochloride
DEA Classification: Not a controlled substance
Preparations: Generally available as 10-, 25-, 50-, 75-, 100-, and 150-mg capsules and as a cream containing 50 mg of doxepin per gram of cream

Clinical Pharmacology

Doxepin prevents the reuptake up norepinephrine and serotonin. It also has H1 and H2 receptor-blocking activity, which is believed to be the basis for its antipruritic effect. It undergoes hepatic metabolism into desmethyldoxepin and nordoxepin (GenDerm 1997). In humans it has a half-life of 8–25 hours (Zeigler et al. 1978; Potter et al. 1995; Nelson 2004). In the dog, it is rapidly absorbed after oral administration with plasma levels peaking in 30–60 minutes, declining thereafter (Hobbs 1969; Kimura et al. 1972). Repeated administration produces higher concentrations than a single dose (Hobbs 1968). Doxepin and some of its metabolites enter various tissues. Initial high levels occur in kidney, liver, spleen, and lung (Hobbs 1969; Kimura et al. 1972). When doxepin is administered to rabbits, concentrations in the heart range from 40 to 200 times more than occur in the plasma at the same time (Elonen et al. 1975). The active metabolite, desmethyldoxepin, also occurs in appreciable amounts in various tissues (Ribbentrop and Schaumann 1965). Only desmethyldoxepin and doxepin enter the brain (Hobbs 1969; Kimura et al. 1972). Dogs excrete various metabolites, including desmethyldoxepin, doxepin-*N*-oxide, a hydroxydoxepin and its glucuronide, as well as doxepin, in their urine (Hobbs 1969).

Doxepin is marketed as a mixture of geometric isomers. The more active *cis*-isomer comprises 15% of a total doxepin dose while the *trans*-isomer comprises 85% of the dose. In human plasma the ratio of the isomers remains the same (*cis*/*trans* = 15:85) or shifts so that the *cis*-isomer is even less than 15%. The ratio of the isomers of the desmethyldoxepin metabolite change so that they are approximately equal or the proportion of the *cis*-isomer is even greater than the *trans*-isomer. There is wide individual variation (Midha et al. 1992; Yan et al. 1997). In the rat, the metabolites are similar to humans, but in the dog, rabbit, and guinea pig the percentage of *cis*-desmethyldoxepin remains proportionately lower than *trans*-desmethyldoxepin, averaging 26% in the dog and 32% in the rabbit and guinea pig (Yan et al. 1997). In horses, the relative composition of the *cis* and *trans* metabolites likewise remain similar to the original ratio (Hagedorn et al. 2001).

In dogs, doxepin and its metabolite, desmethyldoxepin, peak at one to three hours after administration of an oral dose. Approximately 50% of radioactive doxepin is excreted in the urine in this species (Hobbs 1969).

Dogs given 15 mg/kg daily for 30 days show mild sedation and vomiting, while increased heart rate, miosis, sedation, and twitching occur at a dose of 50 mg/kg for 30 days. Dogs given 5 mg/kg daily for a year were almost asymptomatic. Dogs given 25 mg/kg daily for a year exhibited occasional vomiting. Dogs given 50 mg/kg daily for a year exhibit ptosis, sedation, tremors, and vomiting (Brogden et al. 1971).

Both the *cis*- and *trans*-isomers of the metabolite desmethyldoxepin are detectable in horses' urine and plasma up to at least 48 hours after an intravenous injection of 1 mg/kg of doxepin (Hagedorn et al. 2002). When doxepin is given intravenously, the half-life of the more active *cis*-isomer is 3.1 hours, whereas the half-life of the *trans*-isomer is 3.5 hours (Hagedorn et al. 2001).

Uses in Humans

Doxepin is recommended for anxiety and depression in humans. Doxepin cream is used as an antipruritic (Drake et al. 1994; Breneman et al. 1997).

Contraindications

Doxepin is contraindicated in individuals with a history of sensitivity to doxepin or other TCAs. It should not be given in conjunction with MAOIs or within two weeks of administration of MAOIs.

Side Effects

Various CNS-, cardiovascular-, hematologic-, gastrointestinal-, and endocrine-related side effects have been observed in humans (Pfizer 1996). Dogs given 10 mg/kg exhibit some sedative effect (Yan et al. 1997). Rabbits given doxepin by intravenous injection exhibit decreased blood pressure and increased heart rate (Elonen et al. 1974).

In humans, doxepin is considered safe in elderly patients. Reproductive studies conducted in dogs, rats, rabbits, and monkeys have failed to demonstrate adverse effects.

Doxepin is metabolized by the P450 2D6 enzyme system; therefore, levels may be elevated in patients concurrently given other drugs that also use this enzyme system.

Use of the cream may result in stinging or burning sensations or drowsiness (Drake et al. 1994).

Rats given 5, 10, 20, 40, or 80 mg/kg/day PO for 180 days exhibited no adverse effects at 5, 10, or 20 mg/kg/day. At doses of 40 mg/kg/day there was decreased weight gain. No changes were observed in hematology, urine analysis, blood chemistries, or food intake (Noguchi et al. 1972c). In rats, males appear to be more susceptible to toxic effects than females (Noguchi et al. 1972b). The oral LD_{50} in the dog is 200 mg/kg whereas the intravenous LD_{50} is 16 mg/kg in this species. In mice the oral LD_{50} is 117–178 mg/kg and the intravenous LD_{50} is 14.6–30 mg/kg. In rats the oral LD_{50} is 114–460 mg/kg and the intravenous LD_{50} is 12.7–19 mg/kg. In rabbits, the intravenous LD_{50} is 8–14 mg/kg (Noguchi et al. 1972a; Ribbentrop and Schaumann 1965).

Overdose

There is no antidote for doxepin. Decontaminate and provide supportive therapy. Emesis is contraindicated.

Effects Documented in Nonhuman Animals

Dogs

Doxepin centrally and dose-dependently inhibits 2-deoxy-D-glucose-stimulated gastric acid secretion in dogs (Leitold et al. 1984; Shimatani et al. 2001).

Parrots

Johnson (1987) reported successful use of doxepin in the treatment of destructive preening and mutilation, postshipment stress, and as a general aid to taming and handling birds.

Horses

Doxepin is banned in competition horses where it may be used to attempt to calm excited horses. When given at a dose of 1 mg/kg IV, it can be detected up to at least 48 hours later in both blood and urine. Higher concentrations are present in the blood than in the urine. It is therefore recommended that blood be used for assaying the presence of doxepin metabolites in competition horses (Hagedorn et al. 2002).

After administration of 1 mg/kg IV, respiratory rate remains stable, heart rate decreases, and body temperature decreases slightly but returns to normal within five hours. Heart rate also returns to normal within five hours. Within the first hour after injection, horses may appear to be moderately sedated (Hagedorn et al. 2001).

V. Imipramine

Chemical Compound: 5-[3-(Dimethylamino)propyl]-10, 11-dihydro-5-*H*-dibenz [b,f]azepine monohydrochloride

DEA Classification: Not a controlled substance

Preparations: Generally available as 10-, 25-, and 50-mg tablets; 75-, 100-, 125-, and 150-mg capsules; and ampules for intramuscular injection.

Clinical Pharmacology

Imipramine primarily blocks reuptake of norepinephrine at adrenergic synapses and, to a lesser degree, blocks reuptake of serotonin.

When given orally, imipramine is substantially demethylated in the liver during first-pass metabolism, resulting in higher blood levels of desipramine as opposed to the parent molecule. The other active metabolite is norimipramine. When imipramine is injected, the absence of first-pass metabolism results in higher blood levels of imipramine than desipramine (Dencker et al. 1976; Gram and Christiansen 1975; Nagy and Johansson 1977). In humans, it has a half-life of 5–30 hours (Potter et al. 1995; Nelson 2004).

In cattle, imipramine has a terminal elimination half-life of 140 ± 15 minutes. It has extensive peripheral distribution, probably due to high lipid solubility and low plasma binding (Cordel et al. 2001).

MAO-A and MAO-B activity are both inhibited in the brains of the dog, mouse, rat, and monkey in a dose-dependent fashion. In the rat and mouse, imipramine inhibits MAO-B more potently than MAO-A. In the dog and monkey, MAO-B activity is more inhibited than MAO-A activity at low concentrations, while MAO-A activity is more inhibited than MAO-B activity at relatively higher concentrations (Egashira et al. 1999).

Uses in Humans

Imipramine is used in humans to treat depression and childhood enuresis.

Contraindications

Imipramine should not be given to patients with a history of sensitivity to imipramine or other TCAs. It should not be given in conjunction with an MAOI or within two weeks of giving an MAOI. In humans, imipramine can cause cardiac arrhythmias. While studies of cardiac function in normal dogs given clomipramine and amitriptyline have revealed that this species does not have the same sensitivity to cardiac effects that humans do, similar studies have not been conducted on the use of imipramine in dogs. It should be avoided in patients with cardiac arrhythmias (Ciba-Geigy 1996).

Imipramine is metabolized by the P450 2D6 cytochrome; therefore, levels may be elevated if drugs that are also metabolized by this pathway are given concurrently.

Side Effects

Side effects in humans include various cardiovascular problems, anticholergic effects, gastrointestinal effects, and endocrine changes.

In humans, children are known to be more sensitive to overdose than adults. While it is not known if the same sensitivity occurs in other species, imipramine should be used cautiously in juveniles.

When imipramine is given to mice and rats at 2.5 times the maximum human dosage and to the rabbit at up to 25 times the maximum human daily dose, there is no teratogenic effect. There is some evidence of embryotoxic effect, as shown by a reduced litter size, an increase in the stillborn rate, and a reduction in the mean birth weight. Acute oral LD_{50} is 100–215 mg/kg in the dog and 355–682 mg/kg in the rat (Ciba-Geigy 1996).

Cattle and horses given 2 mg/kg may exhibit generalized weakness and ataxia. Hemolysis and discolored urine may also occur (McDonnell et al. 1987; McDonnell and Odian 1994; Cordel et al. 2001).

In guinea pigs, potency for QTC prolongation is 1.7-fold greater with imipramine than with fluvoxamine, an SSRI (Ohtani et al. 2001).

Overdose

There is no specific antidote for imipramine. Decontaminate and provide supportive therapy. Emesis is contraindicated.

Effects Documented in Nonhuman Animals

Cats

Cats that were known mouse-killers but that had consistently deferred to another cat when competing for access to a mouse, that is, were considered to be subordinate by the experimenters, rose in rank when injected intramuscularly with 12.5 or 25 mg of imipramine (Zagrodzka et al. 1985).

Dogs

Imipramine is used for nocturnal enuresis in human children and may be particularly helpful for treatment of submissive and excitement urination in dogs, although no controlled studies addressing this specific use have been published. Research on dogs has shown that 1 mg/kg imipramine decreases the responses of the urethra and bladder to pelvic nerve stimulation. It also reduces response of the bladder, but not the urethra, to histamine, and causes some reduction in bladder and urethra responses to acetylcholine and 5-hydroxytryptamine. It is possible that imipramine acts selectively as a local anesthetic agent in the urinary tract of the dog (Creed and Tulloch 1982). Imipramine also causes increased tone of the urethral sphincter of the dog (Khanna et al. 1975; Tulloch and Creed 1979).

A golden retriever given imipramine (1.85 mg/kg PO q24h) for the treatment of storm phobia initially had no problems. However, after two weeks of treatment, the owner removed the three-month-old tick collar and replaced it with a new one. The collar contained amitraz, a nonspecific MAOI that is commonly used in the treatment of demodicosis and that is present in some collars designed to prevent tick bites. The dog subsequently became lethargic, weak, anorexic, ataxic, and bradycardic. After the collar was removed, clinical signs resolved within eight hours (Simpson 1996).

Dogs given imipramine intramuscularly at doses ranging from 1.4 to 6.25 mg/kg exhibit decreased motor activity in open field tests. Improved learning and decreased fear also occurred in some dogs (Zagrodzka et al. 1981).

Horses

In horses, imipramine commonly induces mild sedation, erection, and masturbation. Intravenous injection of imipramine (2.0 mg/kg), with or without supplemental injection of xylazine (0.3 mg/kg), may be effective in the treatment of ejaculatory dysfunction in stallions (McDonnell et al. 1987; McDonnell and Odian 1994). It can also be given orally as 500 to 1000 mg added to the grain two to four hours before breeding (McDonnell 1999).

Imipramine has also been used to assist in the treatment of urospermia in a stallion with a dysfunctional bladder (Turner et al. 1995a).

Rodents

Single doses of imipramine have been shown to decrease digging behavior, aggressive behavior, and social investigation in mice, while chronic dosing results in increased social investigation indicative of anxiolytic effects (Gao and Cutler 1994).

VI. Nortriptyline

Chemical Compound: 1-Propanamine, 3-(10, 11-dihydro-5*H*-dibenzo[*a,d*]cyclohepten-5-ylidene)-*N*-methyl-,hydrochloride

DEA Classification: Not a controlled substance

Preparations: Generally available in 10-, 25-, 50-, and 75-mg capsules

Clinical Pharmacology

Nortriptyline is antihistaminic and blocks the reuptake of serotonin and norepinephrine. In humans it has a half-life of 20–55 hours (Nelson 2004).

Nortriptyline is excreted in the milk. In rabbits given carbon-14-labeled nortriptyline, the concentration of radioactivity in the milk is equivalent to concentrations in the serum. Concentrations of radioactivity in neonates consuming the milk are substantially lower than concentrations in the equivalent organs in the mother (Aaes-Jørgensen and Jørgensen 1977).

Uses in Humans

Nortriptyline is used to treat depression in humans.

Contraindications

Nortriptyline is contraindicated in patients with a history of sensitivity to nortriptyline or other TCAs. It should not be used concurrently with MAOIs or within two weeks of using an MAOI.

Nortriptyline is metabolized by the P450 2D6 cytochrome system. Therefore, concurrent administration of nortriptyline with other drugs metabolized by this system may result in increased blood levels (Sandoz Pharmaceuticals 1996).

Side Effects

Side effects reported in humans have included various cardiovascular, neurologic, anticholinergic, gastrointestinal, and endocrine effects.

Rabbits given nortriptyline by intravenous injection exhibit decreased blood pressure and increased heart rate (Elonen et al. 1974).

Overdose

There is no specific antidote for nortriptyline. Decontaminate and provide supportive therapy. Emesis is contraindicated.

Effects Documented in Nonhuman Animals

Dogs

Nortriptyline is one of the most effective drugs in the treatment of cataplexy in dogs (Mignot et al. 1993).

Important Information for Owners of Pets Being Placed on Any TCA

The following should be considered when placing an animal on a TCA.

1. It is essential that owners inform their veterinarian of all other medication, herbal supplements, and nutritional supplements they are giving their pet because some of these may interact with the medication.
2. While their pet may respond within a few days, it may be a month before their pet begins responding. They must be patient.
3. If their pet exhibits mild sedation in the beginning, they will probably return to normal levels of activity in two or three weeks as their body adjusts to the medication.
4. If their pet should experience any adverse events such as vomiting, diarrhea, or seizures, they should contact their veterinarian immediately.
5. With the exception of Clomicalm being used in combination with behavior modification for the treatment of separation anxiety in dogs, all use of the medication for nonhuman animals is extra-label use. This does not mean that the drug is not indicated for the problem. In fact, there may be an extensive body of scientific and clinical evidence supporting the use of this drug for their pet's problem. It means that the extensive testing required by the FDA for on-label usage of the drug for their particular species of pet and their particular pet's problem has not been conducted, or, if in progress, been completed. Exceptions to this may occur after the publication of this book if the FDA subsequently approves any of the TCAs for treatment of various behavior problems in domestic animals or approves Clomicalm for uses other than separation anxiety in dogs.

Clinical Examples

Case 1

Signalment

Whiskey was a neutered, mixed-breed female dog weighing 16.5 kg that appeared to be primarily keeshond.

Presenting Complaint

Whiskey was presented for storm phobia. She was also afraid of all humans except her current owner.

History

Whiskey had survived being in a house that had been hit by a tornado and had been pulled from the wreckage of the house after the tornado had passed. She had been subsequently adopted by the owner who presented her. The owner also reported that Whiskey had been both physically and mentally abused by her previous owners, but the specifics of that alleged abuse could not be confirmed other than that the dog had been beaten. Upon examination, Whiskey exhibited behaviors characteristic of abused dogs; she was timid and avoided all attempts by clinic personnel to interact with her, and she would not accept treats or petting. Her ears were frequently pinned back and her tail was held low. She was not aggressive, however. At the time the owner had adopted her, she had heartworms, but these had been treated, and she had successfully recovered from the treatment.

Whiskey had been afraid of storms since the owner had adopted her three years previously. Signs of fear began about 30 minutes before storms began and continued for at least one hour after the abatement of the storm. Her score on the Georgia Storm Phobia Assessment Scale (SPA; Crowell-Davis et al. 2003) was 29.5 out of 50. Her most severe behaviors were persistent whining, which continued long after storms discontinued, pacing, panting, trembling, and alternately hiding or remaining near the owner.

At the time of presentation, the owner did not get any sleep on stormy nights. Instead, she and other dogs that lived in the same household would take Whiskey to a closet and shut themselves in, surrounding Whiskey. If they did this, Whiskey still exhibited fright, but it was less intense than when out in the house or alone.

The owner had attempted treatment with Benadryl and diazepam, consoling Whiskey, ignoring her, and playing thunderstorm tapes.

Diagnosis

Whiskey was diagnosed with storm phobia and fear of humans. It was not known if she had had some degree of storm phobia prior to surviving the tornado, but it was probable that the tornado was a significant contributor to the severity of Whiskey's problem, if not the entire cause. Based on the known and suspected history, the fear of humans was probably due to abuse.

Treatment Plan

The initial treatment plan did not include treatment of the fear of humans because Whiskey was not afraid of her current owner, and her fear of other people was dealt with by avoiding contact. Whiskey was placed on clomipramine (Clomicalm) 2 mg/kg b.i.d. and alprazolam, 0.02 mg/kg to be given 30–60 minutes prior to storms. The owner was instructed to not comfort Whiskey during storms or to punish her (which she hadn't been doing). Whiskey's response to audio recordings of storms was tested in the clinic, and she exhibited a mild response of fear. Significantly less intense fear in the clinic as opposed to the home environment is common. The owner was instructed in desensitization and counterconditioning of Whiskey to the sounds of rain and thunder using various audio recordings.

Follow-up

Sixty days after treatment was initiated, Whiskey's SPA score had decreased from 29.5 to 7. The owner considered her to be substantially improved, but not resolved. At 120 days (four months) after initiation of treatment, Whiskey's SPA score had decreased to 0.5. All that remained was a small amount of panting. The owner considered the problem to be resolved. She also reported that Whisky had, overall, become much calmer and self-confident. She went out during a rainstorm to eliminate without being accompanied. Her fear of humans had also significantly abated. During this visit, she accepted petting and treats from clinic staff and lay down to nap during playing of storm CDs.

References

Aaes-Jørgensen T and Jørgensen A 1977. Studies of excretion in rabbit milk after administration of carbon-14 labelled amitriptyline and nortriptyline. *Archives Internationales de Pharmacodynamie et de Therapie* 227(2): 294–301.

Benfield DP, Harries CM and Luscombe DK 1980. Some pharmacological aspects of desmethylclomipramine. *Postgraduate Medical Journal* 56 (Suppl 1.): 13–18.

Bolden-Watson C and Richelson E 1993. Blockade of newly developed antidepressants of biogenic amine uptake into rat brain symaptosomes. *Life Sciences* 52: 1023–1029.

Breneman DL, Dunlap FE, Monroe EW, Schupbach CW, Shmunes E and Phillips SB 1997. Doxepin cream relieves eczema-associated pruritus within 15 minutes and is not accompanied by a risk of rebound upon discontinuation. *Journal of Dermatological Treatment* 8: 161–168.

Broadhurst AD, James HD, DellaCorte L and Heeley AF 1977. Clomipramine plasma level and clinical response. *Postgraduate Medical Journal* 53: 139–145.

Brogden RN, Speight TM and Avery GS 1971. Doxepin: A review. *Drugs* 1: 194–226.

Chew DJ, Buffington CAT, Kendall MS, DiBartola SP and Woodworth BE 1998. Amitriptyline treatment for severe recurrent idiopathic cystitis in cats. *Journal of the American Veterinary Medical Association* 213(9): 1282–1286.

Ciba-Geigy 1996. Tofranil® product information. *1997 Physician's Desk Reference*. Medical Economics Co. Montvale, NJ pp. 876–878.

Cordel C, Swan GE, Mülders MSG and Bertschinger HJ 2001. Pharmacokinetics of intravenous imipramine hydrochloride in cattle. *Journal of Veterinary Pharmacology and Therapeutics* 24(2): 143–145.

Creed KE and Tulloch AGS 1982. The action of imipramine on the lower urinary tract of the dog. *British Journal of Urology* 54: 5–10.

Crowell-Davis SL, Seibert LM, Sung W, Parthasarathy V and Curtis TM 2003. Use of clomipramine, alprazolam and behavior modification for treatment of storm phobia in dogs. *Journal of the American Veterinary Medical Association* 222:744–748.

Dehasse J 1997. Feline urine spraying. *Applied Animal Behaviour Science* 52: 365–371.

Dencker H, Dencker S-J, Green A and Nagy A 1976. Intestinal absorption, demethylation and enterohepatic circulation of imipramine studied by portal catherization in man. *Clinical Pharmacology and Therapeutics* 19: 584–586.

Diamond S 1965. Human metabolization of amitriptyline tagged with carbon 14. *Current Therapeutic Research* 7(3): 170–175.

Drake LA, Fallon JD, Sober A and The Doxepin Study Group 1994. Relief of pruritus in patients with atopic dermatitis after treatment with topical doxepin cream. *Journal of the American Academy of Dermatology* 31(4): 613–616.

Egashira T, Takayama F and Yamanaka Y 1999. The inhibition of monoamine oxidase activity by various antidepressants: Differences found in various mammalian species. *Japanese Journal of Pharmacology* 81(1): 115–121.

Elonen E, Linnoila M, Lukkari I and Mattila MJ 1975. Concentration of tricyclic antidepressants in plasma, heart and skeletal muscle after their intravenous infusion to anesthetized rabbits. *Acta Pharmacologica et Toxicologica* 37: 274–281.

Elonen E, Mattila MJ and Saarnivaara L 1974. Cardiovascular effects of amitriptyline, nortriptyline, protriptyline and doxepin in conscious rabbits. *European Journal of Pharmacology* 28: 178–188.

Evans LEJ, Bett JHN, Cox JR, Dubois JP and Van Hees T 1980. The bioavailability of oral and parenteral chlorimipramine (Anafranil). *Progress in Neuro-psychopharmacology* 4:293–302.

Faigle JW and Dieterle W 1973. The metabolism and pharmacokinetics of clomipramine (Anafranil). *Journal of International Medical Research* 1:281–290.

Falletta JM, Stasney CR and Mintz AA 1970. Amitriptyline poisoning treated with physostigmine. *Southern Medical Journal* 63: 1492–1493.

Fenwick JD 1982. The metabolism of amitriptyline in the horse: A preliminary report. *Scientific Proceedings of the 4th International Conference on the Control of the Use of Drugs in Racehorses,* pp. 182–184, May 11–14, Melbourne, Australia.

Gao B and Cutler MG 1994. Effects of acute and chronic administration of the antidepressants, imipramine, phenelzine and mianserin, on the social behaviour of mice. *Neuropharmacology* 33(6): 813–824.

GenDerm 1997. Zonalon® product information. *1997 Physicians desk reference,* pp. 1042–1043, Medical Economics Co., Montvale, New Jersey.

Goldberger E and Rapoport JL 1991. Canine acral lick dermatitis-response to the antiobsessional drug clomipramine. *Journal of the American Animal Hospital Association* 27(2): 179–182.

Gram LF and Christiansen J 1975. First pass metabolism of imipramine in man. *Clinical Pharmacology and Therapeutics* 17: 555–563.

Grindlinger HM and Ramsay E 1991. Compulsive feather picking in birds. *Archives of General Psychiatry* 48(9): 857.

Gulikers KP and Panciera DL 2003. Evaluation of the effects of clomipramine on canine thyroid function tests. *Journal of Veterinary Internal Medicine* 17(1): 44–49.

Hagedorn H-W, Meiser H, Zankl H and Schulz R 2001. Elimination of doxepin isomers from the horse following intravenous application. *Journal of Veterinary Pharmacology and Therapeutics* 24(4): 283–289.

Hagedorn H-W, Meiser H, Zankl H and Schulz R 2002. The isomeric metabolites of doxepin in equine serum and urine. *Journal of Pharmaceutical and Biomedical Analysis* 29(1–2): 317–323.

Hanno PM, Buehler J and Wein AJ 1989. Use of amitriptyline in the treatment of interstitial cystitis. *The Journal of Urology* 141: 846–848.

Heninger GR and Charney DS 1987. Mechanism of action of antidepressant treatments: implications for the etiology and treatment of depressive disorders. In *Psychopharmacology: The third generation of progress,* pp. 535–545, edited by HY Meltzer, Raven, New York.

Hewson C, Ball RO, Luescher UA, Parent J, Conlon P and Murphy DL 1995. The effect of clomipramine on monoamine metabolites in the normal canine brain. *Proceedings of the 29th International Congress of the International Society for Applied Ethology,* pp. 105–106, August 3–5, Exeter, UK.

Hewson CJ, Conlon PD, Luescher UA and Ball RO 1998a. The pharmacokinetics of clomipramine and desmethylclomipramine in dogs: Parameter estimates following a single oral dose and 28 consecutive daily oral doses of clomipramine. *Journal of Veterinary Pharmacology and Therapeutics* 21: 214–222.

Hewson CJ, Luescher A, Parent JM, Conlon PD and Ball RO 1998b. Efficacy of clomipramine in the treatment of canine compulsive disorder. *Journal of the American Veterinary Medical Association* 213(12): 1760–1766.

Hobbs DC 1968. Distribution and metabolism of doxepin in rat and dog. *Pharmacologist* 10(2): 154.

Hobbs DC 1969. Distribution and metabolism of doxepin. *Biochemical Pharmacology* 18: 1941–1954.

Houpt KA 1994. Animal behavior case of the month. *Journal of the American Veterinary Medical Association* 204(11): 1751–1752.

Johnson CA 1987. Chronic feather picking: A different approach to treatment. *Proceedings of the International Conference on Zoological and Avian Medicine*, pp. 125–142, Oahu, Hawaii.

Jones RB and Luscombe DK 1977. Plasma level studies with clomipramine (Anafranil). *Journal of International Medical Research* 5: 98–107.

Juarbe-Diaz SV 2000. Animal behavior case of the month. *Journal of the American Veterinary Medical Association* 216(10): 1562–1564.

Khanna OP, Heber D, Elkouss G and Gonick P 1975. Imipramine hydrochloride, pharmacodynamic effects on lower urinary tract of female dogs. *Urology* 6(1): 48–51.

Kimura Y, Kume M and Kageyama K 1972. Absorption, distribution and metabolism of doxepin hydrochloride. *Pharmacometrics* 6: 955–971.

King JN, Maurer MP, Altmann BO, and Strehlau GA 2000a. Pharmacokinetics of clomipramine in dogs following single-dose and repeated-dose oral administration. *American Journal of Veterinary Research* 61(1): 80–85.

King JN, Maurer MP, Hotz RP and Fisch RD 2000b. Pharmacokinetics of clomipramine in dogs following single-dose intravenous and oral administration. *American Journal of Veterinary Research* 61(1):74–79.

King JN, Simpson BS, Overall KL, Appleby D, Pageat P, Ross C, Chaurand JP, Heath S, Beata C, Weiss AB, Muller G, Paris T, Bataille BG, Parker J, Petit S, Wren J and The CLOCSA (Clomipramine in Canine Separation Anxiety) Study Group 2000c. Treatment of separation anxiety in dogs with clomipramine: Results from a prospective, randomized, double-blind, placebo-controlled, parallel-group, multicenter clinical trial. *Applied Animal Behaviour Science* 67: 255–275.

King JN, Steffan J, Heath SE, Simpson BS, Crowell-Davis SL, Harrington LJM, Weiss A-B and Seewald W 2004a. Determination of the dosage of clomipramine for the treatment of urine spraying in cats. *Journal of the American Veterinary Medical Association* 225(6): 881–887.

King JN, Overall KL, Appleby D, Simpson BS, Beata C, Chaurand CJP, Heath SE, Ross C, Weiss AB, Muller G, Bataille BG, Paris T, Pageat P, Brovedani F, Garden C and Petit S 2004b. Results of a follow-up investigation to a clinical trial testing the efficacy of clomipramine in the treatment of separation anxiety in dogs. *Applied Animal Behaviour Science* 89: 233–242.

Kuss H-J and Jungkunz G 1986. Nonlinear pharmacokinetics of chlorimipramine after infusion and oral administration in patients. *Progress in Neuro-Psychopharmacology & Biological Psychiatry* 10(6): 739–748.

Landsberg GM 2001. Clomipramine—Beyond separation anxiety. *Journal of the American Animal Hospital Association* 37(4): 313–318.

Leitold M, Fleissig W and Merk A 1984. Anti-ulcer and secretion-inhibitory properties of the tricyclic derivative doxepin in rats and dogs. *Arzneimittel-Forschung/Drug Research* 34–1(4): 468–473.

Lheureux P, Vranckx M, Leduc D and Askenasi R 1992a. Risks of flumazenil in mixed benzodiazepine-tricyclic antidepressant overdose: Report of a preliminary study in the dog. *Journal de Toxicologie Clinique et Expérimentale* 12(1): 43–53.

Lheureux P, Vranckx M, Leduc D and Askenasi R 1992b. Flumazenil in mixed benzodiazepine/tricyclic antidepressant overdose: A placebo-controlled study in the dog. *The American Journal of Emergency Medicine* 10(3): 184–188.

Liljequist R, Linnoila M and Mattila MJ 1974. Effect of two weeks treatment with chlorimipramine and nortriptyline, alone or in combination with alcohol, on learning and memory. *Psychopharmacologia* 39: 181–186.

Litster A 2000. Use of clomipramine for treatment of behavioural disorders in 14 cats—Efficacy and side-effects. *Australian Veterinary Practitioner* 30(2): 50–54.

McDonnell SM 1999. Libido, erection, and ejaculatory dysfunction in stallions. *Compendium of Continuing Education for the Practicing Veterinarian* 21(3): 263–266.

McDonnell SM, Garcia MC, Kenney RM and Van Arsdalen KN 1987. Imipramine-induced erection, masturbation, and ejaculation in male horses. *Pharmacology, Biochemistry and Behavior* 27: 187–191.

McDonnell SM and Odian MJ 1994. Imipramine and xylazine-induced ex copula ejaculation in stallions. *Theriogenology* 41: 1005–1010.

Mealy KL, Peck KE, Bennett BS, Sellon RK, Swinney GR, Melzer K, Gokhale SA and Krone TM 2004. System absorption of amitriptyline and buspirone after oral and transdermal administration to healthy cats. *Journal of Veterinary Internal Medicine* 18: 43–46.

Merck 1998. Elavil® product information. *2001 Physician's desk reference*, pp 626–628, Medical Economics Co., Montvale, New Jersey.

Merrell Pharmaceuticals 2000. Norpramin product information. *2003 Physician's desk reference*, pp. 749–751, Medical Economics Co., Montvale, New Jersey.

Mertens PA and Dodman NH 1996. Medikamentöse Behandlung der akralen Leckdermatitits des Hundes. *Kleintier-Praxis* 41(5): 327–337.

Mertens P and Torres S 2003. The use of clomipramine hydrochloride for the treatment of feline psychogenic alopecia. *Journal of the American Animal Hospital Association* 39: 509–512.

Midha KK, Hubbard JW, McKay G, Hawes EM, Korchinski ED, Gurnsey T, Cooper JK and Schwede R 1992. Stereoselective pharmacokinetics of doxepin isomers. *European Journal of Clinical Pharmacology* 42(5): 539–544.

Mignot E, Renaud A, Nishino S, Arrigoni J, Guilleminault C and Dement WC 1993. Canine cataplexy is preferentially controlled by adrenergic-mechanisms: evidence using monoamine selective uptake inhibitors and release enhancers. *Psychopharmacology* 113(1): 76–82.

Moon-Fanelli AA and Dodman NH 1998. Description and development of compulsive tail chasing in terriers and response to clomipramine treatment. *Journal of the American Veterinary Medical Association* 212(8): 1252–1257.

Nagy A and Johansson R 1977. The demethylation of imipramine and clomipramine as apparent from their plasma kinetics. *Psychopharmacology (Berlin)* 54(2): 125–131.

Nelson JC 2004. Tricyclic and tetracyclic drugs. In *Textbook of psychopharmacology*, pp. 207–230, edited by AF Schatzberg and CB Nemeroff, American Psychiatric Publishing Inc., Washington, DC.

Noguchi Y, Sakai T, Ishiko J and Sugimoto S 1972a. Acute toxicity of doxepin hydrochloride. *Pharmacometrics* (Tokyo) 6(5): 889–897.

Noguchi Y, Sakai T, Arakawa M and Nabata H 1972b. Subacute toxicity of doxepin hydrochloride in rats. *Pharmacometrics* 6(5): 899–928.

Noguchi Y, Sakai T, Arakawa M and Nabata H 1972c. Chronic toxicity of doxepin hydrochloride in rats. *Pharmacometrics* (Tokyo)6(5): 929–954.

Novartis 1998. Anafranil® product information. In *1999 Physician's desk reference*, pp. 1988–1992, Thomson PDR Montvale, New Jersey.

Novartis 2000. Clomicalm® product information.

Nurten A, Yamantürk P and Enginar N 1996. The effects of amitriptyline and clomipramine on learning and memory in an elevated plus-maze test in mice. *European Neuropsychopharmacology* 6: 26.

Ohtani H, Odagiri Y, Sato H, Sawada Y and Iga T 2001. A comparative pharmacodynamic study of the arrhythogenicity of antidepressants, fluvoxamine and imipramine, in guinea pigs. *Biological & Pharmaceutical Bulletin* 24(5): 550–554.

Overall K 1994. Use of clomipramine to treat ritualistic stereotypic motor behavior in three dogs. *Journal of the American Veterinary Medical Association* 205(12): 1733–1741.

Overall K 1998. Animal behavior case of the month. *Journal of the American Veterinary Medical Association* 213(1): 34–36.

Overall KL and Dunham AE 2002. Clinical features and outcome in dogs and cats with obsessive-compulsive disorder: 126 cases (1989–2000). *Journal of the American Veterinary Medical Association* 221(10): 1445–1452.

Petit S, Pageat P, Chaurand J-P, Heude B, Beata C and DeHasse J 1999. Efficacy of clomipramine in the treatment of separation anxiety in dogs: Clinical trial. *Revue de Maédecine Vaétaerinaire* 150 (2): 133–140.

Pfeiffer E, Guy N and Cribb A 1999. Clomipramine induced urinary retention in a cat. *The Canadian Veterinary Journal* 40(4): 265–267.

Pfizer 1996. Sinequan product information. *Physicians' desk reference*, pp. 2028–2030, Thomson PDR, Montvale, New Jersey.

Podberscek AL, Hsu Y and Serpell JA 1999. Evaluation of clomipramine as an adjunct to behavioural therapy in the treatment of separation-related problems in dogs. *The Veterinary Record* 145: 365–369.

Potter WZ 1984. Psychotherapeutic drugs and biogenic amines: Current concepts and therapeutic implications. *Drugs* 28: 127–143.

Potter WZ, Manji HK and Rudorfer MV 1995. Tricyclics and tetracyclics. In *Textbook of psychopharmacology*, pp. 141–160, edited by AF Schatzberg and CB Nemeroff, The American Psychiatric Press, Washington, DC.

Potter WZ, Rudorfer MV, and Manji H 1991. The pharmacologic treatment of depression. *New England Journal of Medicine* 325: 633–642.

Pouchelon JL, Martel E, Champeroux P, Richard S and King JN 2000. Effects of clomipramine hydrochloride on heart rate and rhythm in healthy dogs. *American Journal of Veterinary Research* 61(8): 960–964.

Ramsay ED and Grindlinger H 1992. Treatment of feather picking with clomipramine. *Proceedings of the Association of Avian Veterinarians* 379–382.

Rapoport JL, Ryland DH and Kriete M 1992. Drug treatment of canine acral lick: An animal model of obsessive-compulsive disorder. *Archives of General Psychiatry* 49: 517–521.

Reich M 1999. Animal behavior case of the month. *Journal of the American Veterinary Medical Association* 215(12): 1780–1782.

Reich MR, Ohad DG, Overall KL and Dunham AE 2000. Electrocardiographic assessment of antianxiety medication in dogs and correlation with serum drug concentration. *Journal of the American Veterinary Medical Association* 216(10): 1571–1575.

Ribbentrop A and Schaumann W 1965. Pharmakologische Untersuchungen mit Doxepin, einem Antidepressivum mit zentral anticholinerger und sedierender Wirkung. *Arzneimittel-Forschung* 15: 863–868.

Richelson E and Nelson A 1984a. Antagonism by antidepressants of neurotransmitter receptors of normal human brain in vitro. *Journal of Pharmacology and Experimental Therapeutics* 230(1): 94–102.

Richelson E and Pfenning M 1984b. Blockade by antidepressants and related compounds of biogenic amine uptake into rat brain synaptosomes: Most antidepressants selectively block norepinephrine uptake. *European Journal of Pharmacology* 104: 277–286.

Rudorfer MV and Robins E 1982. Amitriptyline overdose: Clinical effects on tricyclic antidepressant plasma levels. *Journal of Clinical Psychiatry* 43(11): 457–460.

Sandoz Pharmaceuticals 1996. Pamelor® product information. *1997 Physicians desk reference*, pp. 2409–2411, Thomson PDR, Montvale, New Jersey.

Sawyer LS, Moon-Fanelli AA and Dodman NH 1999. Psychogenic alopecia in cats: 11 cases (1993–1996). *Journal of the American Veterinary Medical Association* 214(1): 71–74.

Seibert L 2000. Animal behavior case of the month. *Journal of the American Veterinary Medical Association* 216(10): 1562–1564.

Seibert LM, Crowell-Davis SL, Wilson GH and Ritchie BW 2004. Placebo-controlled clomipramine trial for the treatment of feather picking disorder in cockatoos. *Journal of the American Animal Hospital Association* 40: 261–269.

Seksel K and Lindeman MJ 1998. Use of clomipramine in the treatment of anxiety-related and obsessive-compulsive disorders in cats. *Australian Veterinary Journal* 76(5): 317–321.

Seksel K and Lindeman MJ 1999. Einsatz von clomipramin zur behandlung angstspezifischer und obsessive-kompulsiver Störungen bei Katzen. *Kleintierpraxis 44(12)*: 925–934.

Shanley K and Overall K 1992. Psychogenic dermatoses. In *Current veterinary therapy XI*, pp. 552–558, edited by RW Kirk and JD Bonagura, WB Saunders Co., Philadelphia, Pennsylvania.

Shimatani T, Inoue M, Okajima M, Kawahori K and Fujii K 2001. Doxepin, a tricyclic antidepressant, centrally inhibits gastric acid secretion, acting on the neurons probably located in the medulla oblongata in conscious dogs. *Gastroenterology* 120(5) (Suppl. 1): A157-A157 836.

Simpson B 1996. Concerns about possible drug interactions. *Journal of the American Veterinary Medical Association* 209(8): 1380–1381.

Simpson B for the Clomipramine in Canine Separation-Related Anxiety Study Group. 1997. Treatment of separation-related anxiety in dogs with clomipramine. Results from a multicentre, blinded, placebo-controlled clinical trial. In *Proceedings of the First International Conference on Veterinary Behavioural Medicine,* pp. 143–154, University Federation for Animal Welfare, Potters Bar, United Kingdom.

Slovis TL, Ott JE, Teitelbaum DT and Lipscomb W 1971. Physostigmine therapy in acute tricyclic antidepressant poisoning. *Clinical Toxicology* 4(3): 451–459.

Sulser F, Vetulani J and Mobley PL 1978. Mode of action of antidepressant drugs. *Biochemical Pharmacology* 27: 257–261.

Takeuchi Y, Houpt, KA and Scarlett JM 2000. Evaluation of treatments for separation anxiety in dogs. *Journal of the American Veterinary Medical Association* 217(3): 342–345.

Tatsumi M, Groshan K, Blaekly RD and Richelson E 1997. Pharmacological profile of antidepressants and related compounds at humane monoamine transporters. *European Journal of Pharmacology* 340: 249–258.

Thompson PJ 1991. Antidepressants and memory. Human *Psychopharmacology* 6:79–90.

Thornton LA 1995. Animal behavior case of the month. *Journal of the American Veterinary Medical Association* 206(12): 1868–1870.

Tulloch AGS and Creed KE 1979. A comparison between propantheline and imipramine on bladder and salivary gland function. *British Journal of Urology* 51: 359–362.

Turner RMO, Love CC, McDonnell SM, Sweeney RW, Twitchell, Habecker PL, Reilly LK, Pozor MA and Kenney RM 1995a. Use of imipramine hydrochloride for treatment of urospermia in a stallion with a dysfunctional bladder. *Journal of the American Veterinary Medical Association* 207: 1602–1606.

Turner RMO, McDonnell SM and Hawkins JF 1995b. Use of pharmacologically induced ejaculation to obtain semen from a stallion with a fractured radius. *Journal of the American Veterinary Medical Association* 206(12): 1906–1908.

Vernier VG 1961. The pharmacology of antidepressant agents. *Symposium on depression with special studies of a new antidepressant, amitriptyline,* pp. 7–13, Physicians Postgraduate Press, New York, New York.

Vetulani J and Sulser F 1975. Action of various antidepressant treatments reduces reactivity of noradrenergic cyclic AMP generating system in limbic forebrain. *Nature* 257: 495–496.

Virga V, Houpt KA and Scarlett JM 2001. Efficacy of amitriptyline as a pharmacological adjunct to behavioral modification in the management of aggressive behaviors in dogs. *Journal of the American Animal Hospital Association* 37(4): 325–330.

White MM, Neilson JC, Hart BL and Cliff KD 1999. Effects of clomipramine hydrochloride on dominance-related aggression in dogs. *Journal of the American Veterinary Medical Association* 215(9): 1288–1291.

Yan J-H, Hubbard JW, McKay G and Midha KK 1997. Stereoselective *in vivo* and *in vitro* studies on the metabolism of doxepin and N-desmethyldoxepin. *Xenobiotica* 27(12): 1245–1257.

Zagrodzka J, Fonberg E and Brudnais-Graczyk Z 1985. Predatory dominance and aggressive display under imipramine treatments in cats. *Acta Neurobiologiae Experimentalis* 45: 137–149.

Zagrodzka J, Korczynski R and Fonberg E 1981. The effects of imipramine on socio-emotional and alimentary motivated behavior in dogs. *Acta Neurobiologiae Experimentalis* 41(4): 363–372.

Ziegler VE, Biggs JT, Wylie LT, Rosen SH, Hawf DJ and Coryell WH 1978. Doxepin kinetics. *Clinical Pharmacology and Therapeutics* 23(5): 573–579.

Chapter Twelve
Endogenous Opioid Peptides

Opiates are drugs derived from opium and include morphine, codeine (both alkaloids), and a variety of semisynthetic analogs derived from them or from thebaine, which is another component of opium (Reisine and Pasternak 1996). Opium preparations extracted from poppy seeds have been used for thousands of years to treat pain, cough, and diarrhea, and to produce euphoria. The term *opioid* is more general and is used to describe all drugs, irrespective of structure, with morphine-like activity, including endogenous peptides.

The existence of specific receptors for opiates in mammalian tissues had been suspected since the 1950s, based on strict structure-activity requirements, including stereospecificity, for opiate drugs. In the early 1970s methods developed for the biochemical detection of receptors were applied to the search for specific opiate receptors in brain tissue. Using a radioligand-binding method, Snyder and colleagues identified an opiate receptor in brain and intestinal tissue in 1973 (Snyder 2004). The identified receptor was pharmacologically relevant in that an extensive series of opiate drugs bound with affinities closely matching their analgesic potencies. These opiate receptors were found to be enriched in areas of animal brain known to be involved in the processing of sensory and pain signals, such as the periaqueductal gray, medial thalamus, and the substantia gelatinosa of the spinal cord and brain stem. A very high density of opiate receptors was also found in the locus coeruleus, where opioids exert a regulatory influence on noradrenergic pathways (Snyder 2004). The discovery of these specific receptors for opiates immediately suggested the presence of endogenous opiatelike substances that normally target these receptors. The first description of such endogenous substances was in 1975 with the characterization of substances from porcine brain that had opiate agonist properties (Hughes et al. 1975). These substances consisted of two enkephalin pentapeptides: [Met]enkephalin (Tyr-Gly-Gly-Phe-Met) and [Leu]enkephalin (Tyr-Gly-Gly-Phe-Leu). Subsequent to the identification of these two enkephalin pentapeptides, other investigators characterized several additional endorphins (endogenous opioids) from porcine hypothalamus-neurohypophysis. The endorphins all contain the N-terminal Tyr-Gly-Gly-Phe (Met or Leu) sequence followed by varied C-terminal extensions yielding peptides from 5 to 31 amino acids in length (Akil et al. 1998). Two important members of the endorphin family are β-endorphin, an extremely potent endogenous opioid and dynorphin A, a 17-amino acid peptide with a distinctive neuroanatomical distribution and physiology. In mammals the endogenous opioid peptides are derived from four precursors: proopiomelanocortin (POMC), proenkephalin, prodynorphin, and pronociceptin/orphanin FQ. The characterization of the POMC gene revealed that it codes for the stress hormone ACTH and the opioid peptide β-endorphin. The endogenous opioid peptides and their respective precursors are listed in Table 12.1.

Table 12.1 Mammalian endogenous opioids

Precursor	Endogenous opioid	Amino acid sequence
Proopiomelanocortin	β-Endorphin	Tyr-Gly-Gly-Phe-Met-Thr-Ser-Glu-Lys-Ser-Gln-Thr-Pro-Leu-Val-Thr-Leu-Phe-Lys-Asn-Ala-Ile-Ile-Lys-Asn-Ala-Tyr-Lys-Lys-Gly-Glu
Proenkephalin	[Met]enkephalin	Tyr-Gly-Gly-Phe-Met
	[Leu]enkephalin	Tyr-Gly-Gly-Phe-Leu
Prodynorphin	Dynorphin A	Tyr-Gly-Gly-Phe-Leu-Arg-Arg-Ile-Arg-Pro-Lys-Leu-Lys-Trp-Asp-Asn-Gln
	Dynorphin A (1-8)	Tyr-Gly-Gly-Phe-Leu-Arg-Arg-Ile
	Dynorphin B	Tyn-Gly-Gly-Phe-Leu-Arg-Arg-Gln-Phe-Lys-Val-Val-Thr
	α-Neoendorphin	Tyr-Gly-Gly-Phe-Leu-Arg-Lys-Pro-Lys
	β-Neoendorhin	Tyr-Gly-Gly-Phe-Leu-Arg-Lys-Pro
Pronociceptin/OFQ	Nociceptin	Phe-Gly-Gly-Phe-Thr-Gly-Ala-Arg-Lys-Ser-Ala-Arg-Lys-Leu-Ala-Asn-Gln

The proenkehalin precursor encodes for multiple copies of [Met]enkephalin as well as one copy of [Leu]enkephalin. Similarly, prodynorphin encodes for three opioid peptides of distinct lengths, including dynorphin A, dynorphin B, and the neoendorphins.

The POMC-derived peptides have a limited distribution in the central nervous system (CNS) with high levels found in the arcuate nucleus and pituitary. The prodynorphin and proenkephalin peptides have a wider distribution in the CNS and are frequently found in the same pathways. The proenkephalin peptides are present in areas of the CNS that are involved with the perception of pain such as laminae I and II of the spinal cord, the spinal trigeminal nucleus, and the periaqueductal gray. These peptides are also found in limbic structures regulating affective behavior and reward, such as the amygdala, nucleus accumbens, hippocampus, locus ceruleus, and cerebral cortex. Although there are a few long-axon enkephalinergic tracts in the brain, these peptides are typically expressed in interneurons. One group of long-axon prodynorphin and proenkephalin gene product-containing pathways comprise part of the output neurons of the striatum and accumbens (Akil et al. 1997). In the dorsal striatum the striatonigial neurons contain prodynorphin products, substance P and GABA, whereas the striatopallidal neurons contain enkephalin and GABA. As a result of the limited distribution of β-endorphin in the brain, the enkephalins and dynorphins are considered to be the predominant central opioid peptide neurotransmitters.

It is now well established that these endogenous opioids interact with an opioid receptor family composed of three subtypes. Pharmacological studies using opioid peptides, alkaloids, and synthetic derivatives of opiates indicated multiple subtypes of opioid receptors. This classification of multiple opioid receptors was originally based on the production of distinct syndromes in dogs by derivatives of morphine (Martin et al. 1976). The three drugs used in these early studies were morphine as the prototype for the mu- (μ-) opioid receptor, ketocyclazocine for the kappa- (κ-) opioid receptor, and SKF-10,047 (N-allylnormetazocine) for a sigma-(σ-) receptor. The morphine syndrome (μ) in the dog was characterized by miosis, bradycardia, hypothermia, a general depression of the nociceptive responses, and indifference to environmental stimuli. Ketocyclazocine (κ) constricted pupils, depressed the flexor reflex, and produced sedation, but did not markedly alter pulse rate or the skin-twitch reflex. SKF-10,047 (σ), in contrast to morphine and ketocyclazocine, caused mydriasis, tachypnea, tachycardia, and mania (Martin et al. 1976). The σ site was subsequently demonstrated to not represent an opioid receptor inasmuch as the actions of SKF-10,047 were not blocked by prototypic opioid antagonists such as naloxone and naltrexone. Investigations with both nonpeptide and peptide derivatives led to the demonstration of the delta- (δ-) opioid receptor as the third subtype. In fact, the first opioid receptor to be cloned was the δ receptor (Kieffer et al. 1992), and this was soon followed by successful isolation of cDNA clones for the μ- and κ-receptors. The cloning and sequencing of all three opioid receptors from a variety of species verified that these receptors belonged to the G protein-coupled family of receptors. Opioids exert their characteristic pharmacologic actions through activation of these receptors that mediate hyperpolarizing effects on pre- and postsynaptic neurons and reducing Ca^{2+} influx into presynaptic neurons, which inhibits neurotransmitter release. Opioid receptors are coupled to G proteins that regulate adenylyl cyclase, K^+ channels, and Ca^{2+} channels.

The affinity of endogenous opioid peptides for μ-, δ-, and κ-receptors varies, but none of the peptides bind exclusively to only one receptor. β-Endorphin has similar affinities for μ- and δ-opioid receptors, but has very low affinity for κ receptors. [Met] and [Leu] enkephalins have high affinity for δ-opioid receptors and have approximately 10-fold lower affinity for μ-opioid receptors; these endogenous enkephalins possess negligible affinity for κ receptors. Of the three subtypes of opioid receptors, the subtype with the greatest selectivity for endogenous peptides is unquestionably the κ-opioid receptor. The κ-receptor displays subnanomolar (nM) affinities for the dynorphins, while its affinity for [Leu]enkephalin is 100 nM; a potency difference of 1000-fold (Akil et al. 1997). The endogenous ligands for κ-opioid receptors are the dynorphins. With the exception of the dynorphins, most endogenous opioid peptides have a higher affinity for δ rather than μ receptors. Notwithstanding this pharmacological signature of endogenous opioids, the μ-receptor clearly mediates the analgesic and euphorigenic actions of opioid drugs. The δ-opioid receptor is much less involved in the analgesic and rewarding effects of opioid drugs, while κ-opioid receptors mediate spinal analgesia and dysphoria. The use of transgenic mice that lack μ-opioid receptors has revealed that morphine-induced analgesia, reward, respiratory depression, and constipation are virtually absent in these mice (Keiffer 1999).

A summary of the receptor selectivities and efficacies of opioid drugs is given in Table 12.2. Similar to other drugs, these opioids exert either an agonist, partial agonist, or antagonist action at a given receptor. The term mixed agonist/antagonist is, although confusing, sometimes used to describe the pharmacology of specific opioids such as buprenorphine. This term implies that a given drug may exert agonist or partial agonist activity at one opioid receptor subtype while exerting an antagonist action at a different opioid receptor subtype

As indicated in Table 12.2, compounds such as morphine and etorphine exhibit a preference for μ-opioid receptors but also activate δ- and κ-receptors with lower affinity. Similarly, the opioid receptor antagonists, naloxone, naltrexone, and diprenorphine are promiscuous in the sense that they do not discriminate well between opioid receptor subtypes.

Veterinary pharmacology of opioids is characterized, and complicated, by the dramatic species differences that exist with regard to drug-induced responses. As with hu-

Table 12.2 Actions and selectivities of opioids at the various opioid receptor subtypes

Drug	Receptor		
	μ	δ	κ
Morphine	+++	+	+
Methadone	+++	+	
Etorphine	+++	+++	+++
Fentanyl	+++	+	
Sufentanyl	+++	+	+
Butorphanol	p.a.		++
Buprenorphine	p.a.		ant.
Pentazocine	p.a.		++
Nalbuphine	ant.		+
Diprenorphine	ant.	ant.	ant.
Naloxone	ant.	ant.	ant.
Naltrexone	ant.	ant.	ant.

Note: +, agonist; p.a., partial agonist; ant, antagonist.

mans, morphine produces CNS depression in the dog and monkey, whereas excitation is observed in the cat, horse, goat, sheep, pig, mouse, and cow. The excitatory effects of opioids such as fentanyl have indeed been used illegally in race horses. The physiological basis for these species differences in response to opioids is poorly understood, but is likely a function of the distinct distribution and/or density of opioid receptors in the neurocircuitry of the limbic system. The "morphine mania" that is characteristic in cats is avoided by either repeated administration of small doses or concurrent administration of a neuroleptic or sedative. In all species, however, morphine and related opioids are capable of relieving intense pain associated with injury or surgery.

The chronic administration of opioids such as morphine to laboratory rodents produces a sensitization to the locomotor-enhancing effects of these drugs. This sensitization, or reverse tolerance, also develops to the oral gnawing stereotypy observed in rats (Kornetsky 2004). This sensitization in response to chronic exposure to an opioid indicates that a long-lasting change in opioid receptor-signaling mechanisms develops that is distinct from those mechanisms subserving tolerance development to particular pharmacologic actions of opioids. A hyperactive endogenous opioid neurotransmission caused by opioid receptor sensitization may be involved in the expression of animal behavioral stereotypies. This may have relevance to the effectiveness of opioid antagonists in stereotypic self-licking and self-mutilation behavior in dogs and horses (Dodman et al. 1987, 1988). The effectiveness of opioid antagonists such as naltrexone, naloxone, and diprenorphine may therefore be related to their ability to reverse or attenuate a sensitization that develops to endogenous opioid peptide activation of opioid receptors.

In the context of the treatment of self-mutilation stereotypies, one other aspect of the pharmacology of compounds structurally related to opioids that deserves discussion is the effectiveness of dextromethorphan. This compound is the stereoisomer of levomethorphan, a potent morphinelike analgesic. As described earlier in this chapter, opioid drugs display pronounced stereospecificity with respect to their ability to bind to opioid receptors. Thus, the levorotatory isomer of morphine, l- or (−) morphine, is pharmacologically active, while the dextrorotatory isomer, d- or (+) morphine, is essentially inactive. Similarly, the levorotatory isomer levomethorphan substitutes for morphine, whereas its dextrorotatory isomer dextromethorphan is over 1000-fold less active at opioid receptors. The inactivity of dextromethorphan at opioid receptors does not, however, generalize to the NMDA subtype of glutamate receptor where this compound acts as a potent noncompetitive antagonist (Franklin and Murray 1992). Dextromethorphan is widely used in human medicine as an over-the-counter antitussive drug. Dextromethorphan has been demonstrated to reduce stereotypic cribbing in horses and self-directed mutilation stereotypies in dogs (Rendon et al. 2001; Dodman et al. 2004). This pharmacologic effect of dextromethorphan may be presumed to derive from its ability to antagonize glutamate activation of NMDA receptors in the CNS.

References

Akil H, Owens C, Gutstein H, Taylor L, Curran E, and Watson S 1998. Endogenous opioids: Overview and current issues. *Drug Alcohol Depend.* 51: 127–140.

Dodman NH, Shuster L, Court MH and Dixon R 1987. Investigation into the use of narcotic antagonists in the treatment of a stereotypic behavior pattern (crib-biting) in the horse. *American Journal of Veterinary Research* 48(2): 311–319.

Dodman NH, Shuster L, White SD, Court MH, Parker D and Dixon R 1988. Use of narcotic antagonists to modify stereotypic self-licking, self-chewing, and scratching behavior in dogs. *Journal of American Veterinary Medical Association* 193(7): 815–819.

Dodman NH, Shuster L, Nesbitt G, Weissman A, Lo W-Y, Chang W-W and Cottam, N 2004. the use of dextromethorphan to treat repetitive self-directed scratching, biting, or chewing in dogs with allergic dermatitis. *Journal of Veterinary Pharmacology Therapeutics* 27: 99–104.

Franklin PH and Murray TF 1992. High affinity [3H]dextrorphan binding in rat brain is localized to a noncompetitive antagonist site of the activated N-methyl-D-aspartate receptor-cation channel. *Molecular Pharmacology* 41(1): 134–146.

Hughes J, Smith T, Morgan B, and Fothergill L 1975. Purification and properties of enkephalin—the possible endogenous ligand for the morphine receptor. *Life Sciences* 16: 1753–1758.

Kieffer BL 1999. Opioids: First lessons from knockout mice. *Trends in Pharmacological Science* 20: 19–26.

Kieffer BL, Befort K, Gaveriaux-Ruff C and Hirth CG 1992. The δ-opioid receptor: Isolation of a cDNA by expression cloning and pharmacological characterization. *Proceedings of the National Academy of Science* 89: 12048–12052.

Kornetsky C 2004. Brain-stimulation reward, morphine-induced oral stereotypy, and sensitization: Implications for abuse. *Neuroscience and Biobehavioral Reviews* 27: 777–786.

Martin, WR, Eades CG, Thompson JA, Huppler RE and Gilbert PE 1976. The effects of morphine- and nalorphine-like drugs in the nondependent and morphine-dependent chronic spinal dog. *Journal of Pharmacology and Experimental Therapeutics* 197(3): 517–532.

Pert CB and Snyder SH 1973. Opiate Receptor: Demonstration in Nervous Tissue. *Science* 179:1011–1014.

Reisine T and Pasternak GW 1996. Opioid analgesics and antagonists. In *Goodman & Gilman's the pharmacological basis of therapeutics*, pp 521-556, edited by JG Hardman and LE Limbird, New York, McGraw-Hill.

Rendon RA, Shuster L and Dodman NH 2001. The effect of NMDA receptor blocker, dextromethorphan, on cribbing in horses. *Pharmacology Biochemistry and Behavior* 68: 49–51.

Snyder SH 2004. Opiate receptors and beyond: 30 years of neural signaling research. *Neuropharmacology* 47: 274–285.

Chapter Thirteen
Opioids and Opioid Antagonists

Action

There are multiple theories as to why narcotic antagonists are sometimes effective in the treatment of stereotypies and compulsive disorder in nonhuman animals. One possibility is that stress, such as an overstimulating or understimulating environment, causes an animal to initiate stereotypic behavior. Carrying out the stereotypic behavior then causes the release of endogenous endorphins, which reinforce the behavior. Narcotic antagonists would block this release of the endogenous endorphins, thereby blocking the reinforcement. This results in the animal discontinuing the behavior. If this theory were true, it would be expected that the animal would continue in the stereotypy for awhile before gradually decreasing the behavior, because it would have to learn that carrying out the stereotypy no longer resulted in pleasant sensations. The rapid response exhibited in clinical situations fails to support this hypothesis.

An alternative hypothesis is that opioids are directly involved in the initiation of the stereotypic behavior. The narcotic antagonists then block the opioids, thereby preventing their inducing stereotypic behavior. This hypothesis is supported by the rapid clinical response that occurs when opioid antagonists are administered. Opioids do enhance amphetamine-induced stereotypic behavior, and naloxone blocks this enhancement.

While both morphine (0.1–0.5 mg/kg) and oxymorphone (0.125–0.50 mg/kg) have been reported as alleviating the crying of separation distress in puppies, they also decreased motor activity (Panksepp et al. 1978). Timid beagle/telomian hybrids have also been treated with morphine at 0.25 mg/kg. While they did show some improvement with the combination of morphine and behavior modification, they also became less socially solicitous than placebo-treated dogs, possibly as a consequence of sedative effects (Panksepp et al. 1983). Morphine has also been shown to decrease a variety of aggression types in laboratory animals (Gianutsos and Lal 1978). Nevertheless, these medications are not recommended for these or other problems, which are best treated with safer medications.

Overview of Indications

Indications include stereotypic behavior, compulsive disorder, including lick granulomas and tail-chasing in dogs, and self-mutilation and cribbing in horses. Opiate antagonists have been found to be beneficial in the treatment of some forms of self-injurious behavior in humans as well as nonhuman animals (e.g., Richardson and Zaleski 1983; Herman et al. 1987; Smith and Pittelkow 1989; Sandman et al. 1990).

Contraindications, Side Effects, and Adverse Events

Gastrointestinal effects, especially diarrhea, may occur.

Clinical Guidelines

While opioid antagonists have shown substantial promise in the treatment of stereo-typic behaviors in multiple species, their use is not yet widespread for a number of reasons. Some can only be given parenterally and all are expensive. Also, opioid antagonists may be more effective in the early phases of compulsive disorder, although this phenomenon has not been studied across all species and all manifestations of compulsive disorder. Nevertheless, dramatic results in some cases make them a class of drugs that should be considered in the treatment of any stereotypic behavior.

Diprenorphine, which is not reviewed below, has been used in the treatment of cribbing in horses (Dodman et al. 1987). Cribbing is a behavior that occurs in horses kept in confinement. During cribbing, the horse grabs a horizontal object with its teeth, bites down hard, and flexes its neck. It may or may not swallow air as it does this. Diprenorphine was twice administered to a horse with a problem with cribbing behavior, once at 0.02 mg/kg and the second time at 0.03 mg/kg intramuscularly (IM). In both cases, after a latency period of 30 minutes, injection of diprenorphine resulted in almost total discontinuation of cribbing for periods of 3–5.5 hours. Animal doses and some cost comparisons are given in Tables 13.1 and 13.2.

Specific Medications

I. Nalmefene

Chemical Compound: 17-(Cyclopropylmethyl)-4,5α-epoxy-6-methylenemorphinan-4,14-diol, hydrochloride salt
DEA Classification: Not a controlled substance
Preparations: Generally available as 1-ml ampules containing 100 μg/mL and 2-ml ampules containing 1 mg/mL of a sterile solution suitable for intravenous, intramuscular, and subcutaneous administration (Baker Norton Pharmaceuticals, Inc. 1997)

Table 13.1 Doses of various opiate antagonists inhibitors for dogs, cats, horses, and parrots

Opiate antagonist	Cat	Dog	Parrot	Horse
Naltrexone	25–50 mg/cat q24h	1–2.2 mg/kg q12–24h	1.5 mg/kg q12h	0.7 mg/kg q24h
Naloxone		0.01 mg/kg SC as a test dose		
Pentazocine		2.5 mg/kg q12h		

Note: All doses for naltrexone are oral.
Source: Brown et al. 1987a; Turner 1993; Overall 1997; Nurnberg et al. 1997.

Clinical Pharmacology

Nalmefene reverses and prevents the effects of opioids, including respiratory depression, sedation, and hypotension. It has a longer duration of action than naloxone. It is equally bioavailable if given by intravenous, intramuscular, or subcutaneous routes. Peak levels are reached within minutes if it is given intravenously. However, there is a delay to maximum plasma concentration if it is given subcutaneously (about 1.5 hours in humans) or intramuscularly (about 2.3 hours in humans). If nalmefene is given parenterally, it blocks 80% of brain opioid receptors within five minutes (Baker Norton Pharmaceuticals, Inc. 1997).

Nalmefene is primarily metabolized by glucuronide conjugation, which occurs in the liver, after which the metabolites are excreted in the urine. Less than 5% of the urinary excretion is the parent compound. Fecal excretion accounts for only 17% of a nalmefene dose (Baker Norton Pharmaceuticals 1997).

The pharmacokinetics of nalmefene have been studied in three mixed-breed dogs given 0.5–0.9 mg/kg IV. Elimination half-life was 120–218 minutes (Dodman et al. 1988b).

In the horse, nalmefene has a half-life of 3–5 hours following intramuscular injection of 1 mg/kg. With intravenous injection the half-life is only 50 minutes. After oral administration of 2 mg/kg, no intact nalmefene is detectable in the plasma. High levels of nalmefene glucuronide appear rapidly after oral administration and are detectable for up to 16 hours. In this species, therefore, nalmefene must be administered parenterally, as it has poor oral bioavailability with extensive first-pass metabolism (Dixon et al. 1992).

Uses in Humans

Nalmefene is used in humans for reversal of the effects of opioid medications.

Contraindications

Nalmefene is contraindicated in patients with a known history of intolerance to the medication. In humans with hepatic or renal disease there is a decrease in plasma clearance (Baker Norton Pharmaceuticals 1997).

Side Effects

Side effects have not been reported in non-addicted animals given clinically relevant doses.

Administration of up to 1200 mg/m^2/day to rats has not resulted in any decrease in fertility, reproductive performance or offspring survival. Giving up to 2400 mg/m^2/day orally to rats or up to 96 mg/m^2/day intravenously to rabbits did not result in any harm to the fetuses. Administration of up to 205 mg/m^2/day in rat pups did not cause any adverse events (Baker Norton Pharmaceuticals 1997).

Other Information

Nalmefene has been administered to humans after administration of benzodiazepines with no adverse interactions (Baker Norton Pharmaceuticals 1997).

Effects Documented in Nonhuman Animals

Dogs

Dodman et al. (1988b) studied the use of various narcotic antagonists for the treatment of stereotypic self-licking, self-chewing and scratching in 9 dogs. Nalmefene was injected SC at a dose of 1 to 4 mg/kg after a baseline rate of self-licking, self-chewing and scratching was measured. During the 90-minute period following injection, the amount of time spent in these behaviors was significantly reduced in 6 of the 9 dogs. The problem behaviors were completely suppressed for 75 minutes in 2 dogs. No side effects were reported.

Horses

Dodman et al. (1987) treated five crib-biting horses with nalmefene across 20 trials by a variety of routes, specifically intramuscularly, subcutaneously, intravenously via continuous infusion and via a sustained release implant. Doses for the IM and SC injections ranged from 0.08 to 0.1 mg/kg. A single injection resulted in discontinuation of cribbing for 2.75 to 13 hours. The sustained release preparations resulted in a substantial decrease in cribbing for a minimum of 2 days.

Dodman et al. (1988a) reported a case study of a 500-kg Arabian stallion with a 4-year history of self-mutilation, specifically biting the flank and pectoral region. The stallion was treated, on successive days, with doses of 0.2 mg/kg, 0.4 mg/kg, 0.8 mg/kg, and 1.6 mg/kg given IM as a single dose. There was a dose-specific decrease in acts of self-mutilation or attempted self-mutilation during the four hours following the injection, with a 94% decrease at the highest dose. While this result seems promising, the authors report that, in preliminary pharmacokinetic studies, horses excrete nalmefene rapidly and the bioavailability of nalmefene given to horses is low.

II. Naloxone HCl

Chemical Compound: (-)-17-Allyl-4,5a-epoxy-3, 14-dihydroxy morphinan-6-one-hydrochloride

DEA Classification: Not a controlled substance

Preparations: Generally available as a 0.02 mg, 0.4 mg or 1 mg/ml solution for subcutaneous, intramuscular, or intraenous injection

Table 13.2 Examples of cost for one-month treatment for a 20-kg dog, a 5-kg cat, or a horse

Medication	Example	Cost
Pentazocine 50 mg/naloxone 0.5 mg	1 daily (dog)	$$$
Naltrexone 50 mg	1/2 daily (cat)	$$$$
Naltrexone 50 mg	1 daily (dog)	$$$$$$
Naltrexone 50 mg	5 daily (horse)	$$$$$$

Note: One reason that opiate antagonists are generally not a first drug of choice in the treatment of stereotypies and compulsive disorders is because they are expensive. Nevertheless, they may be effective in patients for which other classes of medication have not been effective.

Clinical Pharmacology

Naloxone is a pure opioid antagonist. As such, it prevents or reverses the effects of opioids, such as respiratory depression, hypotension and sedation. Product literature for humans states that in the absence of opioids or opioid agonists it exhibits essentially no pharmacological activity. However, it is precisely because of its efficacy in some animals exhibiting stereotypic behavior that it is used in veterinary behavior. It does not produce dependence or tolerance. The mechanism of action is not fully understood, but it appears to act by competing with opioids for receptor sites (Endo Pharmaceuticals 2001).

Naloxone undergoes glucuronide conjugation in the liver and is excreted in the urine. In human adults the serum half-life is 30–81 minutes (Endo Pharmaceuticals 2001).

Uses in Humans

In humans, naloxone is used for reversal of opioid depression, including respiratory depression. It is also used as an adjunctive agent in the management of septic shock, in which situation it facilitates the raising of blood pressure (Endo Pharmaceuticals 2001).

Contraindications

Naloxone is contraindicated in patients with a known sensitivity to it. It should be used with caution in patients with preexisting cardiac disease (Endo Pharmaceuticals 2001).

Side Effects

Some decrease in activity has been observed in cats (see below). Studies of reproduction in mice and rats given high doses of naloxone have not resulted in any impairment of reproduction or teratogenicity (Endo Pharmaceuticals 2001).

Chemical impurities in naloxone, specifically noroxymorphone and bisnaloxone, may produce emesis in dogs when administered intravenously at high doses (Endo Pharmaceuticals 2001).

The intravenous LD_{50} (the lethal dose that kills 50% of the animals tested) is 150 mg/kg in rats and 109 mg/kg in mice. Subcutaneous injection of 100 mg/kg/day for three weeks produces transiently increased salivation and partial ptosis. No side effects were observed at 10 mg/kg/day for three weeks.

Overdose

Treat an overdose symptomatically and monitor.

Doses in Nonhuman Animals

Because it is injected and short acting, naloxone is not a practical medication for maintenance treatment of stereotypic behaviors or compulsive disorders. It is best used as a tool for testing whether or not opioid antagonists are likely to be effective in the treatment of a given patient. In this capacity, they can be very useful. The patient should be checked into the hospital and monitored to determine a baseline for exhibition of the stereotypic behavior and to allow the patient time to acclimate to the hospital environment. Naloxone is then injected at a time when the patient can be closely monitored for at least the next two hours, and preferably longer. Ideally, observation should be remote, that is by a video camera, so that responses to humans do not alter the patient's behavior. However, the presence of humans may be irrelevant in many cases.

In the first case the author was involved in treating the patient, a dog, which chased its tail incessantly to the point of exhaustion. It was covered with bruises and lacerations from running into walls. It would not eat or drink unless it was physically restrained and its head was held still in a food or water bowl. When naloxone was injected, it began exploring its environment, interacting with students and clinicians, and voluntarily eating and drinking for the first time since presentation to the hospital (see Brown et al. 1987a, 1987b for further information).

Discontinuation

Since only a few doses should be given to test the patient's response to an opioid antagonist, discontinuation is not an issue.

Effects Documented in Nonhuman Animals

Cats

Cats given 0.4 mg/kg of naloxone IV are somewhat less active than when not given naloxone, but exhibit no cardiac changes (Waldrop et al. 1987).

Dogs

In a case of severe compulsive tail-chasing in a 20-kg Bull terrier, Brown et al. (1987a, 1987b) gave 0.2 mg (0.01 mg/kg) of naloxone SC. This resulted in nearly complete cessation of the tail-chasing behavior within 20 minutes. The effect lasted about three hours. This dose was repeated multiple times over the next two days with the same effect. The patient was sent home on an oral, mixed narcotic agonist-antagonist combination of pentazocine (50 mg, see below) and naloxone (0.5 mg) given b.i.d. The pentazocine/naloxone combination was readily administered by the owners and resulted in a low rate of compulsive tail-chasing in the home environment. Eventually, the dog was weaned off the pentazocine/naloxone combination and maintained fairly normal behavior. It continued to chase its tail during periods of intense excitement, but was otherwise a normal pet.

Horses

Dodman et al. (1987) gave naloxone to one cribbing horse in a series of three trials at 0.02 mg/kg, 0.03 mg/kg, and 0.04 mg/kg IV. After a 12- to 23-minute latent period, crib-biting stopped for an average of 20 minutes.

Pigs

Sows injected with naloxone, 0.64–1.0 mg/kg, exhibit a 57% decrease in the amount of time spent in stereotypic behaviors such as sham chewing, chain chewing, and tether chain chewing. The decrease begins about 10–15 minutes after injection and lasts 2–3 hours (Cronin et al. 1985, 1986).

III. Naltrexone Hydrochloride

Chemical Compound: 17-(Cyclopropylmethyl)-4,5 α-epoxy-3, 14-dihydroxymorphine-6-one hydrochloride

DEA Classification: Not a controlled substance

Preparations: Generally available in 50-mg, scored tablets

Clinical Pharmacology

Naltrexone hydrochloride is an opioid antagonist, with no opioid agonist properties, that acts by competitive binding. It does not produce tolerance or dependence. It is well absorbed orally, after which it undergoes extensive first-pass metabolism. In humans, oral bioavailability ranges from 5 to 40%. Both the parent drug and one of the metabolites, 6-β-naltrexol, are active, with peak plasma levels of both occurring about 1 hour after oral dosing. Most of a dose is excreted as various metabolites, primarily by the kidney. Very little fecal excretion occurs. In humans, the half-life for naltrexone is 4 hours and for 6-β-naltrexol is 13 hours. While hepatic metabolism occurs, there are also extrahepatic sites of metabolism (Mallinckrodt Inc. 2002).

Its pharmacological efficacy in humans is 24–74 hours, depending on the dose (Mallinckrodt Inc. 2002).

Uses in Humans

Naltrexone is used in the treatment of alcoholism and opioid addiction.

Contraindications

A history of sensitivity to naltrexone, liver failure, kidney failure.

Side Effects

Pupillary constriction may occur. The mechanism for this effect is not known (Mallinckrodt Inc. 2002).

Naltrexone can cause hepatocellular injury when given in overdose. In humans, the apparently safe dose of naltrexone and the dose causing hepatic injury is only a five-fold increase. Five of 26 human patients given 300 mg/day exhibited elevated ALT after three to eight weeks of treatment (Mallinckrodt Inc. 2002). This ratio is unknown in dogs, cats, and other veterinary patients.

One case has been reported of naltrexone-induced pruritus in a dog that was being given naltrexone at 1 mg/kg q6h, which is at the high end of the normal clinical dose range (Schwartz 1993). Another dog being medicated with naltrexone at 2.2 mg/kg q24h exhibited drowsiness. This side effect resolved after withdrawal of the medication for 48 hours (White 1990).

Rats given 100 mg/kg/day of naltrexone over two years had a slightly increased incidence of mesotheliomas in males and of vascular tumors in both males and females. A dose of 100 mg/kg/day results in an increase in pseudopregnancy and a decrease in true pregnancy in the rat. Male fertility is unaffected at this dose. Naltrexone is both embryocidal and fetotoxic in rats and rabbits when given at doses of 30 mg/kg/day (rats) or 60 mg/kg/day (rabbits). However, there is no evidence of teratogenicity when pregnant rabbits and rats are given doses of up to 200 mg/kg/day during the period of organogenesis (Mallinckrodt Inc. 2002).

In the mouse, rat, and guinea pig, the oral LD_{50} for each is 1,100 mg/kg, 1,450 mg/kg, and 1,490 mg/kg, respectively. In the mouse, rat, and dog death occurs due to clonic-tonic convulsions and/or respiratory failure when given large doses in acute toxicity studies. In one study, humans given 800 mg daily for up to one week did not exhibit toxicity (Mallinckrodt Inc. 2002).

Overdose

Treat an overdose of naltrexone symptomatically and monitor the situation.

Discontinuation

Patients that have been maintained on naltrexone for treatment of severe stereotypic behavior should undergo gradual discontinuation.

Other Information

The liver function of patients that are maintained on naltrexone for the treatment of stereotypic behavior problems should be monitored regularly.

Uses Documented in Nonhuman Animals

Dogs

Seven of 11 dogs with acral lick dermatitis that were treated with naltrexone, 2.2 mg/kg q12–24h, responded positively to treatment. When naltrexone was discontinued, all responders relapsed after durations of time ranging from one week to three years. Five of these dogs again responded to naltrexone treatment. The other two were euthanized due to unrelated health problems (White 1990).

Dodman et al. (1988b) gave naltrexone, 1 mg/kg SC, to two dogs with stereotypic self-licking, self-chewing, and scratching behavior. Both showed a significant reduction in these behaviors for at least 90 minutes after the injection. No side effects were reported.

Intense pruritus has occurred in one dog given a dose of 1 mg/kg q6h (Schwartz 1993).

Horses

Dodman et al. (1988a) gave naltrexone to three horses with crib-biting behavior at a dose of 0.04–0.4 mg/kg IV. After a brief latent period, crib-biting was substantially decreased or completely suppressed for 1.5–7 hours. One horse was subsequently implanted with a pellet of 0.6 g of naltrexone. Its crib-biting was substantially decreased for two days, with occasional breakthroughs.

A 10-year-old thoroughbred mare with a five-year history of weaving exhibited a 30% reduction in weaving behavior when given naltrexone at 0.7 mg/kg/day PO. Specifically, weaving decreased from 43.5 per minute to 32.3 per minute (Nurnberg et al. 1997).

Parrots

Turner (1993) treated 41 birds with feather-picking with naltrexone, 1.5 mg/kg b.i.d. A solution was created by dissolving a 50-mg tablet of naltrexone, which is highly soluble in water, in 10 ml of sterile water. The species treated were, specifically, 2 eclectus, 6 African grey, 1 cockatiel, 7 Amazons (1 orange wing, 3 yellow nape, 1 red lored, 1 Blue Front, and 1 double), 9 macaws (2 hyacinth, 1 scarlet, 4 blue/gold, 1 green wing, and 1 Catalina) and 16 cockatoos (4 umbrellas, 1 rosebreast, 6 Moluccan, 2 citron, and 3 lesser sulfur). Treatment duration ranged from one to six months. Thirty-five of the 41 birds responded positively to treatment. However, remission often occurred within a few months. Pre- and posttreatment blood panels did not identify any changes. Undesirable behavioral effects were not induced.

Pigs

Naltrexone, at a dose of 1.0–1.3 mg/kg IM, partially blocks the relaxation response in pigs (Grandin et al. 1989).

Other Species

Turner (1993) reported remission of a tail wound in a cougar that was maintained by self-mutilation when the cougar was treated with naltrexone, but did not report the dose. The cougar was monitored for a subsequent two years, with no remission.

Kenny (1994) used naltrexone to treat a variety of psychogenically induced dermatoses in zoo animals, as follows, with variable efficacy.

A 36-kg Amur leopard (*Panthera pardus orientalis*) that was pulling hair out of the dorsal part of its tail and back was initially treated with prednisone, 20 mg PO 124h. After an initial small improvement, the behavior worsened, and naltrexone was added to the treatment at 25 mg (1.4 mg/kg) PO q24h. After one week, no adverse effects had been noted, so the dose was increased to 50 mg (2.8 mg/kg) q24h. The prednisone dose was gradually reduced and discontinued. Relapses occurred after a loud concert was held close to the hospital and subsequent to the keeper discovering the leopard removing the naltrexone tablets from its meat. The tablets were thereafter crushed and mixed into the meat. Total remission of the hair-pulling occurred after this protocol, and the leopard was subsequently maintained on 50 mg of naltrexone daily (Kenny 1994).

A clouded leopard (*Panthera nebulosa*) that was excessively grooming the medial surface of her thighs was treated with prednisone, 25 mg PO q12h for five days, after which the prednisone was discontinued. The behavior relapsed and the leopard was treated with prednisone seven times over the following three years. When the leopard was immobilized for examination, she was found to have a subacute to chronic ulcerative pyogranulomatous dermatitis. She was initially treated with 1.6 mg/kg naltrexone, q24h. When she was immobilized three months later, the lesions were completely resolved. There were no changes in values for alanine transaminase before and after treatment. The dose of naltrexone was then decreased to 0.8 mg/kg, resulting in recurrence of the problem. Returning to the higher dose did not result in improvement until prednisone (40 mg, q24h) was added. Once the prednisone was discontinued she was maintained on 1.6 mg/kg without further relapse (Kenny 1994).

A tricolored squirrel (*Callosciuis prevostii*) had repeated episodes of self-mutilation that responded to treatment with glucocorticoid. Skin scrapings and fungal cultures taken after immobilization were unremarkable. The squirrel was treated with naltrexone at 1.0 mg/kg q24h, which resulted in resolution of the problem. Serum transaminase levels were not notably different before and after 6 weeks and 10 weeks of treatment (Kenny 1994).

An Arctic wolf (*Canis lupus hudsonicus*) with repeat episodes of acute moist dermatitis did not respond to treatment with 1.0 mg/kg PO of naltrexone given q24h. This problem responded only to high doses of glucocorticoids. No adverse events were reported from the treatment attempt with naltrexone (Kenny 1994).

A polar bear (*Ursus maritimus*) mutilated its perineum by rubbing it on concrete as part of ritualized pacing behavior. Treatment with 1.2 mg/kg q24h had no beneficial effect and treatment was discontinued after one month (Kenny 1994). No adverse events were reported.

IV. Pentazocine

Chemical Compound: 1,2,3,4,5,6-Hexahydro-6,11–dimethyl-3-3(3-methyl-2-butenyl)-2,6-methano-3-benzazocin-8-ol hydrochloride
DEA Classification: Schedule IV controlled substance
Preparations: Generally available as a tablet containing 50 mg of pentazocine and 0.5 mg of naloxone (see naloxone)

Clinical Pharmacology

Pentazocine is an analgesic with some opiate antagonistic effects. The naloxone is combined with pentazocine in this medication because at the dose of 0.5 mg it antagonizes both pentazocine and various narcotics; misuse of pentazocine by grinding the tablets up and injecting them as a solution is effectively prevented. Naloxone at this dose does not counteract pentazocine when given orally (Synofi-Synthelabo, Inc. 1999).

In humans, onset of analgesia typically occurs 15–30 minutes after oral administration (Synofi-Synthelabo, Inc. 1999).

Uses in Humans

For humans, pentazocine is for oral use only for cases of moderate to severe pain.

Contraindications

Do not give pentazocine to patients with a history of sensitivity to either naloxone or pentazocine. Use with caution in patients with renal or liver disease.

Side Effects

Seizures may occur in patients with a history of seizures, though the mechanism for this is not known. Various side effects include cardiovascular (e.g., hypotension, tachycardia, syncope), respiratory (respiratory depression), central nervous system (e.g., hallucinations, disorientation, sedation, weakness), gastrointestinal (e.g., emesis, constipation, diarrhea), and decreased white blood cell count (Synofi-Synthelabo, Inc. 1999).

Overdose

In case of overdose, provide supportive therapy and monitor. If respiratory depression occurs, administer naloxone, a specific antagonist.

Discontinuation

Discontinue pentazocine by gradual tapering of dose.

Other Information

Pure opiate antagonists, such as naltrexone, should be the first drug of choice for treatment of pets with stereotypic behavior problems that exhibit a positive response to a naloxone trial. Cost may be an issue, however, particularly in remote rural areas where, due to an absence of a population of drug addicts that are being treated with pure opiate antagonists, local pharmacies do not stock these medications. In this case, the use of pentazocine may be considered after consideration of the potential for human abuse, the risk of side effects, and the fact that pentazocine is not a pure opiate antagonist. While pentazocine has been shown to be effective in at least some cases of stereotypic behaviors, trials comparing the relative efficacy of pentazocine with various pure opiate agonists have not been conducted.

Effects Documented in Nonhuman Animals
Dogs

A dog with severe compulsive tail-chasing responded well to a test treatment with naloxone given subcutaneously (Brown et al. 1987a, 1987b). It was subsequently successfully treated at home with Talwin, at a combination of 50 mg pentazocine and 0.5 mg naloxone given orally b.i.d. The medication was eventually discontinued, and the dog remained relatively normal, exhibiting tail-chasing only during periods of intense excitement.

References

Baker Norton Pharmaceuticals 1997. Revex®. *Physicians desk reference,* pp. 1863–1865. Montvale, New Jersey.

Brown SA, Crowell-Davis S, Malcolm T and Edwards P 1987a. Naloxone-responsive compulsive tail chasing in a dog. *Journal of the American Veterinary Medical Association* 190(7): 884–886.

Brown SA, Crowell-Davis S, Malcolm T and Edwards P 1987b. Correction to naloxone-responsive compulsive tail chasing in a dog. *Journal of the American Veterinary Medical Association* 190: 1434.

Cronin GM, Wiepkema PR and van Ree JM 1985. Endogenous opioids are involved in abnormal stereotyped behaviours of tethered sows. *Neuropeptides* 6: 527–530.

Cronin GM, Wiepkema PR and van Ree JM 1986. Endorphins implicated in stereotypies of tethered sows. *Experientia* 42: 198–199.

Dixon R, Hsiao J, Leadon D, Dodman N and Shuster L 1992. Nalmefene: Pharmacokinetics of a new opioid antagonist which prevents crib-biting in the horse. *Research Communications in Substances of Abuse* 13: 231–236.

Dodman NH, Shuster L, Court MH and Dixon R 1987. Investigation into the use of narcotic antagonists in the treatment of a stereotypic behavior pattern (crib-biting) in the horse. *Journal of the American Veterinary Medical Association* 48(2): 311–319.

Dodman NH, Shuster L, and Court MH. 1988a. Use of a narcotic antagonist (nalmefene) to suppress self-mutilative behavior in a stallion. *Journal of the American Veterinary Medical Association* 192(11): 1585–1586.

Dodman NH, Shuster L, White SD, Court MH, Parker D and Dixon R. 1988b. Use of narcotic antagonists to modify stereotypic self-licking, self-chewing, and scratching behavior in dogs. *Journal of the American Veterinary Medical Association.* 193(7): 815–819.

Endo Pharmaceuticals Inc. 2001. In *2003 Physicians desk reference*, pp.1300–1302, Thomson PDR, Montvale, New Jersey.

Gianutsos G and Lal H 1978. Narcotic analgesics and aggression. In *Modern problems of pharmacopsychiatry: Psychopharmacology of aggression* 13, pp. 114–138, edited by L Valzelli, T Ban, FA Freyhan and P Pichot, Karger, New York.

Grandin T, Dodman N and Shuster L. 1989. Effect of naltrexone on relaxation induced by flank pressure in pigs. *Pharmacology Biochemistry & Behavior* 33: 839–842.

Herman BH, Hammock MK, Arthur-Smith A, Chatoor I and Zelnik N 1987. Naltrexone decreases self-injurious behavior. *Annals of Neurology* 22(4): 550–552.

Kenny DE 1994. Use of naltrexone for treatment of psychogenically induced dermatoses in five zoo animals. *Journal of the American Veterinary Medical Association* 205(7): 1021–1023.

Mallinckrodt Inc. 2002. Depade™. Package insert.

Marder AR. 1991. Psychotropic drugs and behavioral therapy. *Veterinary Clinics of North American: Small Animal Practice* 21(2): 329–342.

Nurnberg HG, Keith SJ and Paxton DM 1997. Consideration of the relevance of ethological animal models for human repetitive behavioral spectrum disorders. *Society of Biological Psychiatry.* 41: 226–229.

Overall, KL 1997. *Clinical Behavioral Medicine for Small Animals,* Mosby, St. Louis, Missouri, 303 pages.

Panksepp J, Herman B, Conner R, Bishop P and Scott JP 1978. The biology of social attachments: Opiates alleviate separation distress. *Biological Psychiatry* 13(5): 607–618.

Panksepp J, Conner R, Forster PK, Bishop P and Scott JP 1983. Opioid effects on social behavior of kennel dogs. *Applied Animal Ethology* 10: 63–74.

Richardson JS and Zaleski WA 1983. Naloxone and self-mutilation. *Biological Psychiatry* 18(1): 99–101.

Sandman CA, Barron JL and Colman H 1990. An orally administered opiate blocker, naltrexone, attenuates self-injurious behavior. *American Journal of Mental Retardation* 95: 93–102.

Schwartz S. 1993. Naltrexone-induced pruritus in a dog with tail-chasing behavior. *Journal of the American Veterinary Medical Association* 202: 278–280.

Smith KC and Pittelkow MR 1989. Naltrexone for neurotic excoriations. *Journal of the American Academy of Dermatology* 20(5): 860–861.

Synofi-Synthelabo, Inc. 1999. Talwin® Nx. 2003 *Physicians's desk reference*, pp. 3012–3013, Thomson PDR, Montvale, New Jersey.

Turner R, 1993. Trexan (naltrexone hydrochloride) use in feather picking in avian species. *Proceedings of the Association of Avian Veterinarians*, pp. 116–118.

Waldrop TG, Bielecki M and Geldon D 1987. Effects of naloxone on cardiovascular responses to static exercise and behavior in conscious cats. *Physiology & Behavior* 40: 1–5.

White SD 1990. Naltrexone for treatment of acral lick dermatitis in dogs. *Journal of the American Veterinary Medical Association.* 196: 1073–1076.

Chapter Fourteen
Hormones

This chapter is included for completeness and historical reference, rather than because progestins or any other hormones are highly recommended for the treatment of behavior problems in nonhuman animals. Progesterone and its metabolites act in various parts of the body (e.g., brain, smooth muscle, uterus, sperm, oocyte) through multiple mechanisms of action (Mahesh et al. 1996). Therefore, its effects are not discrete and specific, but instead are widespread and varied. A variety of side effects, including polydypsia, polyuria, polyphagia, weight gain, sedation, overproduction of growth hormone, suppression of the hypothalamic-pituitary-adrenocortical axis, insulin resistance, and cancer, make their use for the treatment of behavior problems very risky for the patient. Nevertheless, in some cases they can be useful as a treatment of last resort in patients for which safer and more conservative treatments have proven ineffective and for which euthanasia is the next step if significant, rapid improvement does not occur. Behavioral effects are attributable to both an antiandrogenic effect and a calming effect on the limbic system (Henik et al. 1985).

The use of a hormone, methyloestrenolone, which is not currently available commercially, in the treatment of behavior problems of dogs and cats was first reported in 1964 (Gerber and Sulman 1964). It was found that, in bitches and queens, estrus could be postponed or prevented and pseudopregnancy could be terminated with this medication. In male cats, roaming and urine marking were also reported as being effectively treated, as were roaming, urine marking, and mounting in male dogs.

Action

The progestins have a variety of actions. They inhibit the secretion of pituitary gonadotropin, suppress the production of testosterone, alter the binding of transcription factor to DNA, alter membrane fluidity, act on $GABA_A$ receptors to produce effects similar to those caused by benzodiazepines, and possibly increase levels of β-endorphin and met-enkephalin in the hippocampus. There are various mechanisms of action, including an intracellular receptor-mediated mechanism, steroid action involving phospholipids layers, steroid action mediated by second messenger systems, steroid action exerted at the cell membrane, and steroid effects initiated by interaction with GABA receptors and ligand insertion (Mahesh et al. 1996). A detailed discussion of the role of the progestins in reproductive physiology is beyond the scope of this book.

Overview of Indications

In-depth discussion of the use of progestins to modify reproductive status is beyond the scope of this book and is covered elsewhere, for example, Evans and Jemmett (1978). Progestins can be useful in cases of excessive sexual behavior, dominance aggression in dogs and cats, urine marking, persistent mounting by neutered males, excess vocalization in neutered male cats responding to estrous queens, and human-directed sexual aggression in cats. More generally, progestins can be effective in suppressing behaviors that are more predominant in males than in females (Hart 1979c; Hart and Eckstein 1998). These effects occur even with castrated males.

In an early report on 50 cats treated with either medroxyprogesterone acetate (MPA) or megestrol acetate (MA), Hart (1979a) reported that about one-third of 31 spraying cats improved to the client's satisfaction. Two of 11 cats with inappropriate urination resolved, and 5 of 8 aggressive cats showed improvement.

Pemberton (1980, 1983) subsequently reported that progestins were effective in the treatment of a spectrum of behavior problems including territorial aggression, jealousy, dog fighting, hyperkinesis, persistent barking, anorexia nervosa, tail-chasing, timidity, destructiveness, phobias, predatory aggression, viciousness, unacceptable sexual activity, roaming, digging holes, self-mutilation, night howling, attention-seeking behavior, and urine marking. However, no data from either retrospective or prospective clinical surveys were given, except for urine spraying in cats. A success rate of 80% was reported for this problem, a rate that has not been replicated in other studies.

Contraindications, Side Effects, and Adverse Events

The use of progestins is contraindicated in breeding animals and diabetics. There are many side effects. In the author's experience, polyphagia, polydipsia, and sedation are all so common that the owner should be told to expect them. In a retrospective clinical report, 25% of cats treated with progestins for behavior problems exhibited an increased appetite and about 20% of cats exhibited sedation, that is, the owner reported that they were depressed, lethargic, or inactive. Mammary gland enlargement, without tumor development, occurred in 3 of the 50 cats (Hart 1979a).

Various pathological changes have been identified as occurring in the uteruses of both cats and dogs, with the changes being dependent on both dose and duration of medication (e.g., Dow 1958; Anderson et al. 1965; Brodey and Fidler 1966; Withers and Whitney 1967; Cox 1970; Austin and Evans 1972; Teale 1972). Even remnants of reproductive tissue left after neutering have been reported to undergo changes and infection (Jones 1975). Other side effects include elevated blood glucose, mammary hyperplasia (e.g., Hinton 1977), diabetes, endometrial hyperplasia, pyometra, and carcinoma. These side effects, while serious, generally occur when a patient has been on progestins for weeks or months.

Overdose

To treat progestin overdose evacuate stomach if within first 30 minutes and then provide supportive therapy.

Clinical Guidelines

Because of the common and potentially very serious side effects that can occur with progestins, they should be considered a treatment of last resort. They should only be used in patients that have not responded to safer treatments such as selective serotonin reuptake inhibitors combined with behavior modification, and for whom euthanasia is probable or certain if the behavior does not resolve.

In some cases, progestins can produce dramatic improvement, particularly in cases of dominance aggression in male dogs. Safety risks can be minimized if the medication is viewed as providing a brief window of opportunity to make progress with behavior modification, with the goal of having the patient off of medication in two to three months. Patients can learn while on progestins. Thus, for example, if aggressiveness is substantially suppressed in a patient with dominance-motivated aggression, the owners can initiate various behavior modification protocols to teach the dog to defer to humans and reverse the dominance hierarchy, making the dog the omega member of the household. Then the medication can be steadily decreased, typically at two-week intervals until the patient is off of medication.

Some patients respond excellently to progestins but cannot be weaned off of them; for example, while the owners have carried out appropriate behavior modification protocols and the dog has become submissive and nonaggressive, aggression and dominance posturing resurfaces every time the medication is lowered to a certain dose. At this point, the potential for serious risks with long-term use must be reviewed with the owners. Some families who are strongly attached to their pets but who find the behavior problem intolerable may elect long-term use. In this case even if, as is likely, the pet develops a serious medical problem in later years as a consequence of the medication, additional years as an acceptable pet will have been gained. In all such cases, the potential risks and benefits should be discussed in depth with the family.

Delmadinone acetate, which is not discussed further, prevents estrus in queens if given at a dose of 0.25–0.7 mg/kg PO weekly or 2.5–5.0 mg/kg SC every six months. Estrus behavior can be suppressed in queens given 0.5–1.0 mg/kg daily for six days or 2.5–6.75 mg/kg SC as one or two injections, 24 hours apart (Gerber et al. 1973).

Urine marking and wandering by males can potentially be effectively treated by 0.25–1.0 mg/kg of delmadinone acetate given daily for 7–14 days or 10.0–20.0 mg/kg SC given as one or two injections 24 hours apart (Gerber et al. 1973).

Delmadinone acetate given at 0.5–1.0 mg/kg PO daily for six days or as a 2.5–5.0 mg/kg SC injection causes termination of pseudocyesis in bitches. At the same doses, it will also suppress estrus. Attraction for males decreases, but any matings that occur are still fertile. Estrus can be postponed for 6–12 months if it is given once a week at a dose of 0.25–5.0 mg/kg or twice a year at a dose of 1.0–3.0 mg/kg (Gerber et al. 1973).

In male dogs, problems of urine marking, roaming, pack formation, and mounting have been reported to resolve for 3–12 months when they are given 0.5–1.5 mg/kg daily for 7–14 days or 5.0–12.5 mg/kg as one or two subcutaneous injections (Gerber et al. 1973).

Specific Medications

I. Medroxyprogesterone Acetate (MPA)

Chemical Compound: Pregn-4-ene-3,20-dione, 17-(acetyloxy)-6-methyl-,(6α)
DEA Classification: Not a controlled substance
Preparations: Generally available as 2.5-, 5-, and 10-mg tablets and as a 150 mg/ml injectable solution

Clinical Pharmacology

MPA inhibits secretion of gonadotropins. In humans, a single intramuscular injection of MPA results in increasing plasma concentrations of MPA for three weeks, followed by an exponential decrease in plasma concentrations. MPA levels in the plasma become undetectable in 120–200 days (Pharmacia & Upjohn 1999).

Uses in Humans

MPA is used in humans to treat abnormal uterine bleeding, amenorrhea, renal or endometrial cancer and endometrial hyperplasia.

Contraindications

Use of MPA is contraindicated when sensitivity to MPA, pregnancy, liver disease, or mammary tumors are present. Do not use MPA to treat behavior problems in intact females.

Side Effects

Dogs treated with eight doses of MPA at 10 mg/kg SC or proligestone (PROL) at 50 mg/kg SC at three-week intervals exhibited a variety of histologic changes. The adrenal cortex atrophied, foci of hyperplastic ductular epithelium developed in the mammary glands, benign mammary tumors developed, steroid-induced hepatopathy occurred, and the cells of the islets of Langerhans became vacuolated. There were no significant differences between the dogs treated with MPA and the dogs treated with PROL (Selman et al. 1995).

Adverse Drug Interactions

Aminoglutethimide significantly depresses serum concentrations of MPA (Pharmacia & Upjohn 1999).

Effects Documented in Nonhuman Animals

Cats

MPA, given as a single injection of 100 mg to males and 50 mg to females, resulted in successful treatment of urine spraying or urine marking in 29% of cases. Less than 10% of the treated cats exhibited depression and/or increased appetite. Both males and cats from single-cat homes responded better than did females or cats from multicat homes, with males from single-cat homes having the best response. Some cats that were initially treated with MA subsequently responded to MPA (Hart 1980). When used as a treatment for urine spraying or marking in cats, injections of MPA are repeated once per month or as needed.

In a later study of 35 male and 25 female cats, Cooper and Hart (1992) found that MA and MPA were equally effective, with about 42% of cats treated with a progestin showing a positive response to treatment. Progestins were less effective for females than for males and, in females, were less effective than diazepam or buspirone. In males, progestins were about as effective as diazepam or buspirone.

Dogs

Male dogs given MPA at 10–20 mg/kg SC have been observed to exhibit 75–100% improvement of various problems, including aggression toward other males, urine marking, and mounting of dogs, people, or inanimate objects. There was poor efficacy for human-directed aggression in the male and aggression toward other females (Hart 1979b). Three out of four males treated with 10 mg/kg MPA SC for fighting with other males responded to therapy, whereas only one out of seven males given the same treatment for human-directed aggression exhibited improvement. Side effects observed included increased appetite and weight gain (Hart 1981).

MPA was once used as a canine contraceptive. However, this was discontinued in the early 1970s due to problems with endometritis and pyometra. While these problems are most likely to occur when MPA is given during proestrus, estrus, in overdose, or in dogs with genital disease, its use should be avoided in intact females (Stabenfeldt 1974). Spayed female beagles given doses of MPA as low as 3 mg/kg every three months almost invariably develop mammary nodules within four years. At the higher dose of 30 mg/kg there is a threefold increase in the development of nodules. In addition, levels of serum growth hormone and insulin increase in a dose-dependent fashion, while levels of triiodothyronine, cortisol, and 17 β-estradiol decrease (Frank et al. 1979).

Parrots

MPA has been used in the treatment of feather-picking in parrots at a dose of 0.07 mg/g IM as a single dose. Side-effects reported include increased appetite, polydipsia, polyuria, and sedation (Galvin 1983; Ryan 1985).

II. Megestrol Acetate

Chemical Compound: 17α-(acetyloxy)-6-methylpregna-4,6-diene-3,20-dione
DEA Classification: Not a controlled substance
Preparations: Generally available as 40 mg/ml oral suspension and as 5-, 20-, and 40-mg tablets

Clinical Pharmacology

MA is a steroid with rapid onset of action. It has antigonadotropic and antiandrogenic effects and glucocorticoid activity. There is slight mineralocorticoid activity. It does not have anabolic or estrogenic activity and does not have masculinizing effects on the developing fetus (David et al. 1963; Gupta et al. 1978; Muller et al. 1983; Henik et al. 1985).

In humans, the major route of elimination is the urine, although some fecal excretion occurs (Bristol-Myers Squibb 2000). The opposite occurs in the dog. When MA is given to bitches at a dose of 2 mg/kg PO for eight days, it is rapidly eliminated, primarily through the feces (about 87%) and to some degree in the urine (about 9%). One week after the last dose 90% of the medication has been excreted, although there is further gradual elimination up to three weeks later (Chainey et al. 1970).

Uses in Humans

MA is used to treat anorexia, cachexia (e.g., Aisner et al. 1990), and adenocarcinoma of the breast and endometrium in humans.

Contraindications

MA should not be used in dogs with evidence of any disease of the reproductive organs, prior to first estrus, in pregnant dogs, or in dogs with mammary tumors (Schering-Plough 2003).

MA should not be used for treatment of behavior problems in intact females.

Adverse Drug Interactions

Concurrent administration of MA with dofetilide, an antiarrhythmic drug, causes decreased dofetilide elimination and increased dofetilide plasma concentrations. This can result in ventricular arrhythmias (Yamareudeewong et al. 2003).

Side Effects

Side effects reported in cats include mammary hyperplasia, induction of lactation, mammary carcinoma, pyometra, diabetes mellitus, polyphagia with weight gain, adrenocortical atrophy, and personality changes including listlessness and depression (e.g., Aspinall and Turner 1972; Long 1972; Wilkins 1972; Baker 1973; Chesney 1976; Nelson and Kelly 1976; Oen 1977; Nimmo-Wilkie 1979; Hart 1980; Chastain et al. 1981; Gosselin et al. 1981; Tomlinson et al. 1984; Kwochka and Short 1984; Middleton 1986; Middleton et al. 1987).

MA given at 0.25 mg/lb for 32 days during the second half of pregnancy results in decreased litter size and increased mortality in the puppies. No adverse events are reported when it is given during the first half of pregnancy. Dogs treated with 2 mg/kg/day for 64 days exhibit signs of early cystic endometritis. When MA was administered orally at 0.5 mg/kg for 5 months, mild uterine hyperplasia has been observed, which subsequently regresses. MA at 0.1–0.25 mg/kg/day for 36 months also results in cystic endometrial hyperplasia, which likewise reverses if dosing is discontinued (Schering-Plough 2003).

In a two-year chronic toxicity/carcinogenicity study in rats there was evidence of decreased lymphocyte counts, increased neutrophil counts, and increased frequency of respiratory infections (Bristol-Myers Squibb 2001).

MA induced both benign and malignant mammary tumors in female beagles given 0.01, 0.1, or 0.25 mg/kg/day for up to seven years (Nelson et al. 1973; Owen and Briggs 1976). Female monkeys did not develop mammary tumors. Male offspring of females treated with MA during pregnancy exhibit decreased fertility. Additionally, female rats treated with MA had a reduction in the number of live births and fetal weight and feminization of male offspring (Bristol-Myers Squibb 2001).

Overdose

Single doses of up to 5 g/kg in mice and 1600 mg/day in humans have not produced toxic effects. There is no specific treatment. In case of large overdose, monitor the patient and provide supportive therapy.

Effects Documented in Nonhuman Animals

Cats

In a clinical trial of the treatment of urine marking and spraying using megestrol acetate, 13 cats were treated as follows: 5 mg/cat were given daily PO for 7–10 days. If improvement occurred within seven days, the frequency of dosing was decreased to every other day for two weeks. If this dose continued to control the problem, the frequency of dosing was further reduced to twice a week for one month. Frequency of dosing was then further reduced to once a week for two to six months. If the behavior recurred when frequency of dosing was decreased, the client was instructed to return to the previously effective frequency of dosing (Hart 1980).

This treatment resulted in 36% of the patients showing substantial improvement. Both males and cats from single-cat homes responded better than did females or cats from multicat homes, with males from single-cat homes having the best response. Some other cats that were initially treated with MPA subsequently responded to treatment with MA. Over 30% of the cats exhibited increased appetite, while almost 30% of the cats became depressed. In addition, one female developed mammary gland enlargement that regressed when treatment was discontinued (Hart 1980).

In the author's experience, this regimen almost invariably produces decreased activity. Fewer side effects are achieved with a faster regimen of decreasing frequency for cats that are responding to treatment. Specifically, begin with 2.5–5 mg daily for three to five days, giving only 2.5 mg to small cats under eight pounds. Decrease the dosing frequency to every other day for just one week, to twice a week for two weeks, and then to once a week. In this way, the cat is receiving MA once a week in less than a month.

Romatowski (1989) recommends, for behavioral abnormalities, 2 mg/kg/day for five days, followed by 1 mg/kg/day for five days, and then 0.5 mg/kg/day for five days.

Of 244 cats that were given MA to delay estrus, 5 owners reported that their cats exhibited increased aggression while 34 owners reported that their cats were less aggressive (Oen 1977). Additionally, 2 nonaggressive cats have been reported to become aggressive when placed on MA (Baker 1973).

Cats treated with MA at 5 mg/cat/day for eight days exhibit increased fasting blood glucose concentration and decreased glucose excretion rate (Middleton and Watson 1985). Cats treated with MA at a dose of 5 mg/cat/day for two weeks, and then 5 mg/cat three times a week for a total of one year of treatment, have been shown to produce a progressive deterioration in glucose tolerance, an increase in mean fasting plasma glucose concentration, and a decrease in mean plasma glucose clearance rate. There was also a progressive decrease in resting plasma cortisol concentrations and cortisol concentrations subsequent to administration of ACTH. The glucose intolerance resolved three months after discontinuation of treatment (Peterson 1987).

Cats given 1 mg/kg of MA every other day for three weeks did not exhibit changes in plasma glucose or insulin concentrations in response to intravenous glucose administration (Mansfield et al. 1986).

Dogs

MA is used to postpone estrus and disrupt false pregnancy in the dog (Schering-Plough 2003). When given at a dose of 2.2 mg/kg for eight days during proestrus, it suppresses estrus in 92% of bitches (Burke and Reynolds 1975).

Pemberton (1980) has recommended doses as high as 15 mg/kg daily in dogs. This is substantially higher than doses the author has used. When treating dogs with MA, the author has typically used the following schedule: 2.0 mg/kg q24h for 14 days, followed by 1.0 mg/kg q24h for 14 days, followed by 0.5 mg/kg q24h for 14 days, then discontinue. If the problem resumes when the dose is decreased, go back up to the last dose that worked for two to three weeks, then try reducing again. Even on this schedule, decreased activity, polyphagia, and polydypsia may be observed during the initial two weeks of treatment.

Parrots

MA has been used in the treatment of feather-picking at a dose of 1.25 mg PO daily for 7–10 days, then twice weekly (Petrak 1969; Galvin 1983; Ryan 1985).

References

Aisner J, Parnes H, Tait N, Hickman M, Forrest A, Greco FA, and Tchekmedyian NS 1990. Appetite stimulation and weight gain with megestrol acetate. *Seminars in Oncology* 17(6): 2–7.

Anderson RK, Gilmore CE and Schnelle GB 1965. Utero-ovarian disorders associated with the use of medroxyprogesterone in dogs. *Journal of the American Veterinary Medical Association* 146: 1311–1316.

Aspinall KW and Turner WT 1972. Feline miliary dermatitis. *The Journal of Small Animal Practice* 13(12): 709–710.

Austin AR and Evans JM 1972. Pyometritis in spayed cats. *Veterinary Record* 91: 77–78.

Baker KP 1973. Letter to the editor. *Journal of Small Animal Practice* 14:225–226.

Bristol-Myers Squibb 2000. Megace® product description. In 2001 *Physician's desk reference*, pp. 1047–1049, Montvale, New Jersey.

Brodey RS and Fidler IJ 1966. Clinical and pathological findings in bitches treated with progestational compounds. *Journal of the American Veterinary Medical Association* 149: 1406–1415.

Burke TJ and Reynolds HA 1975. Megestrol acetate for estrus postponement in the bitch. *Journal of the American Veterinary Medical Association* 167(4): 285–287.

Chainey D, McCoubrey A and Evans JM 1970. The excretion of megestrol acetate by beagle bitches. *The Veterinary Record* 86(10): 287–288.

Chastain CB, Graham CL and Nichols CE 1981. Adrenocortical suppression in cats given megestrol acetate. *American Journal of Veterinary Research* 42(12): 2029–2035.

Chesney CJ 1976. The response to progestagen treatment of some diseases of cats. *The Journal of Small Animal Practice* 17(1): 35–44.

Cooper LL and Hart BL 1992. Comparison of diazepam with progestin for effectiveness in suppression of urine spraying behavior in cats. *Journal of the American Veterinary Medical Association* 200(6): 797–801.

Cox JE 1970. Progestagens in bitches: A review. *Journal of Small Animal Practice* 11(12): 759–778.

David A, Edwards K, Fellowes KN and Plummer JM 1963. Anti-ovulatory and other biological properties of megestrol acetate. *Journal of Reproduction and Fertility* 5: 331–346.

Dow C 1958. The cystic hyperplasia-pyometra complex in the bitch. *Veterinary Record* 70: 1102–1109.

Evans JM and Jemmett JE 1978. The use of progestogens in dogs and cats. *The Veterinary Annual* 18: 276–284.

Frank DW, Kirton KT, Murchison TE, Quinlan WJ, Coleman ME, Gilbertson TJ, Feenstra ES and Kimball FA 1979. Mammary tumors and serum hormones in the bitch treated with medroxyprogesterone acetate or progesterone for four years. *Fertility and Sterility* 31(3): 340–346.

Galvin C 1983. The feather picking bird. In *Current Veterinary Therapy VIII*, pp. 646–651, edited by RW Kirk. W.B. Saunders, Philadelphia, Pennsylvania.

Gerber HA, Jöchle W and Sulman FG 1973. Control of reproduction and of undesirable social and sexual behaviour in dogs and cats. *Journal of Small Animal Practice* 14: 151–158.

Gerber HA and Sulman FG 1964. The effect of methyloestrenolone on oestrus, pseudo-pregnancy, vagrancy, satyriasis and squirting in dogs and cats. *The Veterinary Record* 76(39): 1089–1092.

Gosselin Y, Chalifoux A and Papageorges M 1981. The use of megestrol acetate in some feline dermatological problems. *Canadian Veterinary Journal* 22(12): 382–384.

Gupta C, Bullock LP and Bardin CW 1978. Further studies on the androgenic, anti-androgenic, and synandrogenic actions of progestins. *Endocrinology* 102(3): 736–744.

Hart B 1979a. Evaluation of progestins therapy for behavioral problems. *Feline Practice* 9(3): 11–14.

Hart B 1979b. Indications for progestin therapy for problem behavior in dogs. *Canine Practice* 6(5): 10–14.

Hart BL 1979c. Problems with objectionable sociosexual behavior of dogs and cats: Therapeutic use of castration and progestins. *Compendium on Continuing Education for the Practicing Veterinarian* 1: 461–465.

Hart BL 1980. Objectionable urine spraying and urine marking in cats: Evaluation of progestin treatment in gonadectomized males and females. *Journal of the American Veterinary Medical Association* 177: 529–533.

Hart BL 1981. Progestin therapy for aggressive behavior in male dogs. *Journal of the American Veterinary Medical Association* 178: 1070–1071.

Hart BL and Eckstein RA 1998. Progestins: Indications for male-typical behavior problems. In *Psychopharmacology of animal behavior disorders*, edited by NH Dodman and L Shuster, pp. 255–263, Blackwell Science, Massachusetts.

Henik RA, Olson PN and Rosychuk RAW 1985. Progestogen therapy in cats. *Compendium on Continuing Education for the Practicing Veterinarian* 7: 132–141.

Hinton M 1977. Nonneoplastic mammary hypertrophy in the cat associated either with pregnancy or with oral progestagen therapy. *The Veterinary Record* 100(14): 277–280.

Jones AK 1975. Pyometra in the cat [letter]. *The Veterinary Record* 97(5): 100.

Kwochka KW and Short BG 1984. Cutaneous xanthomatosis and diabetes mellitus following long-term therapy with megestrol acetate in a cat. *Compendium on Continuing Education for the Practicing Veterinarian* 6: 185–192.

Long RD 1972. Pyometritis in spayed cats. *The Veterinary Record* 91: 105–106.

Mahesh VB, Brann DW and Hendry LB 1996. Diverse modes of action of progesterone and its metabolites. *The Journal of Steroid Biochemistry and Molecular Biology* 56: 209–219.

Mansfield PD, Kemppainen RJ and Sartin JL 1986. The effects of megestrol acetate treatment on plasma glucose concentration and insulin response to glucose administration in cats. *Journal of the American Animal Hospital Association* 22: 515–518.

Middleton DJ 1986. Megestrol acetate and the cat. *The Veterinary Annual* 26: 341–347.

Middleton DJ and Watson ADJ 1985. Glucose intolerance in cats given short-term therapies of prednisolone and megestrol acetate. *American Journal of Veterinary Research* 46(12), 2623–2625.

Middleton DJ, Watson ADJ, Howe CJ and Caterson ID 1987. Suppression of cortisol responses to exogenous adrenocorticotrophic hormone, and the occurrence of side effects attributable to glucocorticoid excess in cats during therapy with megestrol acetate and prednisolone. *Canadian Journal of Veterinary Research* 51: 60–65.

Muller GH, Kirk RW and Scott DW 1983. *Small animal dermatology*, pp. 174–175, W.B. Saunders Co., Philadelphia, Pennsylvania.

Nelson LW and Kelly WA 1976. Progestogen-related gross and microscopic changes in female beagles. *Veterinary Pathology* 13(2): 143–156.

Nelson LW, Weikel JH Jr and Reno FE 1973. Mammary nodules in dogs during four years treatment with megestrol acetate or chlormadinone acetate. *Journal of the National Cancer Institute* 51: 1303–1311.

Nimmo-Wilkie JS 1979. Progesterone therapy for cats. *Canadian Veterinary Journal* 20: 164.

Oen EO 1977. The oral administration of megestrol acetate to postpone oestrus in cats. *Nordisk Veterinaermedicin* 29(6): 287–291.

Owen LN and Briggs MH 1976. Contraceptive steroid toxicology in the beagle dog and its relevance to human carcinogenicity. *Current Medical Research and Opinion* 4: 309–329.

Pemberton PL 1980. Feline and canine behavior control: Progestin therapy. In *Current veterinary therapy VII: Small animal practice,* pp. 845–853, edited by R. Kirk, Saunders, Philadelphia, Pennsylvania.

Pemberton PL 1983. Canine and feline behavior control: Progestin therapy. In *Current veterinary therapy VIII: Small animal practice*, pp. 62–71, edited by R. Kirk, Saunders, Philadelphia, Pennsylvania.

Peterson ME 1987. Effects of megestrol acetate on glucose tolerance and growth hormone section in the cat. *Research in Veterinary Science* 42: 354–357.

Petrak ML 1969. *Diseases of cage and aviary birds.* Lea & Febiger, Philadelphia.

Pharmacia & Upjohn 1999. Depo-Provera® product information. In 2001 *Physicians desk reference*, pp. 2596–3000, Montvale, New Jersey.

Romatowski J 1989. Use of megestrol acetate in cats. *Journal of the American Veterinary Medical Association* 194(5): 700–702.

Ryan TP 1985. Feather picking in caged birds. *Modern Veterinary Practice* 66(3): 187–189.

Schering-Plough 2003. Ovaban® product information. In *The compendium of veterinary products,* pp. 1868–1869, North American Compendiums, Ltd.

Selman PJ, van Garderen E, Mol JA and van den Ingh TS 1995. Comparison of the histological changes in the dog after treatment with the progestins medroxyprogesterone acetate and proligestone. *The Veterinary Quarterly.* 17 (4): 128–133.

Stabenfeldt GH 1974. Physiologic, pathologic and therapeutic roles of progestins in domestic animals. *Journal of the American Veterinary Medical Association* 164(3): 311–317.

Teale ML 1972. Pyometritis in spayed cats. *The Veterinary Record* 91(5): 129.

Tomlinson MJ, Barteaux L, Ferns LE and Angelopoulos E 1984. Feline mammary carcinoma: A retrospective evaluation of 17 cases. *Canadian Veterinary Journal* 25: 435–439.

Wilkins DB 1972. Pyometritis in a spayed cat. *Veterinary Record* 91(1): 24.

Withers AR and Whitney JC 1967. The response of the bitch to treatment with medroxyprogesterone acetate. *Journal of Small Animal Practice* 8(5): 265–271.

Yamareudeewong W, DeBisschop M, Martin LG and Lower DL 2003. Potentially significant drug interactions of class III antiarrhythmic drugs. *Drug Safety* 26(6): 421–438.

Chapter Fifteen
Combinations

Introduction

When a patient fails to respond to a given drug at a given dose, the clinician has three main options. They can (1) increase the dose of the drug currently being given if the maximum dose has not yet been arrived at and the patient is not exhibiting any undesirable side-effects in response to the current dose, (2) change drugs or (3) augment the first drug with a second drug. This chapter will focus on the topic of augmentation of one drug with another.

Sometimes the goal is a synergistic effect, in which the two drugs will, together, be more effective than either alone. An example would be augmentation of a serotonin reuptake inhibitor with a serotonin agonist. The two drugs work together to facilitate serotonin activity. Sometimes the goal is a complementary effect. A common example is treatment of a patient with chronic mild to moderate anxiety that peaks under certain conditions. In this case, daily administration of a maintenance anti-anxiety medication, such as clomipramine or fluoxetine, can be supplemented with context specific administration of a fast-acting, stronger anxiolytic, such as alprazolam. A complementary effect can also be achieved by combining drugs with different speeds of onset and duration of action. For example, dogs are sometimes presented with severe separation anxiety, so that a crisis situation faces the clinician. Owners may be facing eviction if there is one more complaint of their dog howling and barking in their absence, or the dog may be doing itself harm, or doing several hundred dollars worth of damage to the house every time it is left alone. In this situation, waiting for clomipramine or another slow onset of action medication to take effect is not an option. A benzodiazepine may be chosen in the early stages of treatment until the SRI and behavior modification have time to take effect.

Potentially Beneficial Combinations

In cases of serotonin dysregulation leading to behavioral changes, augmentation of a serotonin reuptake inhibitor with an agonist, such as buspirone, a 5-HT$_{1A}$ partial agonist, may be beneficial (Bakish 1991). For example, human patients with major depression who have been unresponsive to fluoxetine (at least 30 mg daily) or citalopram (at least 40 mg daily) have shown better improvement when they received buspirone augmentation of 20 to 60 mg/day vs. placebo. No serious events were observed (Appelberg et al. 2001). Likewise, patients with OCD may respond positively when fluoxetine treatment is supplemented with buspirone (e.g. Jenike et al. 1991). The author has successfully used this combination in cases where some, but insufficient, improvement occurred with fluoxetine. Likewise, augmentation of fluoxetine or lofepramine with lithium in cases of non-responders with major depression has been shown to be more beneficial than augmentation with placebo. The combination of fluoxetine, an SSRI, and desipramine, a TCA, results in more rapid improvement in patients with major depression than treatment with desipramine alone, presumably because of more rapid down-regulation of ß-adrenergic receptors (Baron et al. 1988; Nelson et al. 1991).

There are numerous examples of combining slow onset of action medications, such as SSRIs or TCAs, with fast onset of action medications, especially benzodiazepines. The combination of alprazolam and clomipramine has been shown to be beneficial in the treatment of storm phobia in dogs (Crowell-Davis et al. 2003). Alprazolam and fluoxetine have been combined in the treatment of urine spraying in a cat (Seibert 2004a, 2004b). This logic is also used in human anxiety disorders (e.g., Goddard et al. 2001; Stahl 2002).

Algorithms

An algorithm is "a computational procedure whose application yields a solution to an associated class of problems" (Hartley 1999). Put simply, they are a set of decision-making protocols for patient management at different stages of treatment, depending upon response to given treatments. Algorithms for clinical decision making have become common in psychiatric medicine. They also have a place in veterinary behavioral medicine, although the same disadvantages, as well as advantages, that apply in human psychiatry, apply here. Algorithms that are based on extensive research literature, particularly research that focuses on success or failure of treatments that are initiated after an initial non-response, can be useful in guiding clinicians into decision-making processes that are based on evidence. Unfortunately, the quantity of research on success rates of various primary treatments for veterinary behavior patients, much less second tier treatments, is still small. Nevertheless, this information will hopefully grow with time (Stein and Jobson 1996).

At this time, algorithms in veterinary behavior must be based on clinical experience of specialists, rather than data. However, the development of such algorithms will provide a basis for developing research that tests their veracity. In the long run, this will result in refinement, modification and ultimately improvement of clinical algorithms for veterinary behavior. Even when algorithms have become well developed and well tested, the weakness that exists for such algorithms in human psychiatry today will apply to veterinary behavior algorithms. Algorithms necessarily reduce a complicated situation into a simple decision-making process. In so doing, they may present an oversimplified view, failing to take into consideration all the complicating medical, management and experiential factors that can apply in a given case. Thus, even in two or three decades when veterinary behavior algorithms have been extensively tested, they should be taken as guidelines, rather than irrefutable laws. It is up to the clinician to consider all relevant information in a given case before making a decision as to the best course of treatment (Stein and Jobson 1996).

Cytochrome P450 (CYP)

The cytochrome P450 enzyme system is critical in hormone biosynthesis and catabolism, the biotransformation of toxins and the metabolism of a variety of drugs (He et al. 2001). While the specific distribution and quantities of the various specific enzymes, including mutant variations, have been extensively studied in humans, less research has been conducted in the various species treated by veterinarians (e.g., von Moltke et al. 1995). While there are many similarities, there are also differences which, in many cases, have not been quantitatively identified. This is an area where future research will hopefully clarify important information.

Adverse Interactions

In addition to potential issues of producing overdoses by giving two drugs that either act the same, or are metabolized by the same mechanisms, and thus compete with each other, combining drugs can present the risk of producing adverse consequences specific to the way particular drugs interact with each other.

Serotonin syndrome has been reported in monkeys, rats, rabbits, dogs and humans (e.g., Oates and Sjoerdsma 1960; Hess and Doepfner 1961; Curzon et al. 1963; Grahame-Smith 1971; Sinclair 1973; Brown et al. 1996; Martin 1996). It is a consequence of taking excessive quantities of medications that increase serotonin levels and/or taking certain medications that interact incompatibly in regards to serotonin metabolism. There is no diagnostic test for serotonin syndrome, and diagnosis is based on a history of medication with drugs that may interact incompatibly or a history of medication with excessive quantities of drugs that facilitate serotonin activity, combined with presenting symptoms and the exclusion of other medical conditions. The potential for serotonin syndrome is one reason that it is important to get a complete listing of all herbal medications being given to a patient, as some, such as St. John's Wort, act on serotonin. The mechanism for serotonin syndrome is not fully understood, but most investigators believe the primary mechanism is excess 5-HT_{1A}-receptor stimulation (Brown et al. 1996; Martin 1996).

Signs and symptoms can be grossly grouped into mental changes, neuromuscular changes and autonomic changes. In humans, the problem is usually mild and resolves in 24 to 72 hours, but it can cause death (Beaumont 1973; Mendis et al. 1981; Brennan et al. 1988; Tackley and Tregaskis 1987; Kline et al. 1989; Neuvonen et al. 1993; Kuisma 1995). The most serious cases result when an SSRI has been taken with 1) an MAO inhibitor, which decreases serotonin metabolism, 2) a serotonin receptor agonist, such as buspirone, 3) a tricyclic antidepressant, which is a non-selective serotonin reuptake inhibitor, or 4) meperidine, tryptophan or dextromethorphan. Specific changes in mental status symptoms reported in humans include confusion, agitation, coma, hypomania and anxiety. Motor abnormalities include myoclonus, hyperreflexia, muscle rigidity, restlessness, tremor, ataxia, shivering, nystagmus and seizures. Cardiovascular changes include hypertension, hypotension and sinus tachycardia. Gastrointestinal signs and symptoms include nausea, diarrhea, abdominal pain and excessive salivation. Other signs include diaphoresis, hyperpyrexia, tachypnea, and unreactive pupils (Brown et al. 1996).

Treatment and management includes discontinuation of all serotonergic medications and supportive treatment. Benzodiazepines such as diazepam or lorazepam may be given for myoclonus and the hyperthermia resulting from myoclonus. However, clonazepam is not effective with serotonin syndrome (Nierenberg and Semprebon 1993; Skop et al. 1994; Brown and Skop 1996). In severe cases, 5-HT antagonists such as cyproheptadine, methysergide or propranolol can be given (Goldberg and Huk 1992; Brown et al. 1996; Martin 1996).

Gwaltney-Brant et al. (2000) reported on 21 cases of dogs that had been exposed through accidental poisoning to the nutritional supplement 5-Hydroxytryptophan, which is the immediate precursor to serotonin. The dose consumed ranged from 2.5 mg/kg to 573 mg/kg. The dog that had been exposed to 2.5 mg/kg received no treatment and exhibited no symptoms. One dog, which had consumed a dose of 222 mg/kg, had emesis induced within 30 minutes. This dog exhibited no symptoms. The lowest dose at which signs developed was 23.6 mg/kg. The lowest dose at which death occurred was 128 mg/kg. The time of onset of clinical signs varied from 10 minutes to 4 hours after ingestion. Nineteen of the dogs developed clinical toxicosis. Of these, 3 died. Mental status changes included depression, coma and disorientation. Sensorimotor changes included tremors, hyperesthesia, ataxia, paresis, hyperreflexia, and weakness. Respiratory and cardiovascular signs included tachycardia, cyanosis and dyspnea. Gastrointestinal signs included vomiting, diarrhea, abdominal pain, flatulence, and bloat. Other signs included mydriasis, transient blindness, hypersalivation, hyperthermia, hypothermia and vocalization. Treatment included decontamination by inducing emesis, anticonvulsants, thermoregulation and fluid therapy. The 16 dogs that exhibited clinical toxicosis and recovered all did so within 36 hours of beginning treatment. Clinical blindness, if present, was the last sign to resolve.

Because of their long half-lives, serotonin syndrome has occurred five to six weeks or later after discontinuiation of fluoxetine, paroxetine, sertraline or irreversible MAOIs (Pato et al. 1991; Coplan et al. 1993; Martin 1996).

Interactions That Can Affect Dosing

Some drugs interact in a way that can affect dosing schedules or specific drug selections within a class when it is desired to use two or more classes of drugs. For example, in adult male humans, fluoxetine impairs the clearance of alprazolam by microsomal oxidation, but does not affect the rate of clearance of clonazepam by nitroreduction. Thus, in adult human males, fluoxetine can be administered with clonazepam without affecting clonazepam's efficacy, while co-administration of fluoxetine and alprazolam will result in significantly prolonged half-life of alprazolam (Lasher et al. 1991; Greenblatt et al. 1992). Similarly, fluvoxamine results in a significantly longer half-life for alprazolam (Fleishaker and Hulst 1994). As with many other aspects of the application of psychopharmacology to veterinary science, these detailed interactions remain to be studied in the veterinary population. For this reason we must proceed cautiously with combinations while beginning by extrapolating from human clinical trial data.

Conclusion

Combining medications can be useful in particular situations and for patients that do not respond to treatment with any one drug. However, there are potential risks to this approach, including competition between drugs for metabolic pathways and direct, adverse interactions between drugs. Ongoing research in the use of psychoactive medications for the treatment of behavior problems in nonhuman animals will continue to provide a stronger knowledge base for these decisions.

References

Appelberg BG, Syvälahti EK, Koskinen TE, Mehtonen O-P, Muhonen TT and Naukkarinen HH 2001. Patients with severe depression may benefit from buspirone augmentation of selective serotonin reuptake inhibitors: Results from a placebo-controlled, randomized, double-blind, placebo wash-in study. *Journal of Clinical Psychiatry* 62 (6): 448–452.

Bakish D 1991. Fluoxetine potentiation by buspirone: three case histories. *Canadian Journal of Psychiatry* 36 (10): 749–750.

Baron BM, Ogden AM, Siegel BW, Stegeman J, Ursillo RC and Dudley MW 1988. Rapid down regulation of ß-adrenoceptors by co-administration of desipramine and fluoxetine. *European Journal of Pharmacology* 154: 125–134.

Beaumont G 1973. Drug interactions with clomipramine (Anafranil). *Journal of International Medical Research* 1: 480–484.

Brennan D, MacManus M, Howe J and McLoughlin J 1988. "Neuroleptic malignant syndrome" without neuroleptics [letter] *British Journal of Psychiatry* 152: 578–579.

Brown TM and Skop BP 1996. Nitroglycerin in the treatment of the serotonin syndrome (letter). *Annals of Pharmacotherapy* 30:191.

Brown TM, Skop BP and Mareth TR 1996. Pathophysiology and management of the serotonin syndrome. *The Annals of Pharmacotherapy* 30: 527–533.

Coplan JD and Gorman JM 1993. Detectable levels of fluoxetine metabolites after discontinuation: An unexpected serotonin syndrome [letter]. *American Journal of Psychiatry* 150 (5): 837.

Crowell-Davis SL, Seibert LM, Sung WL, Parthasarathy V and Curtis TM 2003. Use of clomipramine, alprazolam, and behavior modification for treatment of storm phobia in dogs. *Journal of the American Veterinary Medical Association* 222(6): 744–748.

Curzon G, Ettlinger G, Cole M and Walsh J 1963. The biochemical, behavioral and neurologic effects of high L-tryptophan intake in the rhesus monkey. *Neurology* 12: 431–438.

Fleishaker JC and Hulst LK 1994. A pharmacokinetic and pharmacodynamic evaluation of the combined administration of alprazolam and fluvoxamine. *European Journal of Clinical Pharmacology* 46(1): 35–39.

Goddard AW, Brouette T, Almai A, Jetty P, Woods SS and Charney D 2001. Early coadministration of clonazepam with sertraline for panic disorder. *Archives of General Psychiatry* 58(7): 681–686.

Goldberg RJ and Huk M 1992. Serotonin syndrome from trazodone and buspirone. *Psychosomatics* 33(2): 235–236.

Grahame-Smith DC 1971. Studies in vivo on the relationship between brain tryptophan, brain t-HT synthesis and hyperactivity in rats treated with a monoamine oxidase inhibitor and L-tryptophan. *Journal of Neurochemistry* 18: 1053–1066.

Greenblatt DJ, Preskorn SH, Cotreau MM, Horst WD and Harmatz JS 1992. Fluoxetine impairs clearance of alprazolam but not of clonazepam. *Clinical Pharmacology and Therapeutics* 52(5): 479–486.

Gwaltney-Brant SM, Albretsen JC and Khan SA 2000. 5-Hydroxytryptophan toxicosis in dogs: 21 cases (1989–1999). *Journal of the American Veterinary Medical Association* 216: 1937–1940.

Hartley DS 1999. The language of algorithms. In *Textbook of Treatment Algorithms in Psychopharmacology*, pp. 15–32, edited by J Fawcett, DJ Stein and KO Jobson, John Wiley & Sons, Chichester.

He Y-Q, Roussel F and Halpert JR 2001. Importance of amino acid residue 474 for substrate specificity of canine and human cytochrome P450 3A enzymes. *Archives of Biochemistry and Biophysics* 389(2): 264–270.

Hess SM and Doepfner W 1961. Behavioral effects and brain amine contents in rats. *Archives Internationales de Pharmacodynamie et de Therapie* 134(1–2): 89–99.

Jenike MA, Baer L and Buttolph L 1991. Buspirone augmentation of fluoxetine in patients with obsessive compulsive disorder. *Journal of Clinical Psychiatry* 52(1): 13–14.

Katona CLE, Abou-Saleh MT, Harrison DA, Nairac BA, Edwards DRL, Lock T, Burns RA and Robertson MM 1995. Placebo-controlled trial of lithium augmentation of fluoxetine and lofepramine. *British Journal of Psychiatry* 166: 80–86.

Kline SS, Mauro LS, Scala-Barnett DM and Zick D 1989. Serotonin syndrome versus neuroleptic malignant syndrome as a cause of death. *Clinical Pharmacology* 8: 510–514.

Kuisma MJ 1995. Fatal serotonin syndrome with trismus [letter]. *Annals of Emergency Medicine* 26(1): 108.

Lasher TA, Fleishaker JC, Steenwyk RC and Antal EJ 1991. Pharmacokinetic pharmacodynamic evaluation of the combined administration of alprazolam and fluoxetine. *Psychopharmacology* 104(3): 323–327.

Martin TG 1996. Serotonin syndrome. *Annals of Emergency Medicine* 28(5): 520–526.

Mendis N, Pare CMB, Sandler M, Glover V and Stern GM 1981. Is the failure of L-deprenyl, a selective monoamine oxidase B inhibitor, to alleviate depression related to freedom from the cheese effect? *Psychopharmacology* 73(1): 87–90.

Nelson JC, Mazure CM, Bowers MB and Jatlow PI 1991. A preliminary, open study of the combination of fluoxetine and desipramine for rapid treatment of major depression. *Archives of General Psychiatry* 48(4): 303–307.

Neuvonen PJ, Pohjola-Sintonen S, Tacke U and Vuori E 1993. Five fatal cases of serotonin syndrome after moclobemide-citalopram or moclobemide-clomipramine overdoses [letter]. *Lancet* 342(8884): 1419.

Nierenberg DW and Semprebon M 1993. The central nervous system serotonin syndrome. *Clinical Pharmacology & Therapeutics* 53: 84–88.

Oates JA and Sjoerdsma A 1960. Neurologic effects of tryptophan in patients receiving monoamine oxidase inhibitor. *Neurology* 10: 1076–1078.

Overall KL 1995. Animal Behavior Case of the Month. *Journal of the American Veterinary Medical Association* 206(5): 629–632.

Pato MT, Murphy DL and DeVane CL 1991. Sustained plasma concentrations of fluoxetine and/or norfluoxetine four and eight weeks after fluoxetine discontinuation [letter]. *Journal of Clinical Pharmacology* 11(3): 224–225.

Seibert LM 2004a. Animal behavior case of the month. *Journal of the American Veterinary Medical Association* 224(10): 1594–1596.

Seibert LM 2004b. Correction: Animal behavior case of the month. *Journal of the American Veterinary Medical Association* 225(1): 71.

Sinclair JG 1973. Dextromethorphan-monoamine oxidase inhibitor interaction in rabbits. *Journal of Pharmacy and Pharmacology* 25: 803–808.

Skop BP, Finkelstein J, Mareth TR, Magoon M and Brown TM 1994. The serotonin syndrome associated with paroxetine, an over-the-counter cold remedy, and vascular disease: a case report and review. *American Journal of Emergency Medicine* 12: 642–644.

Stahl SM 2002. Don't ask, don't tell, but benzodiazepines are still the leading treatments for anxiety disorders. *Journal of Clinical Psychiatry* 63(9): 756–757.

Stein DJ and Jobson KO 1996. Psychopharmacology Algorithms: Pros and Cons. *Psychiatric Annals* 26 (4): 190–191.

Tackley RM and Tregaskis B 1987. Fatal disseminated intravascular coagulation following a monoamine oxidase inhibitor/Tricyclic interaction. *Anaesthesia* 42: 760–763.

Von Moltke LL, Greenblatt DJ, Schmider J, Harmatz JS and Shader RI 1995. Metabolism of drugs by cytochrome P450 3A isoforms. *Clinical Pharmacokinetics* 29(Suppl. 1): 33–44.

Appendix

Below are brand names of some psychoactive medications that are actively marketed in selected countries. Some medications are available in multi-ingredient forms, which are not listed. Specific drugs may not be available in all sizes in some countries. Most drugs are marketed for human use. Brand names that specifically apply to veterinary use are indicated by (V). DI means that a product with the same name but a different ingredient exists or has existed in another country.

Alprazolam

Argentina: Alplax Digest, Alplax Net, Becede, Bestrol, Krama (DI), Novo Begestabil, Prenadona, Prinox, PTA, Retan, Tensium (DI), Thiprasolan, Tranquinal, Tranquinal Soma, Xanax
Australia: Alprax, Kalma (DI), Xanax
Austria: Alprastad, Alpratyrol, Xanor
Belgium: Alpraz, Xanax
Brazil: Apraz, Frontal, Tranquinal
Canada: APO-Alpraz, NOVO-Alprazol, Nu-Alpraz, Xanax,
Chile: Adax, Grifoalpram, Prazam, Sanerva, Tricalma Retard, Zotran
Denmark: Alprox, Tafil
Finland: Alprox, Xanor
France: Xanax
Germany: Cassadan, Esparon, Tafil, Xanax
Greece: Antanax, Saturnil, Xanax
Hong Kong: Xanax
Hungary: Frontin, Xanax
India: Alprax, Alprocontin, Pacyl, Zolam
Ireland: Alprox, Calmax, Gerax, Xanax
Israel: Alpralid, Alprox, Xanagis, Xanax
Italy: Alprazig, Frontal, Mialin, Valeans, Xanax
Malaysia: APO-Alpraz, Xanax
Mexico: Neupax, Tafil
Netherlands: Xanax
New Zealand: Xanax
Norway: Xanor
Portugal: Alpronax, Pazolam, Prazam, Unilan, Xanax
Singapore: Alzolam, APO-Alpraz, Dizolam, Xanax, Zacetin
South Africa: Alzam, Anxirid, Azor, Drimpam, Xanolam, Xanor, Zopax
Spain: Trankimazin

Sweden: Xanor
Switzerland: Xanax
Thailand: Alcelam, Alnax, Anpress, Farmaline, Dizolam, Marzolam, Mitranax, Pharnax, Siampraxol, Xanacine, Xanax, Xiemed
United Kingdom: Xanax
United States: Xanax

Amitriptyline

Australia: Amitrip, Amitrip M, Endep, Laroxyl, Saroten, Tryptanol
Austria: Limbitrol, Saroten, Tryptizol
Belgium: Redomex, Tryptizol
Brazil: Amytril, Limbitrol, Protanol, Tripsol, Tryptanol
Canada: APO-Amitriptyline, Elatrol, Elavil, Elavil Plus, Levate, NOVO-Triptyn, Triavil
Chile: Antalin, Morelin
Denmark: Saroten, Tryptizol
Finland: Klotriptyl, Limbitrol, Pertriptyl, Saroten, Triptyl
France: Elavil, Laroxyl
Germany: Amineurin, Euplit Dragee, NOVOprotect, Saroten, Syneudon
Greece: Maxivalet, Minitran (DI), Saroten, Stelminal
Hong Kong: Tryptanol
Hungary: Teperin
India: Tryptizol
Ireland: Lentizol
Israel: Elatrol, Elatrolet, Tryptal
Italy: Adepril (DI), Diapatol, Laroxyl, Limbitryl, Mutabon, Sedans, Triptizol
Japan: Adepress, Amiprin
Malaysia: Endep, Tripta, Tryptanol
Mexico: Adepsique, Anapsique, Tryptanol
Netherlands: Sarotex, Tryptizol
New Zealand: Amitrip
Norway: Sarotex, Tryptizol
Portugal: ADT (DI), Mutabon, Tryptizol
Singapore: Tripta
South Africa: Limbitrol, Trepiline, Tryptanol
Spain: Deprelio, Mutabase, Nobritol, Tryptizol
Sweden: Saroten, Tryptizol
Switzerland: Limbitrol, Saroten, Tryptizol
Thailand: Anxipress-D, Neuragon, Polytanol, Tripsyline, Tripta, Triptyline, Tryptanol
United Kingdom: Domical, Elavil, Lentizol, Triptafen, Tryptizol
United States: Amavil, Amitid, Amitril, Elavil, Emtrip, Endep, Limbitrol, Limbitrol, SK-Amitriptyline, Triavil

Atomoxetine

Australia: Strattera
United Kingdom: Strattera
United States: Strattera

Buspirone

Argentina: Ansial
Australia: Buspar
Austria: Buspar
Belgium: Buspar
Brazil: Ansienon, Ansitec, Buspanil
Canada: Buspar, Buspirex
Chile: Paxon
Denmark: Buspar, Stesiron
Finland: Buspar, Stesiron
France: Buspar
Germany: Anxut, Bespar, Busp
Greece: Anchocalm, Antipsichos, Bergamol, Bespar, Boronex, Epsilat, Hiremon, Hobatstress, Kolmasin, Lanamont, Lebilon, Ledion, Loxapin, Nadrifor, Nervostal, Neurorestol, Norbal, Pendium, Stressigal, Svitalark, Tendan, Tensispes, Trafuril, Umolit
Hong Kong: Buspar, Kalmiren
Hungary: Anxiron, Spitomin
India: Buscalm
Ireland: Buspar
Israel: Buspirol, Sorbon
Italy: Axoren, Buspar, Buspimen
Mexico: Buspar
Netherlands: Buspar
New Zealand: Biron, Buspar
Norway: Buspar, Stesiron
Portugal: Ansiten, Busansil, Buscalma, Buspar, Establix
South Africa: Buspar, Pasrin
Spain: Effiplen
Sweden: Buspar
Switzerland: Buspar
Thailand: Anxiolan
United Kingdom: Buspar
United States: Buspar

Chlordiazepoxide

Brazil: Menotensil, Psicosedin

Canada: APO-Chlorax, APO-Chlordiazepoxide, Librax, Librium, Medilium-5, Medilium-10, NOVO-Poxide, Solium

Chile: Aerogastrol, Aero Itan, Antalin, Garceptol, Gaseofin, Gastrolen, Lerogin, Libraxin, Lironex, Morelin, No-Ref, Profisin, Sedogastrol, Tensoliv, Tranvagal

Denmark: Klopoxid, Risolid

Finland: Librax, Risolid

France: Librax

Germany: Klimax-H, Klimax-N, Librium, Multum (DI), Radepur

Greece: Librax, Oasil

Hong Kong: Bralix, Librax, Librium, Medocalum

Hungary: Elenium, Librium

India: Librium

Ireland: Librium

Israel: Nirvaxal

Italy: Diapatol, Librax, Librium, Limbitryl, Reliberan, Sedans

Japan: Consun, Contol

Malaysia: APO-Chlorax, Benpine, Klorpo, Liblan

Mexico: Kalmocaps

Portugal: Librax, Paxium

Singapore: APO-Chlorax, Benpine, Chlobax, Klorpo, Librax, Medocalum

South Africa: Librax, Librium

Spain: Hyberplex, Omnalio, Psico Blocan

Switzerland: Librax

Thailand: Benpine, Epoxide, Kenspa, Librax, Pobrax, Tumax, Zepobrax

United Kingdom: Librium, Tropium

United States: A-Poxide, Chlordiazachel, Clindex, Librax, Libritabs, Librium, Murcil, Reposans-10, SK-Lygen

Citalopram hydrobromide

Australia: Celapram, Cipramil, Talam, Talohexal

Austria: Apertia, Cipram, Citalhexal, Citalon, Citarcana, Citor, Pram, Sepram, Seralgan, Seropram

Belgium: Cipramil

Brazil: Cipramil, Denyl

Canada: Celexa

Chile: Actipram, Cimal (DI), Cipramil, Finap, Prisma, Semax, Setronil, Temperax, Zebrak, Zentius

Denmark: Akarin, Cipramil

Finland: Cipramil

France: Seropram

Germany: Cipramil, Citadura, Sepram

Greece: Seropram

Hong Kong: Cipram, Clomicalm (V)
Hungary: Seropram
Ireland: Cipramil
Israel: Cipramil, Recital
Italy: Elopram, Seropram
Malaysia: Cipram
Mexico: Seropram
Netherlands: Cipramil
New Zealand: Cipramil
Norway: Cipramil
Singapore: Cipram, Clomicalm (V)
South Africa: Cipramil
Spain: Genprol, Prisdal, Seropram
Sweden: Cipramil
Switzerland: Seropram
Thailand: Cipram
United Kingdom: Cipramil
United States: Celexa

Clomipramine hydrochloride

Australia: Anafranil, Clopram, Placil, Clomicalm (V)
Austria: Anafranil, Clomicalm (V)
Belgium: Anafranil, Clomicalm (V)
Brazil: Anafranil
Canada: Anafranil, APO-Clomipramine, CO Clomipramine, NOVO-Clopamine, Clomicalm (V)
Chile: Anafranil, Atenual, Ausentron
Denmark: Anafranil, Clomicalm (V)
Finland: Anafranil, Clomicalm (V)
France: Anafranil, Clomicalm (V)
Germany: Anafranil, Clomicalm (V), Hydiphen
Greece: Anafranil
Hong Kong: Anafranil, Zoiral
Hungary: Anafranil
India: Anafranil
Ireland: Clomicalm (V)
Israel: Anafranil, Maronil, Maronil SR
Italy: Anafranil, Clomicalm (V)
Japan: Anafranil, Clomicalm (V)
Malaysia: Anafranil, Clopress
Mexico: Anafranil
Netherlands: Anafranil, Clomicalm (V)
New Zealand: Anafranil, Clomicalm (V)
Norway: Anafranil, Clomicalm (V)
Portugal: Anafranil, Clomicalm (V)

Singapore: Anafranil
South Africa: Anafranil, Equinorm, Clomicalm (V)
Spain: Anafranil, Clomicalm (V)
Sweden: Anafranil, Clomicalm (V)
Switzerland: Anafranil, Clomicalm (V)
Thailand: Anafranil, Clofranil
United Kingdom: Anafranil, Anafranil SR, Clomicalm (V)
United States: Anafranil, Clomicalm (V)

Clonazepam

Australia: Paxam, Rivotril
Austria: Rivotril
Belgium: Rivotril
Brazil: Rivotril
Canada: APO-Clonazepam, Clonapam, Med Clonazepam, NOVO-Clonazepam, PHL-
    Clonazepam, Ratio-Clonazepam, Rhoxal-Clonazepam, Riva-Clonazepam, Rivotril
Chile: Acepran, Clonapam, Clonazil, Crismol, Neuryl, Ravotril, Valpax
Denmark: Rivotril
Finland: Rivatril
France: Rivotril
Germany: Antelepsin, Rivotril
Greece: Rivotril
Hong Kong: Rivotril
Hungary: Clonapam, Clonogal, Rivotril
Ireland: Rivotril
Israel: Clonex, Rivotril
Italy: Rivotril
Mexico: Kenoket, Kridex, Rivotril
Netherlands: Rivotril
New Zealand: Rivotril
Norway: Rivotril
Portugal: Rivotril
South Africa: Rivotril
Spain: Rivotril
Sweden: Iktorivil
Switzerland: Rivotril
Thailand: Rivotril
United Kingdom: Rivotril
United States: Klonopin

Clozapine

Australia: Clopine, Clozaril
Austria: Lanolept, Leponex

Belgium: Leponex
Brazil: Leponex, Zolapin
Canada: Clozaril, Gen-Clozapine, PMS-Clozapine
Chile: Leponex
Denmark: Leponex
Finland: Froidir, Leponex
France: Leponex
Germany: Elcrit, Leponex
Greece: Leponex
Hong Kong: Clozaril
Hungary: Leponex
Ireland: Clozaril
Israel: Leponex, Lozapine
Italy: Leponex
Malaysia: Clozaril
Mexico: Clopsine, Leponex
Netherlands: Leponex
New Zealand: Clopine, Clozaril
Norway: Leponex
Portugal: Leponex
Singapore: Clozaril
South Africa: Leponex
Spain: Leponex
Sweden: Leponex
Switzerland: Leponex
Thailand: Clozaril
United Kingdom: Clozaril
United States: Clozaril

Clorazepate dipotassium

Australia: Tranxene
Austria: Tranxilium
Belgium: Tranxene, Uni-Tranxene
Brazil: Tranxilene
Canada: APO-Clorazepate, NOVO-Clopate, Nu-Clopate, Tranxene
Chile: Calner, Modival, Tranxilium
France: Noctran, Tranxene
Germany: Tranxilium
Greece: Tranxene
Hong Kong: Tranxene
Ireland: Tranxene
Israel: Tranxal
Italy: Transene
Malaysia: Sanor
Mexico: Tranxene

Netherlands: Tranxene
Portugal: Medipax (DI), Tranxene
South Africa: Tranxene
Spain: Dorken, Tranxilium
Switzerland: Tranxilium
Thailand: Anxielax, Cloramed (DI), Cloraxene, Diposef, Dipot, Flulium (DI), Manotran, Polizep, Pomadom, Posene, Sanor, Serene, Transcap, Tranclor, Trancon, Tranxene, Zetran (DI)
United Kingdom: Tranxene
United States: Azene, Gen-Xene, Tranxene, Tranxene-SD, Tranxene-SD Half Strength, Tranxene T-Tab

Desipramine

Australia: Pertofran
Austria: Pertofran
Belgium: Pertofran
Canada: APO-Desipramine, Norpramin, Pertofrane, Ratio-Desipramine
Chile: Distonal
Germany: Pertofran, Petylyl
Israel: Deprexan
Italy: Nortimil
Mexico: Norpramin (DI)
Netherlands: Pertofran
New Zealand: Pertofran
United Kingdom: Pertofran, Pertofrane
United States: Norpramin

Diazepam

Australia: Antenex, Diazemuls, Ducene, Pro-Pam, Valium, Valpam
Austria: Betamed, Gewacalm, Harmomed, Psychopax, Stesolid, Umbrium, Valium
Belgium: Valium
Brazil: Ansilive, Calmociteno, Compaz, Dialudon, Diazepan, Dienpax, Kiatrium, Moderine, Noan, Pazolini, Somaplus, Uni-Diazepax, Valium, Valix
Canada: APO-Diazepam, Diastat, Diazemuls, Diazepam Parenteral, E-Pam, Meval, NOVO-Dipam, PMS-Diazepam, Rival, Valium, Vivol
Chile: Calmosedan, Cardiosedantol, Diapam, Elongal, Mesolona, Multisedil, Pacinax, Promidan, Sedantol, Sedilit
Denmark: Apozepam, Hexalid, Stesolid, Valaxona, Valium
Finland: Diapam, Gastrodyn Comp, Medipam, Relapamil, Stesolid, Vertipam
France: Novazam, Valium
Germany: Diazep, Faustan, Lamra, Stesolid, Tranquase, Valiquid, Valium, Valocordin-Diazepam
Greece: Apollonset, Atarviton, Distedon, Stedon, Stesolid

Hong Kong: Diazemuls, Kratium, Stesolid
Hungary: Seduxen, Stesolid
India: Valium
Ireland: Anxicalm, Diazemuls, Stesolid, Valium
Israel: Assival, Diaz, Stesolid
Italy: Aliseum, Ansiolin, Diazemuls, Gamibetal Plus, Micronoan, Noan, Spasen Somatico, Spasmeridan, Spasmomen, Somatico, Tranquirit, Valium, Valpinax, Valtrax, Vatran
Japan: Cercine
Malaysia: Diapine, Diapo
Mexico: Adepsique, Alboral, Alboral GD, Arzepam, AT-V, Diapanil, Diatex, Esbelcaps, Freudal, Ifa-Fonal, Laxyl, Numencial, Onapan, Ortopsique, Prizem, Qual, Relazepam, Tandial, Valium, Zeprat
Netherlands: Valium
New Zealand: Diazemuls, Propam, Stesolid
Norway: Stesolid, Valium, Vival
Portugal: Bialzepam, Gamibetal Compositum, Metamidol, Stesolid, Unisedil
Singapore: Diapine, Stesolid
South Africa: Betapam, Calmpose, Doval, Pax, Valium
Spain: Aneurol (DI), Ansium, Aspaserine B6 Tranq, Complutine, Diazepan, Gobanal, Pacium, Sico Relax, Stesolid, Tepazepan, Tropargal, Valium, Vincosedan
Sweden: Apozepam, Stesolid
Switzerland: Paceum, Psychopax, Stesolid, Valium
Thailand: Azepam, Diano, Diapam, Diapine, Dizan, Dizepam, Dizan, DizepamSipam, Stesolid, Valenium, Valium, V Day Zepam, Zopam
United Kingdom: Atensine, Dialar, Diazemuls, Rimapam, Stesolid, Tensium (DI), Valclair, Valium
United States: Diastat, Diazepam Intensol, Dizac, Q-Pam, T-Quil, Valcaps, Valium, ValRelease, Vazepam

Doxepin

Australia: Deptran, Quitaxon, Sinequan
Austria: Sinequan
Belgium: Sinequan
Canada: APO-Doxepin, NOVO-Doxepin, Sinequan, Triadapin, Zonalon
Denmark: Sinequan
Finland: Doxal (DI)
France: Quitaxon
Germany: Aponal, Aponal Dragee, Aponal Orange, Doneurin, Depia, Mareen, Sinquan
Greece: Sinequan
Hong Kong: Sinequan
India: Sinequan
Ireland: Sinequan, Xepin
Israel: Gilex, Zonalon

Mexico: Sinequan
Netherlands: Sinequan
New Zealand: Anten
Norway: Sinequan
Spain: Sinequan
Switzerland: Sinquane
Thailand: Sinequan
United Kingdom: Sinequan, Xepin
United States: Adapin, Sinequan

Fluoxetine hydrochloride

Australia: Auscap, Erocap, Lovan, ProzacZacin
Austria: Felicium, Fluctine, Fluohexal, Fluoxibene, Fluoxistad, Fluoxityrol, Flux (DI), Fluxil, Fluxomed, Mutan, Nufluo, Poxitivum
Belgium: Fontex, Prozac
Brazil: Daforin, Deprax (DI), Depress, Eufor, Fluxine, Nortec, Prozac, Prozen, Psiquial, Verotina
Canada: Alti-Fluoxetine, APO-Fluoxetine, CO Fluoxetine, Dom-Fluoxetine, FXT 10, FXT 20, FXT 40, Gen-Fluoxetine, Med Fluoxetine, PHL Fluoxetine, PMS-Fluox, PMS-Fluoxetine, Prozac, Ratio-Fluoxetine, Rhoxal-Fluoxetine
Chile: Actan, Anisimol, Clinium, Dominium, Pragmaten, Prozac, Sostac, Tremafarm
Denmark: Afeksin, Flutin, Fluxantin, Folizol, Fondur, Fonigen, Fontex, Fonzac
Finland: Fluxantin, Fontex, Seromex, Seronil
France: Prozac
Germany: Fluctin, Fluneurin, Fluox, Fluoxa, Fluoxemerck, Fluoxgamma, Fluox-Puren, Fluxet, Fyxionorm
Greece: Dagrilan, Dinalexin, Exostrept, Flonital, Fludaxir, Fokeston, Orthon, Sartuzin, Stephadilat-S, Stressless (DI), Zinovat
Hong Kong: Deprexin, Fluxil, Magrilan, Nopres, Provatine, Prozac
Hungary: Deprexin, Fefluzin, Floxet, Prozac
Ireland: Affex, Biozac, Gerozac, Norzac, Prozac, Prozamel, Prozatan, Prozit
Israel: Affectine, Flutine, Prizma, Prizma Forte, Prozac
Italy: Deprexen, Diesan, Flotina, Fluoxeren, Fluoxin, Grinflux, Prozac, Serezac, Zafluox
Malaysia: Prozac
Mexico: Auroken, Axtin, Flocet, Florexal, Fluoxac, Prozac, Siquial
Netherlands: Prozac
New Zealand: Fluox, Plinzene, Prozac
Norway: Fontex
Portugal: Digassim, Nodepe, Prozac, Psipax, Salipax, Selectus, Tuneluz
Singapore: Deprexin, Fluxetil, Fluxetin, Magrilan, Prozac, Zactin
Slovenia: Portal
South Africa: Lorien, Nuzak, Prohexal, Prozac, Sanzur
Spain: Adofen, Astrin, Lecimar, Nodepe, Prozac, Reneuron
Sweden: Fluxantin, Fontex, Seroscand

Switzerland: Fluctine, Flucim, Fluox-Basan, Fluoxifar, Flusol

Thailand: Actisac, Anzac, ATD, Deproxin, Flumed, Fluoxine, Flusac, Flutine, Fluxetil, Fluxetin, Fluzac, Hapilux, Loxetine, Magrilan, Oxetine (DI), Oxzac, Prodep, Prozac, Unprozy

United Arab Emirates: Flutin

United Kingdom: Prozac, Prozit

United States: Prozac, Sarafem, Symbyax

Flurazepam

Austria: Staurodorm

Belgium: Staurodorm

Brazil: Dalmadorm

Canada: APO-Flurazepam, Dalmane, Lupam, NOVO-Flupam, Somnol, Som-Pam

Germany: Dalmadorm, Staurodorm Neu

Hong Kong: Dalmadorm

Ireland: Dalmane

Italy: Dalmadorm, Felison, Flunox (DI), Remdue, Valdorm

Netherlands: Dalmadorm

Portugal: Dalmadorm, Morfex

Singapore: Dalmadorm

South Africa: Dalmadorm

Spain: Dormodor

Switzerland: Dalmadorm

Thailand: Dalmadorm

United Kingdom: Dalmane

United States: Dalmane, Durapam

Fluvoxamine

Australia: Faverin, Luvox, Movox

Austria: Felixsan, Floxyfral

Belgium: Dumirox, Floxyfral

Brazil: Luvox

Canada: APO-Fluvoxamine, Gen-Fluvoxamine, Luvox, NOVO-Fluvoxamine, PMS-Fluvoxamine, Ratio-Fluvoxamine, Rhoxal-Fluvoxamine, Riva-Fluvox

Chile: Luvox

Denmark: Fevarin

Finland: Fevarin, Fluvosol

France: Floxyfral

Germany: Desifluvoxamin, Fevarin, Fluvohexal, Fluvoxadura, Myroxim

Greece: Dumyrox, Myroxine

Hong Kong: Faverin

Hungary: Fevarin

Ireland: Faverin
Israel: Favoxil
Italy: Dumirox, Fevarin, Maveral
Malaysia: Luvox
Mexico: Luvox
Netherlands: Fevarin
Norway: Fevarin
Portugal: Dumyrox
Singapore: Faverin
South Africa: Luvox
Spain: Dumirox
Sweden: Fevarin
Switzerland: Flox-Ex, Floxyfral
Thailand: Faverin
United Kingdom: Faverin
United States: Floxyfral, Luvox

Haloperidol

Australia: Pacedol, Serenace
Austria: Haldol
Belgium: Haldol, Haoldol Decanoas IM, Vasalium, Vesalium
Brazil: Haldol, Halo, Haloper, Loperidol, Uni Haloper, Uni Haloper
Canada: Alti-Haloperidol, APO-Haloperidol, APO-Haloperidol LA, Haldol, Haloperidol-LA, Haloperidol Long Acting, NOVO-Peridol, Peridol, PMS-Haloperidol, Ratio-Haloperidol
Chile: Alternus, Haldol
Denmark: Serenase (DI)
Finland: Serenase (DI)
France: Haldol, Vasdol, Vesadol
Germany: Duraperidol, Haldol, Haloneural, Haloper, Sigaperidol
Greece: Aloperidin, Sevium
Hong Kong: Serenace
India: Serenace
Ireland: Haldol, Serenace
Israel: Haldol, Haloper, Pericate, Peridor
Italy: Haldol, Serenase (DI)
Malaysia: Avant, Serenace
Mexico: Haldol, Haloperil
Netherlands: Haldol
New Zealand: Haldol, Serenace
Norway: Haldol
Portugal: Serenelfi
Singapore: Serenace
South Africa: Serenace
Sweden: Haldol

Switzerland: Haldol, Sigaperidol

Thailand: Halomed, Halo-P, Halopol, Haricon, Haridol, H-Tab, Perida, Polyhadol, Schizopol, Tensidol

United Kingdom: Dozic, Haldol, Serenace

United States: Haldol, Haloperidol Decanoate Novaplus, Haloperidol Intensol, Halperon

Imipramine

Australia: Imiprin, Melipramine, Tofranil

Austria: Tofranil

Belgium: Tofranil

Brazil: Depramina, Imipra, Praminan, Tofranil

Canada: APO-Imipramine, Impril, NOVO-Pramine, Tofranil

Denmark: Imiprex

France: Tofranil

Germany: Pryleugan, Prylevgan

Hong Kong: Tofranil

Hungary: Melipramin

India: Tofranil

Ireland: Tofranil

Israel: Primonil, Tofranil

Italy: Tofranil

Japan: Chrytemin

Mexico: Talpramin, Tofranil

Netherlands: Tofranil

New Zealand: Tofranil

Portugal: Tofranil

South Africa: Ethipramine, Tofranil

Spain: Tofranil

Sweden: Tofranil

Switzerland: Tofranil

Thailand: Celamine, Sermonil, Topramine

United Kingdom: Tofranil

United States: Antipress, Imavate, Imiprin, Janamine, Presamine, SK-Pramine, Tofranil, Tofranil-PM, W.D.D.

Lorazepam

Australia: Ativan

Austria: Merlit, Somnium (DI), Temesta

Belgium: Loridem, Optisedine, Serenas (DI), Temesta, Vigiten

Brazil: Loraz (DI), Lorazepan, Loridem, Max-Pax, Mesmerin

Canada: APO-Lorazepam, Ativan, Dom-Lorazepam, NOVO-Lorazem, Nu-Loraz, PMS-Lorazepam, Riva-Lorazepam

Chile: Abinol, Amparax
Denmark: Lorabenz, Temesta
Finland: Temesta
France: Equitam (DI), Temesta
Germany: Durazolam, Laubeel, Somagerol, Tavor (DI), Tolid
Greece: Aripax, Cicletan, Dorm, Modium, Nifalin, Novhepar, Proneurit, Tavor (DI),
  Titus, Trankilium
Hong Kong: Ativan, Lorans, Lorivan
India: Ativan
Ireland: Ativan
Israel: Lorivan
Italy: Control (DI), Lorans, Tavor (DI)
Malaysia: Ativan, Lorans
Mexico: Ativan, Sinestron
Netherlands: Temesta
New Zealand: Lorapam
Portugal: Ansilor, Lorenin, Lorsedal
Singapore: Ativan
Slovenia: Loram
South Africa: Ativan, Tranqipam
Spain: Donix, Idalprem, Orfidal, Orfidal, Placinoral, Sedicepan
Sweden: Temesta
Switzerland: Lorasifar, Perixol, Sedazin, Somnium (DI), Temesta
Thailand: Anta, Anxira, Ativan, Lonza, Lora (DI), Loramed, Lorapam, Lorazene,
  Lorazep, OraTranavan
United Kingdom: Ativan
United States: Alzapam, Ativan, Lorax, Lorazepam Intensol

Methylphenidate

Australia: Attenta, Concerta, Lorentin, Ritalin
Austria: Ritalin
Belgium: Rilatine
Brazil: Ritalina
Canada: Concerta, PMS-Methylphenidate, PMS-Methylphenidate SR, Riphenidate,
  Ritalin, Ritalin SR
Chile: Aradix, Elem, Nebapul, Ritalin, Ritrocel
Denmark: Ritalin
France: Ritaline
Germany: Ritalin
Hong Kong: Ritalin
India: Ritalin
Ireland: Ritalin
Israel: Metadate, Ritalin
Malaysia: Ritalin
Mexico: Ritalin

Netherlands: Ritalin
New Zealand: Ritalin, Rubifen
Norway: Ritalin
Singapore: Ritalin, Rubifen
South Africa: Ritalin, Ritaphen
Spain: Rubifen
Sweden: Concerta
Switzerland: Ritaline
Thailand: Rubifen
United Kingdom: Concerta, Equasym, Ritalin
United States: Concerta, Focalin, Metadate, Metadate CD, Metadate ER, Methylin, Methylin ER, Methylphenidate ER, Methylphenidate IR, Mthylin, Ritalin, Ritalin LA, Ritalin SR

Nalmefene

United States: Revex

Naloxone hydrochloride

Australia: Narcan
Austria: Narcanti
Belgium: Narcan
Brazil: Narcan
Canada: Narcan
Denmark: Narcanti
Finland: Narcanti
France: Nalone, Narcan
Germany: Narcanti
Greece: Narcan
Hong Kong: Mapin, Narcan
Hungary: Narcanti
Ireland: Narcan
Israel: Narcan
Italy: Narcan
Malaysia: Narcan
Mexico: Narcanti
New Zealand: Narcan
Norway: Narcanti
Portugal: Narcan, Naxan, Naxolan
Singapore: Narcan
South Africa: Narcan
Sweden: Narcanti
Switzerland: Narcan
Thailand: Narcan

United Kingdom: Narcan
United States: Narcan, Narcan Neonatal

Naltrexone hydrochloride

Australia: Revia
Austria: Ethylex, Nalone (DI), Naltrexin, Nemexin, Revia
Brazil: Revia
Canada: Revia
Chile: Nalonera
Denmark: Revia
Finland: Revia
France: Nalorex, Revia
Germany: Nemexin
Greece: Nalorex
Hong Kong: Revia
Hungary: Antaxon, Nemexin, Revia
Ireland: Nalorex, Revia
Israel: Revia
Italy: Antaxone, Nalorex, Narcoral
Mexico: Revia
New Zealand: Revia
Norway: Revia
Portugal: Antaxone, Basinal, Destoxican, Nalorex
South Africa: Revia
Spain: Antaxone, Cellupan, Revia
Sweden: Revia
Switzerland: Nemexin
Thailand: Revia
United Kingdom: Nalorex
United States: Depade, Revia, Trexan

Nortriptyline

Australia: Allegron, Nortab, Nortrip
Austria: Nortrilen
Belgium: Nortrilen
Canada: Alti-Nortriptyline hydrochloride, APO-Nortriptyline, Aventyl, Norventyl,
    Ratio-Nortriptyline
Chile: Motitrel
Denmark: Noritren
Finland: Noritren
Germany: Nortrilen
Greece: Nortrilen
Hong Kong: Nortrilen

Israel: Nortylin
Italy: Dominans, Noritren, Vividyl
Netherlands: Nortrilen
New Zealand: Norpress
Norway: Noritren
Portugal: Norterol, Nortrix
Spain: Norfenazin, Paxtibi, Tropargal
Sweden: Sensaval
Switzerland: Nortrilen
Thailand: Norline, Nortrilen, Nortyline, Ortrip
United Kingdom: Allegron, Aventyl
United States: Aventyl, Pamelor

Oxazepam

Australia: Alepam, Benzotran, Murelax, Serepax
Austria: Adumbran, Anxiolit, Anxiolit Plus, Oxahexal, Praxiten
Belgium: Seresta, Tranquo (DI)
Canada: APO-Oxazepam, NOVO-Xapam, Oxpam, Serax, Zapex
Chile: Novalona, Serepax
Denmark: Alopam, Oxabenz, Oxapax, Serepax
Finland: Alopam, Opamox, Oxamin, Oxepam
France: Seresta
Germany: Adumbran, Azutranquil, Durazepam, Mirfudorm, Oxa (DI), Noctazepam,
    Praxiten, Sigacalm, Uskan
Israel: Vaben
Italy: Limbial, Serpax
Netherlands: Seresta
New Zealand: Ox-Pam
Norway: Alopam, Sobril
Portugal: Sedioton, Serenal (DI)
South Africa: Noripam, Purata, Serepax
Spain: Adumbran, NOVO Aerofil Sedante, Suxidina
Sweden: Oxascand, Sobril
Switzerland: Anxiolit, Seresta
United States: Serax, Zaxopam

Paroxetine hydrochloride

Australia: Aropax, Oxetine, Paxtine
Austria: Allenopar, Aparo, Ennos, Glaxopar, Paluxetil, Paroxat, Parocetan, Paroglax,
    Seroxat
Belgium: Aropax, Seroxat
Brazil: Aropax, Cebrilin, Pondera
Canada: Paxil

Chile: Aroxat, Bectam, Posivyl, Seretran, Traviata
Denmark: Oxetine (DI), Seroxat
Finland: Seroxat
France: Divarius
Germany: Euplix, Paroxat, Paroxedura, Seroxat, Tagonis
Greece: Seroxat
Hong Kong: Seroxat
Hungary: Paroxat, Rexetin, Seroxat
Ireland: Meloxat, Parox, Seroxat
Israel: Paxxet, Paxxet 20, Paxxet 30, Seroxat
Italy: Sereupin, Seroxat
Malaysia: Seroxat
Mexico: Aropax, Paxil
Netherlands: Seroxat
New Zealand: Aropax
Norway: Seroxat
Portugal: Paxetil, Seroxat
Singapore: Seroxat
South Africa: Aropax
Spain: Casbol, Frosinor, Motivan (DI), Seroxat
Sweden: Seroxat
Switzerland: Deroxat
Thailand: Seroxat
United Kingdom: Seroxat
United States: Paxil, Paxil CR, Pexeva

Selegiline

Australia: Anipryl (V), Eldepryl, Selgene
Austria: Amboneural, Cognitiv (DI), Jumex, Regepar, Xilopar
Belgium: Eldepryl
Brazil: Anipryl (V), Deprilan, Elepril, Jumexil, Niar, Parkexin
Canada: Anipryl (V), APO-Selegiline, DOM-Selegiline, Eldepryl, MED Selegiline, NOVO-Selegiline, PMS-Selegiline
Chile: Selgina
Denmark: Eldepryl
Finland: Eldepryl
France: Deprenyl, Otrasel
Germany: Amindan (DI), Antiparkin, Maotil, Movergan, Selegam, Selemerck, Selepark, Selgimed, Xilopar
Greece: Cosmopril, Feliselin, Procythol
Hong Kong: Julab, Jumex, Sefmex, Selegos
Hungary: Jumex, Primulex
India: Egibren
Ireland: Eldepryl
Israel: Jumex

Italy: Jumex, Selecom, Seledat, Xilopar
Malaysia: Ginex, Jumex, Selegos
Mexico: Niar
New Zealand: Eldepryl, Selgene
Norway: Eldepryl
Portugal: Jumex, Xilopar
Singapore: Jumex, Selegos
South Africa: Anipryl (V), Eldepryl
Spain: Plurimen
Sweden: Eldepryl
Switzerland: Jumexal, Selecim
Thailand: Elegilin, Julab, Jumex, Kinline, Sefmex, Seline
United Kingdom: Eldepryl, Zelapar
United States: Anipryl (V), Atapryl, Carbex (DI), Eldepryl

Sertraline hydrochloride

Australia: Zoloft
Austria: Gladem, Tresleen
Belgium: Serlain
Brazil: Novativ, Sercerin, Tolrest, Zoloft
Canada: APO-Sertraline, DOM-Sertraline, GEN-Sertraline, NOVO-Sertraline, PMS-Sertraline, Ratio-Sertraline, Rhoxal-Sertraline, RIVA-Sertraline, Sertraline-25, Sertraline-50, Sertraline-100, Zoloft
Chile: Altruline, Deprax, Elrval, Emergen, Implicane, SerivoLowfin, Sedoran
Denmark: Zoloft
Finland: Zoloft
France: Zoloft
Germany: Gladem, Zoloft
Greece: Zoloft
Hong Kong: Zoloft
Hungary: Stimuloton, Zoloft
Ireland: Lustral
Israel: Lustral
Italy: Zoloft
Malaysia: Zoloft
Mexico: Altruline
Netherlands: Zoloft
New Zealand: Zoloft
Norway: Zoloft
Portugal: Zoloft
Singapore: Zoloft
South Africa: Zoloft
Spain: Aremis, Besitran, Sealdin
Sweden: Zoloft
Switzerland: Gladem, Zoloft

Thailand: Zoloft
United Kingdom: Lustral
United States: Zoloft

Triazolam

Australia: Halcion
Austria: Halcion
Belgium: Halcion
Brazil: Halcion
Canada: ALTI-Triazolam, APO-Triazo, Halcion, NOVO-Triolam, NU-Triazo
Chile: Balidon, Somese
Denmark: Halcion, Rilamir
Finland: Halcion
France: Halcion
Germany: Halcion
Greece: Halcion
Hong Kong: Halcion
Ireland: Halcion, Trilam
Israel: Halcion
Italy: Halcion, Songar
Malaysia: Somese
Mexico: Halcion
Netherlands: Halcion
New Zealand: Halcion
Portugal: Halcion
South Africa: Halcion
Spain: Halcion
Sweden: Halcion
Switzerland: Halcion
Thailand: Halcion, Trycam
United Kingdom: Halcion
United States: Halcion

References

Data on file at Novartis Animal Health US 2005, Greensboro, North Carolina.
Martindale Sweetman SC, editor, *The Complete Drug Reference*. Pharmaceutical Press, London. Electronic version, Thomson Micromedex, Greenwood Village, Colorado, (Edition expires [2005]).
Pfizer Animal Health Database 2005, New York, New York.

Index